Hydro-Economic Models for Sustainable Water Resources Management

Hydro-Economic Models for Sustainable Water Resources Management

Guest Editors

Joaquín Melgarejo Moreno
Borja Montaño Sanz

MDPI

Basel • Beijing • Wuhan • Barcelona • Belgrade • Novi Sad • Cluj • Manchester

Guest Editors

Joaquín Melgarejo Moreno
University Institute of Water
and Environmental Sciences
University of Alicante
Alicante
Spain

Borja Montaño Sanz
University Institute of Water
and Environmental Sciences
University of Alicante
Alicante
Spain

Editorial Office
MDPI AG
Grosspeteranlage 5
4052 Basel, Switzerland

This is a reprint of the Special Issue, published open access by the journal *Water* (ISSN 2073-4441), freely accessible at: https://www.mdpi.com/journal/water/special_issues/L8KYRJFYK2.

For citation purposes, cite each article independently as indicated on the article page online and as indicated below:

Lastname, A.A.; Lastname, B.B. Article Title. *Journal Name* **Year**, *Volume Number*, Page Range.

ISBN 978-3-7258-7048-6 (Hbk)
ISBN 978-3-7258-7049-3 (PDF)
https://doi.org/10.3390/books978-3-7258-7049-3

Contents

About the Editors

Joaquín Melgarejo Moreno

Joaquín Melgarejo Moreno is Professor of Applied Economics at the University of Alicante. His academic career focuses on water economics, hydrological planning, water resource management under scarcity conditions, and the analysis of water-related public policies. He has led and participated in numerous research projects funded at regional, national, and European levels and has actively collaborated with public administrations and international organizations on issues related to water governance. He is the author of a large number of scientific publications in high-impact journals and has made significant contributions to academic and technical debates on water sustainability, economic efficiency, and climate change adaptation.

Borja Montaño Sanz

Borja Montaño Sanz is an Associate Professor at the University of Alicante and a researcher at the University Institute of Water and Environmental Sciences, where he carries out academic work in the fields of water economics, water governance, and the historical analysis of hydraulic infrastructures. His main research interests include hydro-economic modeling, water system resilience, desalination, water reuse, and the interaction between public policies and water-dependent strategic sectors. He has participated in competitive national and European research projects focused on sustainability, water and agriculture, industrial resilience, and public policy analysis. He is the author of several scientific articles published in international indexed journals, and his research is characterized by an interdisciplinary approach that integrates economics, history, water management, and institutional analysis.

water

MDPI

Editorial

Hydro-Economic Models for Managing Sustainable Water Resources

Joaquín Melgarejo and Borja Montano *

University Institute of Water and Environmental Sciences, University of Alicante, 03690 Alicante, Spain; jmelgar@ua.es
* Correspondence: borja.montano@ua.es

1. Introduction

Understanding water in the twenty-first century requires acknowledging that it can no longer be analysed from a single disciplinary perspective. The tensions between availability, demand, quality, ecosystem value, and governance compel the construction of bridges between hydrology, economics, ecology, and the social sciences. This Special Issue assembles ten studies which, despite their diverse geographical settings, converge in demonstrating that hydro-economic models are now an essential component for translating the complexity of water resources into informed and sustainable decisions.

One of the most striking commonalities across the contributions is the renewed appreciation of water as a provider of ecosystem services. The proposal to measure the *Gross Ecosystem Product* of the Lishui wetlands at finer spatial scales (contribution 1)—capable of capturing local nuances lost in macro-approaches—aligns with studies estimating the willingness to pay for river beaches in the Peruvian Amazon (contribution 3) and for natural pools in Sri Lanka (contribution 5). All of these studies reach the same conclusion: aquatic ecosystems generate tangible and intangible benefits that are seldom fully reflected in planning processes. By giving voice to the social and recreational value of water, these investigations broaden the focus beyond conventional uses and show how incorporating social preferences can strengthen water management.

Water also underpins critical economic activities whose vulnerability often remains invisible until quantified. The study on low-flow episodes in the Elbe River (contribution 2) reveals that a recurrent hydrological phenomenon can directly affect freight and tourist navigation, disrupting entire logistical chains. At the other end of the water cycle, the techno-economic assessment of advanced technologies to remove emerging contaminants (contribution 8) demonstrates that water quality conditions both the sanitary feasibility and the economic viability of wastewater treatment systems. The historical analysis of the Spanish desalination industry (contribution 4) illustrates how a strategic sector can evolve, innovate, and withstand regulatory and market changes when supported by an appropriate incentive structure. Taken together, these studies underscore that water security is inseparable from economic security.

2. Overview of the Contributions to This Special Issue

The Special Issue also underscores the importance of institutional models and economic incentives in water management. The analysis of the La Marina Baja Water Consortium (contribution 6) shows how cooperation among municipalities sustained the tourism-driven development of Benidorm under conditions of acute water stress, anticipating governance arrangements that have since become essential in many Mediterranean regions.

Likewise, the collaborative model for agricultural water-rights trading (contribution 7) highlights how price reforms and uncertainty influence users' willingness to exchange resources, shaping the system's efficiency and equity. Both studies converge on the same lesson: governance and rules matter as much as the physical availability of water.

A systemic perspective is especially evident in the study analysing the five northwestern provinces of China (contribution 9), where coordination among economic, hydrological, and ecological dimensions is not merely a theoretical aspiration but a structural necessity. The integrated methodology proposed by the authors offers a valuable tool for regions simultaneously facing scarcity, environmental degradation, and uneven development.

Completing the picture, the bibliometric review on household water conservation behaviours (contribution 10) reminds us that no institutional or technological strategy can be effective without a deep understanding of people's habits, psychological barriers, and motivations. Ultimately, sustainability is also determined within households.

3. Conclusions

Read collectively, these ten papers trace a coherent narrative: sustainable water management is only possible when ecological knowledge, economic evaluation, technological innovation, governance, and social behaviour are aligned. None of these dimensions is sufficient on its own; all, however, reinforce one another when integrated through rigorous models that connect the local with the global, the scientific with the political, and the environmental with the economic.

This Special Issue is therefore more than a collection of studies: it is an invitation to understand water as a complex, interdependent, and profoundly human system.

Author Contributions: Conceptualization, B.M.; methodology, B.M.; validation, B.M.; formal analysis, B.M.; resources, B.M.; data curation, B.M.; writing—original draft preparation, B.M.; writing—review and editing, B.M.; visualization, B.M.; supervision, J.M.; project administration, J.M.; funding acquisition, J.M. All authors have read and agreed to the published version of the manuscript.

Funding: This research was partially supported by Vice-Rectorate for Research and Knowledge Transfer of the University of Alicante, by the Water Chair of the University of Alicante-Diputación de Alicante, by the University Institute of Water and Environmental Sciences of the University of Alicante, and by the CDTI through the project "Sustainability, water and agriculture in the 21st century, SOS-AGUA-XXI" (Science and Innovation Missions 2021, Recovery, Transformation and Resilience Plan, NextGenerationEU) and the R&D&I project "Resilience and public policies in the evolution of Spanish industry, 1950–2019" (PID2022-138464NB-I00), funded by MCIN/AEI/10.13039/501100011033 and by ERDF A way of doing Europe.

Conflicts of Interest: The authors declare no conflicts of interest.

List of Contributions

1. Zhu, Z.; Wu, K.; Zhou, S.; Wang, Z.; Chen, W. Multi-Scale Gross Ecosystem Product (GEP) Valuation for Wetland Ecosystems: A Case Study of Lishui City. *Water* **2024**, *16*, 3554. https://doi.org/10.3390/w16243554.
2. Folkens, L.; Bachmann, D.; Satzinger, U.; Schneider, P. The Hydro-Economic Modeling of Low-Flow Events on the Middle Elbe: Assessing Socio-Economic Impacts on River Navigation. *Water* **2024**, *16*, 3497. https://doi.org/10.3390/w16233497.
3. Alarcon-Aguirre, G.; Del Águila Romero, Y.; Vela-Dafonseca, M.; Zevallos Pollito, P.A.; Rodriguez Achata, L.; Ramos Enciso, D.; Cardozo Soarez, J.; Diaz Revoredo, J.L.; Canahuire-Robles, R.; Garate-Quispe, J. Valuation of Ecosystem Services of Fluvial Beaches in the Southeastern Peruvian Amazon. *Water* **2024**, *16*, 3474. https://doi.org/10.3390/w16233474.
4. Montano, B. Historical Analysis of Resilience in Spanish Desalination Companies: Period 1980–2024. *Water* **2024**, *16*, 3318. https://doi.org/10.3390/w16223318.

5. Udugama, M.; Alhafi Alotaibi, B.; Navoda, M.; Najim, M.M.M.; Udayanga, L.; Traore, A. Willingness-to-Pay for Blue Ecosystem Services of Natural Pools in Sri Lanka: A Discrete Choice Experiment. *Water* **2024**, *16*, 2437. https://doi.org/10.3390/w16172437.
6. Sánchez-Pérez, C.; López-Ortiz, M.-I.; Fernández-Aracil, P. La Marina Baja Water Consortium (1950–1978): Hydro-Economic Model of Water Governance behind Tourism Development in Benidorm (Spain). *Water* **2024**, *16*, 1832. https://doi.org/10.3390/w16131832.
7. Song, L.; Wang, H.; Ding, L. Multi-Dimensional Collaborative Optimization Model for Agricultural Water Rights Based on Water Price Reform under Changing Environment. *Water* **2024**, *16*, 1262. https://doi.org/10.3390/w16091262.
8. Fabregat, V.; Pagán, J.M. Technical–Economic Feasibility of a New Method of Adsorbent Materials and Advanced Oxidation Techniques to Remove Emerging Pollutants in Treated Wastewater. *Water* **2024**, *16*, 814. https://doi.org/10.3390/w16060814.
9. Shi, J.; Yang, H.; Wang, F.; Sun, D.; Run, Y. Comprehensive Evaluation and Coupled Coordinated Development Study of Water–Economic–Ecological Systems in the Five Northwestern Provinces of China. *Water* **2023**, *15*, 4260. https://doi.org/10.3390/w15244260.
10. Sanchez, C.; Rodriguez-Sanchez, C.; Sancho-Esper, F. Barriers and Motivators of Household Water-Conservation Behavior: A Bibliometric and Systematic Literature Review. *Water* **2023**, *15*, 4114. https://doi.org/10.3390/w15234114.

water

MDPI

Article

Historical Analysis of Resilience in Spanish Desalination Companies: Period 1980–2024

Borja Montano

Institute of Water and Environmental Sciences, University of Alicante, Carretera San Vicente del Raspeig s/n, 03690 Alicante, Spain; borja.montano@ua.es

Abstract: This article analyzes the evolution and resilience of the Spanish desalination industry in response to shifting market conditions and technological challenges. Initially focused on domestic projects, Spanish companies leveraged the AGUA Program (Actions for the Management and Use of Water; the acronym does not correspond exactly in English, as it is translated from Spanish) to build expertise, which later facilitated their successful international expansion as local demand declined. The industry has adapted to diverse international regulations and local conditions, demonstrating both flexibility and competitiveness. In recent years, there has been an increasing focus on integrating renewable energy into desalination processes to mitigate rising energy costs and address environmental concerns. This shift not only reduces CO_2 emissions but also stabilizes operational costs, underscoring the sector's ongoing innovation and adaptability.

Keywords: desalination industry; renewable; energy integration; water-energy nexus; seawater desalination; resilience strategies

1. Introduction

The group of Spanish desalination companies has gone through several phases, each characterized by clearly differentiated economic and industrial contexts. In fact, the current context is also marked by a shift in market demands, with greater emphasis on the use of green energy, particularly in Western markets. It should be noted that although we refer to the desalination market, there are actually multiple markets with distinct contexts, all sharing the common factor of relative water scarcity [1]. The objective of our study is to answer the following question: what strategies have these companies employed to adapt to the various challenges they have encountered?

Moreover, the reader may notice from the tone of this introduction that we are operating under an initial assumption. We are analyzing the Spanish companies in this sector with the assumption that there are, to some extent, homogeneous patterns within the group, which indeed is the case [2].

The approach of this work does not align with the typical business history case studies that are common in the field of economic history. Two aspects make this case particularly distinctive. First, it is important to emphasize that the desalination industry has a far greater future than past, making it a highly dynamic field. However, this does not diminish the importance of understanding its history and the factors that have shaped the current landscape. Second, the water treatment sector has been largely understudied within the broader context of economic history. For this reason, this work will feature fewer citations and references than is usual in a scientific article published in this journal. In other words, while there may be a temptation to force citations by including articles that tangentially address related topics, the truth is that there are only a limited number of citations that can be coherently and genuinely included.

In the last decade, a group of Spanish companies specializing in the construction and operation of desalination plants has positioned itself among the elite competitors in the global market. Industry rankings are often presented based on total installed capacity or by calculating contracted capacity for a given year. Typically, if we consider the top ten companies in these rankings, depending on the period, it is common to find that around four of them are Spanish. One of the key objectives of this study is to provide a detailed account of the trajectory these companies have followed to reach this position. Since the 1980s, these companies have faced numerous challenges; yet, as is characteristic of a success story, this business group has demonstrated remarkable resilience [1]. The challenges and resilience strategies of Spanish desalination companies are highlighted by Younos and Lee (2019) [1], Navarro (2018) [2], and Vera (2021) [3], providing essential context for understanding the historical trajectory of the industry and its remarkable ability to adapt and thrive in the global market.

2. Historical Overview of the Water Sector Prior to the AGUA Program (1980–2007)

The history of desalination extends much further back than is commonly believed. The earliest references date to Aristotle and Pliny the Elder, who conducted studies on desalination, and to Egyptian alchemists who used stills for distillation. Later, Roman legions utilized solar evaporation to obtain water during their campaigns in Africa, storing water in shallow basins and collecting the condensed liquid afterward. The Vikings also employed "fog-catching" techniques, using their ship sails to gather moisture from the atmosphere during sea voyages. This method is still in use today in some desert regions, including parts of the Andes mountain range.

In Spain, Arab scientific advancements in distillation and evaporation technologies, many of which involved the use of stills, were introduced through institutions like the University of Toledo [4]. Numerous references also exist to the production of water on ships between the 15th and 17th centuries using rudimentary stills powered by wood or coal. With the Industrial Revolution and the development of the steam engine, desalination by evaporation was introduced on ships in a more technological manner and eventually expanded to industrial applications and small desalination plants.

The use of membranes is relatively recent. In 1748, the French cleric and physicist Jean Antoine Nollet studied the passage of water through semipermeable membranes. Years later, Henri Dutrochet, a French physician, biologist, and physiologist, founded the cell theory and discovered the process of osmosis. However, none of these studies had practical applications and remained almost as laboratory curiosities until the 1960s, when researchers Sydney Loeb and Srinivasa Sourirajan developed the first flat Reverse Osmosis membranes made of cellulose acetate in California. This opened the way for the development of commercial membranes, which expanded on a large scale from the 1980s.

In Spain, the first land-based desalination plant was a small seawater desalination plant built in Lanzarote in 1964. This event marked the beginning of desalination development in the Canary Islands, which later extended to the Balearic Islands and eventually to the mainland. In the 1970s, several desalination plants were installed in the Canary Islands, initially for hotels and tourist areas, and then in the 1980s also for agriculture. These installations employed technologies such as Reverse Osmosis (for seawater and brackish water) and electrodialysis reversal (for brackish and wastewater). In the 1980s, potable water desalination plants began to be built on the mainland, both for seawater and brackish water, which progressively increased in size. In the provinces of Almería, Murcia, and Alicante, during the drought of the 1990s, around 300 small private desalination units (500–5000 m^3/day) were installed for agriculture [5]. At that time, agriculture relied heavily on water transfers, and with the drought, alternatives such as desalination were sought for the survival of the sector. Generally, these were plants desalinating brackish groundwater, although some seawater plants were installed in the Canary Islands. Most of these installations used Reverse Osmosis technology, although around 20 electrodialysis reversal plants were built in the Canary Islands, with capacities ranging from 1000 to 5000 m^3/day [5]. Farmers in southeastern Spain continued increasing desalination capacity until they built large-scale plants, such as those of the Irrigation Communities of Cuevas de Almanzora, Mazarrón, and Rambla Morales.

Between 2004 and 2011, the Spanish government, through the Ministry of Environment (now the Ministry for the Ecological Transition), developed the AGUA program to implement numerous desalination projects (around 25 plants with a capacity close to 700 Hm^3/year) along the Mediterranean coast to address the region's water deficit, as opposed to the water transfer policy promoted by previous governments. This led to a massive expansion of desalination, reaching the current installed capacity, estimated at around 5 million m^3 per day, which, if fully dedicated to drinking water production, could supply a population of 34 million people.

Currently, it is estimated that Spain has more than 770 desalination plants with capacities exceeding 100 m^3/day, of which more than 100 have capacities greater than 10,000 m^3/day (AEDyR, 2018). The largest seawater desalination plants in Spain are Torrevieja (240,000 m^3/day) and Águilas (210,000 m^3/day). Regarding brackish water desalination plants, notable examples include the El Atabal plant in Málaga (200,000 m^3/day) and the Abrera plant in Barcelona (200,000 m^3/day), the latter being the largest plant in the world using electrodialysis reversal technology. Today, most large desalination plants are in operation, though not at full capacity. Some facilities, like Águilas, have important agreements with farmers that ensure a high level of productivity (mainly for agriculture, benefiting the Irrigation Communities of Lorca, Pulpí, and Águilas). However, other plants, such as Muchamiel or Sagunto, are significantly underutilized [6]. Most small desalination plants built by Irrigation Communities or private farmers in the 1990s are no longer operational due to various reasons (lack of permits, brine management issues, etc.). However, in recent years, groups of agricultural entrepreneurs from Murcia and Almería have been planning the construction of several large private seawater desalination plants to reduce their reliance on water transfers.

In addition to seawater facilities, the increasing implementation of desalination membranes for the improvement of surface water (including large plants such as the Tajo, El Atabal, and Abrera drinking water treatment plants) and also for tertiary wastewater treatments (such as the Rincón de León wastewater treatment plant in Alicante or the Benidorm wastewater treatment plant) is noteworthy.

If we go back to 1980, desalination was a technology whose cost per cubic meter was substantially higher than it is today. Moreover, it is important to note that there are two major groups of desalination technologies: thermal and membrane-based. In recent decades, membrane plants have become increasingly prevalent because their energy efficiency is substantially higher. However, the further back we go in time, the more common thermal plants become. Thus, unlike in 2024, during the 1980s, desalination was a technology undergoing significant improvements.

At this point, it is important to differentiate between the global desalination sector and the specific characteristics of the group of Spanish companies dedicated to desalination. This section, therefore, focuses on the sector before the AGUA Program. We must understand that the launch of the AGUA Program marked a radical change for Spanish companies. In fact, one could say that before the AGUA Program, Spanish desalination companies did not represent a consolidated business sector.

Before the AGUA Program, this sector consisted of companies that represented diversification strategies for various construction companies. Many emerged as subsidiaries of larger business groups, such as Acciona Agua (part of the Acciona group) or Sadyt (part of Sacyr). In fact, at their inception, their function was predominantly that of construction companies undertaking water projects, among which desalination was just one of many services offered. Naturally, even after the AGUA Program, these companies continue to develop other types of infrastructure, but it is in the field of desalination where we can observe their greatest competitiveness and their presence in international markets.

Therefore, we can say that desalination in Spain before the AGUA Program had a moderate presence, allowing for the execution and operation of existing plants without leading to significant growth in the business sector we are studying.

However, it is important to note that water scarcity had already necessitated enough action to begin creating a group of companies. Generally, it is large public projects that generate demand in the water treatment sector.

A Technology Yet to Mature

Water desalination has emerged as an increasingly utilized solution to address potable water scarcity, particularly in arid and coastal regions. However, despite its apparent benefits, this technology continues to face several significant challenges that limit its widespread adoption. High energy consumption, operational costs, and the environmental impact of brine disposal are key factors indicating that desalination is a technology that still requires maturation. While efforts are underway to optimize these processes and mitigate their drawbacks, desalination remains a last resort rather than a comprehensive solution to the global water crisis.

Currently, technical advancements in desalination have stabilized to the extent that, in recent years, most sector proposals have focused on the integration of renewable energy sources. This shift aims to reduce indirect CO_2 emissions and decouple the energy consumption costs of desalination plants from fluctuating energy market prices. However, if we look back to the 1980s, we find a technology that had significant room for improvement. The degree of technological advancement can be measured by the energy consumption required to produce one cubic meter of desalinated water.

Due to energy considerations, thermal technologies have gradually been phased out in favor of membrane technologies. For readers less familiar with desalination, thermal technologies separate salt from water through an evaporation process, which typically requires more energy than membrane technologies. In contrast, membrane technologies force saltwater through membranes capable of generating a separation process between water and salt. The most widely used membrane technology is known as Reverse Osmosis. The reduction in energy consumption from the 1980s to the present in membrane technologies has been substantial, contributing to the exponential growth of Reverse Osmosis plants.

It is important to note that while we mentioned a reduction in energy consumption for desalination in the previous paragraph, we did not reference the economic implications of that energy consumption. This omission is significant. Given that energy prices fluctuate, an increase in energy costs could lead to higher operational costs for desalination plants. Since energy costs account for nearly half of the total expenses associated with desalination, rising energy prices would ultimately increase the cost of desalinated water.

Therefore, we can conclude that the period from the 1980s to the implementation of the AGUA Program is characterized by a reduction in product costs due to technological advancements, alongside a significant increase in total desalination capacity worldwide. During this period, desalination transitioned from being a novel and uncommon option to a widely implemented technology in countries where water scarcity and economic capacity coexist.

There are four key areas of improvement in which this technology is expected to continue progressing, and indeed, advancements are still being made in these areas today. Table 1 outlines these areas of improvement.

Table 1. The Four Areas of Improvement in Desalination.

	Description	Areas of Improvement
Energy Consumption	Desalination has higher energy consumption compared to other methods of water acquisition. Energy consumption has decreased over the past decades. Currently, between 3 and 4 kWh are required to produce one cubic meter of desalinated water.	- RO membranes are already approaching their thermodynamic limit, and it has been demonstrated that materials have a relatively insignificant impact on increasing energy efficiency [7]. It seems complicated to further reduce energy consumption, which, if possible, would be a considerable technological improvement. - Integration of renewable energies: utilize renewable energy sources, such as solar or wind power, to operate desalination plants, thereby reducing dependence on fossil fuels and minimizing the carbon footprint of the process. - Energy recovery: implement energy recovery techniques in the desalination process, such as pressure exchange technologies, to reuse energy and increase overall efficiency. Energy recovery systems are already used in nearly all RO desalination plants worldwide. However, the device itself can be improved to recover more pressure at low mixing rates - A significant reduction in energy consumption in Saudi Arabia's desalination processes, particularly in Reverse Osmosis (RO), has been achieved primarily through design optimization and improved technology. Over the past decade, Saudi Arabia has reduced the energy required for desalination by about 87%, a remarkable feat given the traditionally high energy demands of this process. This was accomplished through innovations in membrane technology and enhanced operational efficiency in RO systems [8]).
Costs	Costs range between $0.50 and $3 per cubic meter, depending on the type of water, year of construction, and plant size.	- Reduction of operational costs: invest in operational and maintenance improvements that reduce long-term costs, such as using more durable materials and optimizing filtration and pumping processes. - Economies of scale: increase the capacity of desalination plants and promote regional cooperation to leverage economies of scale and reduce unit costs of water production. - Financial innovation: develop financing models and subsidies that facilitate initial investment in desalination infrastructure, making the technology more accessible to developing countries. - New technologies create opportunities for improvement through AI and ML to optimize plant operations, which could reduce energy and chemical consumption.
Environmental Impact	Generation of brine that can harm marine ecosystems. Energy consumption may lead to CO_2 emissions.	- Sustainable brine management: develop more effective methods for brine management, such as dilution before discharge or the use of brine in other industries (e.g., mining) to reduce its environmental impact. - Development of green desalination: innovate in technologies that minimize environmental impact, such as solar thermal desalination, which could reduce the generation of harmful by-products. - Regulation and control: implement stricter regulations and monitoring systems to control brine discharge and protect marine ecosystems. - The CO_2 generated during the energy production process could be utilized in the RO system to mitigate environmental impact. [9]
Global Capacity	More than 16,000 plants in operation, producing less than 1% of total freshwater consumption.	- Capacity expansion: invest in the construction of new desalination plants in strategic regions, particularly in areas with chronic water scarcity, to increase desalination's contribution to the global potable water supply. - Optimization of existing infrastructure: modernize and enhance the efficiency of current desalination plants to maximize water production with the same resources. - Development of advanced technologies: encourage the research and development of new desalination technologies, such as electrodialysis or advanced membrane desalination, which could increase capacity and reduce costs in the future.

3. Current Challenges and Developments in the AGUA Program (2007–2011)

The AGUA Program (Actions for the Management and Utilization of Water) was a key initiative implemented in Spain in 2004 by the government of José Luis Rodríguez Zapatero in response to the growing water scarcity, particularly in the most arid regions of the country, such as the southeastern peninsula. This program marked a paradigm shift in water resource management in Spain, prioritizing sustainability and the optimization of water use over the traditional policy of large-scale water transfers, such as the controversial Ebro River transfer that had been promoted earlier.

One of the fundamental pillars of the AGUA Program was the promotion of desalination as a strategic solution to ensure the supply of potable water in coastal regions with the greatest water deficits. Prior to the program, desalination in Spain was an emerging and scarcely implemented technology, primarily focused on small plants serving isolated or tourist urban centers.

With the implementation of the AGUA Program, desalination experienced exponential growth. The government promoted the construction of new desalination plants along the entire Mediterranean coast, from Catalonia to Andalusia, with the goal of significantly increasing the production capacity of desalinated water. This effort resulted in the creation of infrastructures such as the Torrevieja desalination plant, one of the largest in Europe, capable of producing up to 80 cubic hectometers of water annually.

The AGUA Program also drove innovation in desalination technologies, fostering the development of more efficient and cost-effective techniques, and promoting research into the use of renewable energy sources to reduce the environmental impact of the desalination process. As a result of these policies, Spain became a global leader in desalination, ranking among the countries with the highest installed capacity, not only within Europe but also on a global scale.

During the years of the AGUA Program, there were no significant global changes in the desalination market or in its technological development. However, this program did transform the national landscape. The demand for desalination plants surged abruptly, and this demand was entirely met by domestic companies. This large-scale demand, concentrated over a few years, caused these small water treatment companies to grow substantially. The AGUA Program was also a primary driver of these companies' internationalization because, although they had expanded due to the Spanish market, it had become saturated. Once the AGUA Program's plants were built, the national market was considered exhausted, as the installed desalination capacity meant that no additional water would be required.

Many experts argue that the focus on desalination was disproportionate, a result of the "water war" that occurred at the political level. What was the water war? The Popular Party advocated for the importance of water transfers, particularly a potential transfer from the Ebro River, while the Socialist Party promoted desalination as the most suitable solution for addressing specific water scarcity issues.

The Socialist Party's commitment to desalination was so strong that they ended up constructing more plants than what seemed advisable from a technical perspective. This increased demand, which in turn led to greater competitiveness. Furthermore, given the government's association with desalination, strict environmental requirements were imposed. Any environmental damage caused by a desalination plant would have been used by the opposition as evidence of government failure. This resulted in higher environmental standards than those typically encountered by Spanish desalination companies abroad. However, this also enabled these companies to develop greater competitiveness due to the stringent demands. According to some industry executives, the demand environment in Spain was very challenging due to political and media scrutiny. This, in turn, better prepared these companies with the necessary expertise and know-how when they entered the international market.

3.1. Technological Refinement

The refinement of desalination technology over recent decades has resulted in substantial improvements in efficiency. The desalination plants constructed under Spain's AGUA Program were markedly advanced compared to earlier facilities, with the most significant change being the considerable reduction in energy consumption. These new plants were also designed to minimize negative externalities, provided it was cost-effective from a cost-benefit analysis perspective. Like any industrial or technological process, desalination technologies have continuously improved, although these advancements have predominantly focused on reducing energy consumption. However, while significant energy reductions were achieved in the initial decades, progress has since slowed and plateaued. The current trend within the industry appears to favor partially powering plants with renewable energy sources, rather than further reducing the energy demands of the desalination process.

Reverse Osmosis (RO) remains the most widely adopted desalination method globally. Traditionally, RO required substantial energy to generate the high pressure necessary to force water through semipermeable membranes, which retained the salts. One of the most significant advancements in this technology has been the development of low-pressure Reverse Osmosis, utilizing more efficient membranes that allow desalination to occur at lower pressures, significantly reducing both energy consumption and operational costs.

Another key advancement has been the implementation of energy recovery systems. In Reverse Osmosis plants, the pressure exerted during the process can be recovered and reused, decreasing the overall energy demand of the system. Devices such as pressure exchangers and turbochargers have played a pivotal role in enhancing energy efficiency in desalination.

The integration of renewable energy into desalination processes is also a rapidly advancing field. Notable progress has been made in utilizing solar and wind energy to power desalination plants. For example, solar thermal energy has been successfully applied in solar distillation systems, where the sun's heat vaporizes water, separating it from salts. This approach not only reduces reliance on fossil fuels but also lowers the carbon footprint of desalination plants.

A transformative advancement in the field is the development of nanotechnology membranes. These membranes, which incorporate nanoparticles or nanotubes, offer superior permeability and selectivity, enhancing desalination efficiency while further reducing energy requirements. Additionally, ongoing research on graphene membranes and other advanced materials holds the potential to revolutionize Reverse Osmosis in the near future.

Although less common, freeze desalination is an emerging technology that offers energy efficiency advantages in colder climates. This process involves freezing saline water, where the resulting ice is essentially pure water, leaving the salt behind during solidification. Freeze desalination requires less energy than thermal distillation and is particularly suited for regions with access to natural cold sources.

Finally, hybrid technologies, which combine different desalination methods, are gaining popularity. For example, combining Reverse Osmosis with membrane distillation enhances process efficiency and flexibility, adapting to varying conditions and types of saline water. These hybrid systems optimize resource use and allow for greater control over the quality of the produced water.

3.2. The Water War: The Spanish Case

Water is a scarce resource, and Spain is no exception in experiencing what some have called "the water war". However, this conflict is of particular interest due to its somewhat peculiar nature. In this case, a planned inter-basin water transfer, known as the Ebro Transfer, was never constructed. During the 1980s, 1990s, and early 21st century, the National Hydrological Plan (PHN) generated intense tensions between the autonomous communities of Aragon and Catalonia, on one side, and southeastern regions of Spain, such as Murcia and Valencia, on the other [10]. The plan proposed transferring water from the Ebro River to other areas of Spain, which sparked significant opposition in Aragon and Catalonia, where there were fears that such transfers would negatively impact the Ebro's ecosystem and local water needs. José Marco, President of the General Deputation of Aragon in 1997, stated: "We will not allow the Ebro's water, which is our lifeblood, to be taken from our land to serve interests outside our community". The opposition to the Ebro Transfer culminated in its repeal in 2004, following the election of José Luis Rodríguez Zapatero's government, which promoted an alternative policy based on desalination. The Popular Party in Spain favored the water transfer and largely opposed desalination, while the Socialist Party supported desalination. It is important to note that at that time, the country's political reality was much closer to bipartisanship than it is today. The conflict was so intense that slogans were created, with "water for everyone" as the pro-transfer slogan and "water forever" as the pro-desalination slogan.

This political polarization did not contribute to rational decision-making from a technical standpoint. In 2004, the Socialist Party won the election, significantly increasing the number of desalination plants in the country. However, it is also important to recall that the opposition (the Popular Party) was against desalination. This led to stricter control and oversight of desalination plants than of any other public works. Paradoxically, this increased the competitiveness of Spanish desalination companies, as they were forced to meet strict environmental, aesthetic, economic, and energy demands.

Proponents of the Ebro Transfer heavily criticized the desalination plants of the AGUA Program. Their main argument was the high energy consumption of these plants, which collectively would account for 1% of Spain's total energy consumption. It is not surprising, then, that from the outset, the primary focus of desalination development efforts has been on reducing its energy intensity. Although significant progress has been made, energy consumption remains relatively high [11].

Today, controversies and territorial disputes persist, although the transfer currently at the center of the debate is the Tajo–Segura Transfer. The Tajo–Segura Transfer is an aqueduct built in 1979 to carry water from the Tajo River basin to the arid regions of southeastern Spain, such as Murcia, Alicante, and Almería. This transfer has been a constant source of conflict between the water-receiving communities and those in the source basin, particularly Castilla-La Mancha, which argues that the transfer significantly reduces its own water resources. José Bono, then President of Castilla-La Mancha, stated in 2004: "The Tajo–Segura Transfer is a bleeding scar, a historical injustice that must be reviewed to ensure that water stays where it is needed". Over the years, the transfer has been the subject of multiple debates and regulatory modifications and remains a highly controversial issue in Spanish politics.

4. International Expansion or Decline: 2006–2019

The AGUA Program was like a wave that came and went. When it receded (metaphorically speaking), it left behind an industrial sector that previously did not exist and no longer had opportunities to generate revenue in Spain, as all the necessary plants had already been constructed [12] At this point, Spanish desalination companies began seeking opportunities in other countries [13] The degree of success these companies achieved was substantial, largely due to the experience and competitiveness they had developed in the Spanish market.

The internationalization of Spanish desalination companies following the AGUA Program is a well-documented phenomenon, with various data and examples highlighting how these companies began expanding their global presence during this period.

Starting in 2006, Spanish desalination companies began securing significant contracts abroad, particularly in water-scarce regions such as the Middle East, North Africa, and Latin America. The effects of the AGUA Program were already evident, and the exhaustion of the domestic market in Spain was a clear reality; companies had to internationalize or face extinction. The Spanish company Acciona Agua became a global leader in desalination. Acciona began its international expansion with projects in Algeria, the United Arab Emirates, and Australia. In 2007, it won a contract to build the Adelaide desalination plant in Australia, one of the largest in the world at the time, with a capacity of 300,000 m^3/day.

Another Spanish company, Tedagua, a subsidiary of ACS, also began to gain ground internationally. In 2007, Tedagua was awarded the construction and operation of the Barka II desalination plant in Oman, with a capacity of 120,000 m^3/day.

In 2006, the Spanish company Abengoa started its expansion into the international desalination market, winning contracts in regions such as North Africa and the Middle East. In 2009, Abengoa secured a major contract to build the Beni Saf desalination plant in Algeria, with a capacity of 200,000 m^3/day. Sacyr Vallehermoso, through its subsidiary Sadyt, also began operating internationally in desalination projects. In 2007, Sadyt was selected to develop a desalination plant in Israel, demonstrating the ability of Spanish companies to compete in highly competitive markets.

By 2006, Spanish companies accounted for approximately 20% of the world's installed desalination capacity, establishing themselves as leaders in Reverse Osmosis technology, according to data from the Spanish Desalination and Reuse Association (AEDyR). From 2006 onwards, it is estimated that Spanish companies participated in the construction of more than 50% of the new desalination plants in the Middle East and North Africa.

The Spanish government, through the Spanish Institute for Foreign Trade (ICEX), began actively supporting the internationalization of its water sector companies, including those specializing in desalination, by promoting Spanish technology in strategic markets. These data and examples illustrate how, starting in 2006, Spanish desalination companies not only began to compete internationally but also established themselves as global leaders in the industry, contributing to addressing water challenges in various parts of the world.

5. The Imperative of Energy Sustainability: Challenges and Prospects for 2022–2024

As mentioned earlier, the Spanish desalination sector is an international leader, with numerous companies among the world's top performers. This strength is not solely due to large constructors and operators but also includes suppliers, engineering firms, consultancies, small and medium-sized enterprises, entrepreneurs, public companies, and research centers.

In Spain, there are numerous research centers and universities that are internationally recognized for their research on desalination. Generally, research trends in this sector are focused on energy efficiency and reducing the carbon footprint [6,13], minimizing the environmental impacts of desalination, and improving equipment (membranes) and facilities. In summary, these research efforts are typically applied and more focused on cost and impact reduction than on developing new processes or technologies.

In the field of energy efficiency and CO_2 footprint reduction, there is a growing emphasis on research and the implementation of renewable energy sources. These sources are used both to produce the electricity needed for desalination and to attempt direct integration with desalination systems. However, the expansion of renewable energy for desalination faces several challenges, such as the high concentrations of power required in certain locations (large desalination plants), the technical or economic infeasibility of energy storage (since desalination plants must operate continuously to remain viable), or the fact that the location of the desalination plant does not always coincide with the best site for renewable energy production. This latter issue has been resolved in some countries, such as Spain and Australia, by supplying the necessary renewable energy equivalently from parks located hundreds of kilometers away from the desalination plant, thereby offsetting their emissions.

In earlier sections, we mentioned that the energy consumption of desalination has decreased over the decades. However, does this mean that the cost of desalination has decreased at the same rate? No, and it is important to note that academics highlighted this fact years before it became a reality. It is crucial to understand that the economic cost associated with energy consumption is not the same as the energy consumption itself. The key difference here is that the economic cost linked to energy consumption depends on the price of energy, which can fluctuate. This reality has always been present, but it seems that until what is theoretically certain becomes a fact, it is not approached with the same seriousness.

In 2022, a conflict erupted between Russia and Ukraine, leading to numerous consequences, one of which was a significant increase in energy prices. This resulted in a substantial rise in the economic cost of desalination, given that nearly half of its cost is attributed to energy consumption. Since then, the desalination sector has begun to exhibit a new trend in projects, with growing demand for the use of renewable energy sources in desalination plants.

The integration of renewable energy into desalination offers three key advantages:

- It reduces CO_2 emissions, aligning with the environmental goals of many countries.

- It stabilizes the cost of water by reducing variability, as the portion of energy supplied by renewable sources is linked to a fixed investment cost that does not fluctuate.
- It decreases dependence on external energy sources, as imported energy is subject to a range of variables largely beyond the control of any single country.

Significant advancements have been made in desalination technologies. Reverse Osmosis, the most widely used process, now consumes less energy and, consequently, emits less CO_2 compared to thermal processes. This improvement is the result of several decades of enhanced energy efficiency in the technologies employed. Since 1970, the energy consumption of Reverse Osmosis plants has been reduced tenfold. However, challenges remain, particularly in protecting membranes from salt damage, as well as in further improving the cost-effectiveness and energy efficiency of the process. Most market leaders maintain active research and development (R&D) departments dedicated to this field.

Despite these tangible improvements, Reverse Osmosis desalination remains energy-intensive, which explains the gradual development of its integration with low-carbon energy sources, primarily renewable energies, whose implementation costs have significantly decreased in recent years, and even nuclear energy.

Solar energy is considered to have the greatest potential as a long-term renewable energy source for sustainable desalination [14,15]. There are two main types of solar-powered desalination: Concentrated Solar Power (CSP) and Photovoltaic (PV). CSP generates direct heat and is generally used to evaporate water in thermal desalination. PV uses solar panels to produce electricity, which powers pumps for Reverse Osmosis. For example, the Al Khafji plant in Saudi Arabia produces 60,000 m^3 of desalinated water each day using Reverse Osmosis powered by photovoltaic panels.

A study published in the International Journal of Economic and Management Sciences highlights the potential of solar desalination, showing that a Reverse Osmosis plant powered by photovoltaics can produce water at a cost of $1.213/$m^3$, while the current cost of producing desalinated water using energy from a fossil fuel-based power plant varies considerably, ranging between USD 1.118 and USD 1.555.

The record production cost of 1.75 cents per kWh for the Sakaka project in Saudi Arabia demonstrates that renewable energy can compete broadly with fossil fuels in financial terms.

At this stage, most large-scale desalination projects powered by renewable energy utilize wind power. Wind-powered desalination is particularly suitable for coastal and island communities due to the proximity of the energy source, water supply, and the user population. Wind energy is employed in the Canary Islands of Gran Canaria and Fuerteventura in Spain, where climatic conditions are especially favorable. In Australia, the Perth plant is powered by electricity from the 80 MW Emu Downs wind farm. Each year, this wind farm supplies 270 gigawatt-hours (GWh) to the grid, exceeding the 180 GWh per year requirement of the desalination plant.

Wave energy is more challenging to harness. In Australia, an innovative project was launched in 2014 to produce drinking water and electricity from the ocean. Cape Verde is also on the verge of launching a wave-powered desalination project.

Desalination plants can also be coupled with nuclear generators, and the ongoing installation of three nuclear plants in the United Arab Emirates' grid opens the possibility of coupling them with desalination facilities. Thus, solar and wind coupling has highly promising potential [16,17].

However, currently, only 1% of desalination plants use renewable energy. The Global Clean Water Alliance, founded by the International Desalination Association, has set a goal for at least 20% of new desalination plants to operate on renewable energy between 2020 and 2025. In Australia, all new desalination plants are required to operate on renewable energy.

Nevertheless, obstacles remain. The first is the issue of intermittency, meaning the mismatch between energy supply and demand due to the dependence of production on weather conditions. This is particularly problematic for solar (PV) and wind-powered desalination.

Energy storage is becoming essential for the uninterrupted and reliable operation of desalination plants, yet batteries remain an expensive option that is not always a suitable solution [18] Several approaches can be considered to address the intermittency problem: coupling solar and wind energy wherever possible, supplemented by a grid connection (with more green electricity); and thermal storage, as found in concentrated solar power (CSP) plants that can store heat to continue operating for several hours even without sunlight.

"Currently, most thermal storage systems have an efficiency between 8% and 16%. It is expected that in 10 or 20 years, technical improvements will increase efficiency by 15–25%", according to the World Bank (2019). Another alternative is to increase water storage capacity. Water towers can also be built to store excess water produced during the day and release it at night [13].

6. Conclusions

In the introduction, we posed the question of how Spanish desalination companies have adapted to the multiple changes in the sector. We have observed a business sector with strong resilience, from which we can highlight the following key adaptations to the evolving context:

1. Initial phase. Spanish desalination companies began by undertaking various projects, such as desalination plants, wastewater treatment plants, and brackish water treatment plants. Given the size of the market, these companies initially maintained a small structure with limited staff, and their focus was primarily on the domestic market.
2. Efficient response to the opportunity presented by the AGUA Program. Spanish companies successfully constructed and operated the plants under this program, gaining significant experience and expertise in the process [19].
3. Internationalization. Perhaps the greatest display of resilience occurred when local demand was exhausted. By then, these companies had grown considerably and faced the choice of either internationalizing or dismantling a significant part of their structure. Spanish desalination companies embarked on a successful process of internationalization.
4. Adaptation to the varying conditions of each country. Resilience did not end with internationalization. Desalination plants are not a product that can be manufactured in the home country and exported; rather, they are facilities built on-site, where they must be adapted to local laws and conditions. Spanish desalination companies showed a strong capacity to adapt to the requirements of each tender, allowing them to win contracts against larger, but less flexible, competitors.
5. The most recent demonstration of resilience has been seen in how the sector's companies have adapted to new trends in renewable energy. This change is mainly driven by environmental considerations, but it also brings other benefits. For instance, it allows for more predictable energy supply costs by reducing dependence on the energy market.

Funding: This publication is part of the R&D&I project "Resilience and public policies in the evolution of Spanish industry, 1950–2019" (PID2022-138464NB-I00), funded by MCIN/AEI/10.13039/501100011033/ and by ERDF A way of doing Europe.

Data Availability Statement: Data is contained within the article.

Conflicts of Interest: The author declares no conflict of interest.

References

1. Alsubhi, A.; Balabaid, A.; Al-Qahtani, K.; Al-Gazlan, O.; Shams, A.; Al-Athel, K. The Prospect of Nuclear Power Integrated Desalination Plants in Saudi Arabia. In *Challenges and Recent Advancements in Nuclear Energy Systems*; Shams, A., Al-Athel, K., Tiselj, I., Pautz, A., Kwiatkowski, T., Eds.; SCOPE 2023. Lecture Notes in Mechanical Engineering; Springer: Cham, Switzerland, 2024. [CrossRef]
2. Altmann, T.; Das, R. Process improvement of sea water reverse osmosis (SWRO) and subsequent decarbonization. *Desalination* **2021**, *499*, 114791. [CrossRef]
3. Apolinário, R.; Castro, R. Solar-Powered Desalination as a Sustainable Long-Term Solution for the Water Scarcity Problem: Case Studies in Portugal. *Water* **2024**, *16*, 2140. [CrossRef]
4. Cabreram, E.; Estrela, T.; Lora, J. Desalination in Spain. Past, present and future. *La Houille Blanche* **2019**, *105*, 85–92. [CrossRef]
5. De Miguel, J. Situación actual y futuras actuaciones en las desaladoras gestionadas porAcuamed. In Proceedings of the Congreso Nacional del Agua. Depuración, Reutilización y Desalinización, Orihuela, Spain, 22 February 2019.
6. Eyl-Mazzega, M.C.; Élise Cassignol, E. *The Geopolitics of Seawater Desalination*; Études de l'Ifri, Ifri: Paris, France, 2022.
7. Gabbrielli, E. La desalinización desde el comienzo hasta el final de la Edad Media. In Proceedings of the XIICongreso Internacional de la Asociación Española de Desalación y Reutilización (AEDyR), Toledo, Spain, 23–25 October 2018.
8. García, F. Evaluación de la Viabilidad y Desarrollo de la Innovación de Sistemas Energéticos Híbridos para la Desalinización una Aplicación a las Pequeñas y Medianas Empresas. Ph.D. Thesis, Universidad de León, León, Spain, 2023.
9. Montaño, B. Una visión cooperativa de las medidas ante el posible daño ambiental de la desalación. In *Documentos de Trabajo*; FUNCAS: Madrid, España, 2008; Núm 393.
10. Montaño, B. Análisis Económico de la Desalinización. Ph.D. Thesis, Universidad de Alicante, San Vicente del Raspeig, Spain, 2011.
11. Navarro, T. Water Reuse and Desalination in Spain: Challenges and Opportunities. *J. Water Reuse Desalination* **2018**, *8*, 153–168. [CrossRef]
12. Santos, A. La desalación en España y su proyección internacional. *Econ. Exter. Estud. De La Rev. Política Exter. Sobre La Int. De La Econ. Española* **2007**, *41*, 141–148.
13. Galán, E.S.; Gascón, C.T. Oportunidades de negocio en el sector de la desalación. Mercado mundial en el período 2005–2015. *Ing. Química* **2005**, *423*, 127–130.
14. Straits Research. *Water Desalination Market Size, Share & Trends Analysis Report By Technology (Membrane Technology, Thermal Technology, Other Renewable Technologies), By Applications (Municipal, Industrial, Others), By Water Source (Seawater, Brackish Water, Groundwater and Surface Water) and By Region (North America, Europe, APAC, Middle East and Africa, LATAM) Forecasts, 2023–2031*; Straits Research: Pune, India, 2024.
15. Vera, D. *Spanish Desalination Expertise: A Global Benchmark*; Smart Water Magazine: Madrid, Spain, 2021.
16. Zolghadr-Asli, B.; McIntrye, N.; Djordjevic, S.; Farmani, R.; Pagliero, L.; Martínez, V.; Maestre, J. A review of limitations and potentials of desalination as a sustainable source of water. *Environ. Sci. Pollut. Res.* **2021**, *28*, 15130–15145.
17. Younos, T.; Lee, J. Desalination: Opportunities and Challenges. *WaterWorld*, 10 September 2019.
18. Zarzo, D.; Campos, E.; Terrero, P. Spanish experience in desalination for agriculture. *Desalination Water Treat.* **2013**, *51*, 53–66. [CrossRef]
19. Zarzo, D. La Desalación del Agua en España. *Estud. Sobre La Econ. Española* **2020**, *101*, 169–188.

water

Article

Multi-Scale Gross Ecosystem Product (GEP) Valuation for Wetland Ecosystems: A Case Study of Lishui City

Zhixin Zhu [1,2,*], Keyue Wu [3], Shuyue Zhou [4], Zhe Wang [4,5] and Weiya Chen [6]

1 Department of Environmental Design, Lishui University, Lishui 323060, China
2 Liangshan College (Lishui) China, Lishui University, Lishui 323060, China
3 Lishui Natural Resources and Planning Bureau, Lishui 331100, China; sccdwky@tom.com
4 College of Engineering, Lishui University, Lishui 323060, China; studyzsy@126.com (S.Z.); wangzhe@lsu.edu.cn (Z.W.)
5 Housing and Urban Rural Development Bureau of Lishui, Lishui 323099, China
6 East China Inventory and Planning Institute, NFGA, Hangzhou 310019, China; amilychengood@163.com
* Correspondence: zzx@lsu.edu.cn

Abstract: Traditional gross ecosystem product (GEP) accounting methods often operate at macro scales, failing to reflect the localized and nuanced values of wetland ecosystems. This study addresses these challenges by introducing a fine-grained classification system based on a localized adaptation of international standards. The framework integrates high-precision national land surveys and remote sensing quantitative analysis while incorporating fisheries resource models, climate regulation beneficiary mapping, and visitor interpolation to address data scarcity related to human activities. This approach refines the spatial calculation methods for functional quantity accounting at fine scales. The results demonstrate that the refined classification maintains consistency with traditional methods in total value while adapting to multi-scale accounting, filling gaps at small and medium scales and providing a more accurate representation of localized wetland characteristics. Additionally, the study highlights the dominance of cultural services in GEP, emphasizing the need to balance cultural and regulatory services to ensure fairness in decision-making. Finally, a village-scale decision-support model is proposed, offering actionable guidance for wetland management and sustainable development planning.

Keywords: wetland ecosystem services; gross ecosystem product (GEP); wetland classification; multi-scale accounting; wetland management planning

1. Introduction

Wetlands, often termed the "kidneys of the Earth," are among the most valuable ecosystems due to their high productivity and diverse ecosystem services [1]. As global wetland degradation intensifies, there is increasing recognition of the need for conservation, acknowledging wetlands as essential environmental assets and vital safeguards for the future [2,3]. In response, the gross ecosystem product (GEP) framework has emerged as a promising tool for quantifying ecosystems' economic value, facilitating the integration of ecological benefits into national and local economic planning [4]. In China, the "Two Mountains" theory, which emphasizes that "lucid waters and lush mountains are invaluable assets," guides development policy, promoting the use of GEP to balance economic growth with ecological preservation [5].

As GEP practice advances, there is growing recognition that GEP should not remain merely a policy metric; its valuation results ultimately need to be integrated into concrete urban and rural development as well as specific construction initiatives [6]. Traditional classification methods for large-scale assessments, however, increasingly fall short of current needs [7]. For example, conventional single-label classifications of waterbodies, designed for broad spatial scales, often result in redundant ecosystem service valuations and overlook the functional diversity and specific values of different wetland types. These limitations reduce their effectiveness for contemporary water resource management and planning projects. Addressing these challenges requires developing fine-scale wetland ecosystem service value (WESV) accounting models to enhance GEP's utility as a policy and planning tool. This involves updating and refining WESV methods for GEP by incorporating detailed wetland classifications, implementing adaptive adjustments across spatial scales, and improving accuracy and reliability to better support the practical demands of wetland conservation and management [8].

Assessments of wetland ecosystem services (WESs) have long sought to enhance the diversity of wetland units by employing varied methods to improve the objectivity of functional quantification and evaluation. The integration of diverse geological and statistical data has become widely accepted, as it minimizes reliance on qualitative processes [9]. Studies analyze the impact of human activities on wetlands using Land Use and Land Cover (LULC) [10,11], Nighttime Light (NTL) data [12,13], multispectral indices [14,15] and hydrological modeling [16,17] to assess production and living characteristics at wetland boundaries. However, from the perspective of gross ecosystem product (GEP), the monetary value of wetlands reflects specific societal preferences and demands for wetland products and services [18,19]. Incorporating wetland classification into research improves functional specificity, linking classifications directly with ecosystem product catalogs and statistical data and allowing flexibility in methodological adaptation. Despite numerous studies exploring wetland ecological functions through targeted classifications, inconsistencies in technical standards and guiding principles have led to variability in classification approaches. Many methods classify wetlands by traditional waterbody types, focusing on the influence of these types on dominant ecosystem functions; however, these broad categories can aggregate waterbodies with distinct functions [20–22], risking issues such as double counting. More specific classification methods yield refined insights; for example, Yan and Xia utilized machine learning to subdivide waterbodies, calculating equivalent factors for each type and adjusting biomass values regionally via the Thornthwaite Memorial model [23,24]. Wang's evaluation of ecosystem service values categorizes wetlands into five major types based on waterbody morphology, aligning with the Ramsar Convention but lacking detailed subcategories [25]. Similarly, Dang's GEP study on coastal wetlands applied the MONRE classification system—a RAMSAR convention-based framework—that categorizes coastal wetlands into 19 types, aligning with global standards while incorporating regional attributes to enhance practical relevance [26]. In contrast, Rooney's study used the Alberta Wetland Rapid Evaluation Tool-Actual (ABWRET-A) for Canadian wetlands, offering detailed classifications and water-level subcategories tailored for strong localization [27].

Each classification method for value assessment has unique limitations and focal points, yet all highlight the advantage of linking wetland types with their specific functions, moving beyond the constraints of traditional "one-size-fits-all" accounting. Future research should aim to adopt globally standardized classification frameworks while accommodating localized standards or developing quantitative subcategories to capture regional diversity. This approach allows researchers to choose valuation methods that suit specific wetland types, addressing data gaps, improving accounting efficiency, and enhancing the practical relevance of evaluation results at the regional scale.

Therefore, this study aims to develop a tailored classification system and quantitative analysis methods for the GEP valuation of wetlands in Lishui. Specifically, the objectives are to: (1) optimize a localized wetland classification by integrating new ground survey data and high-resolution remote sensing, grounded in the RAMSAR Convention framework and national wetland classification standards; (2) refine wetland ecosystem service metrics and innovate spatial computation methods for a functional metrics base map across various scales; and (3) publish multi-scale, visualized accounting results to analyze wetland contributions across multiple administrative levels, linking these insights to decision-making models to enhance the practical applications of these results, particularly at small and medium scales.

2. Materials and Methods

2.1. Research Area

Lishui City is located in the southwestern part of Zhejiang Province, China, between 27°25′ to 28°57′ N and 118°41′ to 120°26′ E. The city includes one central urban area and eight counties, covering approximately 1.73 million hectares, with waterbodies totaling 41,285.18 hectares (Figure 1). Situated in a mountainous region with a subtropical monsoon climate, Lishui has diverse wetlands influenced by its varied terrain.

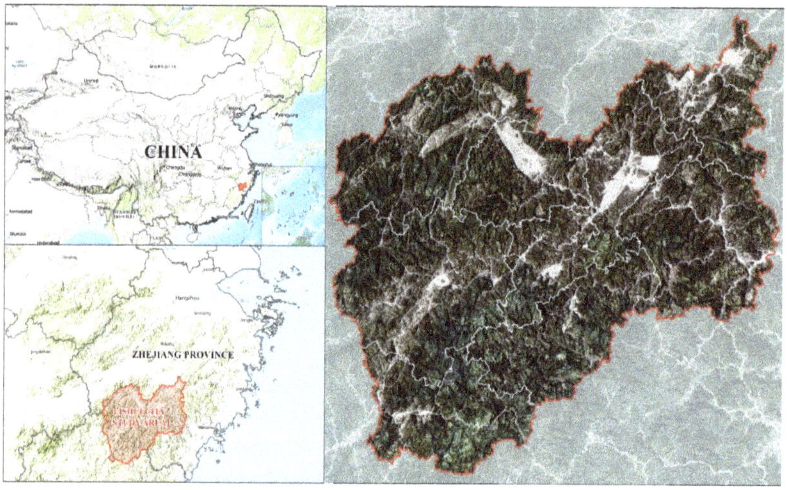

Figure 1. Layout of study area.

Lishui is a leading area in China's ecological development, particularly known for its implementation of the "Two Mountains" theory, which emphasizes the value of ecological resources. Unlike other cities in Zhejiang Province, Lishui prioritizes ecological preservation, focusing on sustainable development instead of GDP growth. The city also released the "Guidelines for Ecological Product Value Accounting," specifically for mountainous regions, demonstrating its commitment to valuing the ecological services provided by wetlands.

2.2. Data and Materials

The integration of satellite imagery and unmanned aerial vehicle (UAV) technology has greatly enhanced wetland surveys, offering detailed visualizations of water features. However, accurately mapping and classifying diverse wetland types remains challenging due to their similarities. To address this, the study utilized the third national land resource survey data(3rd-NLS), provide by the Lishui Natural Resources and Planning Bureau. These datasets, derived from high-resolution satellite imagery (<1 m), combine digital mapping with manual validation to outline waterbodies and provide foundational information. While primarily for government use, 3rd-NLS data have proven instrumental in recent GEP studies. To update these maps, Gaofen-2 multispectral imagery and Google Maps were used alongside 3rd-NLS data, employing eCognition multi-scale segmentation and water index threshold analysis to detect changes and refine vector boundaries.

Additional data sources included public government databases and inter-departmental coordination. Vector data encompassed boundaries of major waterbodies, nature reserves, national parks, scenic areas, and fishing restriction zones, provided by the Municipal Natural Resources and Planning Bureau, Agricultural and Rural Affairs Bureau, and Water

Resources Bureau. Raster data, such as IFSAR (1 m vertical accuracy, 5 m resolution), supported distance cost calculations, and water rendering. Statistical data, including functional indicators and value references, were obtained from sources such as the Lishui Statistical Yearbooks [28], China Population Census Data by Township [29], and reservoir datasets. Interpolation connected spatial positions with tabular data to ensure precise predictive imputation.

2.3. Wetland Mapping

Wetland GEP accounting relies on refined classification of digital waterbody data. However, traditional land classification systems often narrowly define wetlands, excluding many waterbodies and failing to account for the diverse wetland types that are essential from a water resources perspective. China's national standard for wetland classification (GB/T 24708-2009) [30], grounded in the Ramsar Convention's core principles, addresses these shortcomings. It provides comprehensive coverage of waterbodies tailored to China's diverse conditions, aligning with international standards through long-term research and practice. The Wetland Protection Law of the People's Republic of China(WPL-PRC) [31] further underscores the ecological significance of wetlands and excludes waterbodies used exclusively for production purposes. In this study, we adhered to GB/T 24708-2009 [30], excluding farmland and breeding ponds per WPL-PRC guidelines while retaining unique cultural heritage types such as rice–fish co-culture systems and uncultivated paddy fields as wetland types.

Based on Lishui's local wetland origins, geomorphology, hydrological characteristics, and vegetation, we structured the wetlands into three hierarchical levels comprising 13 wetland types, following national standards. The 3rd-NLS dataset, which references the Current Land Use Classification (GB/T 21010-2017) [32], separates wetlands and waterbodies into independent primary categories [33]. Waterbodies were classified as rivers, reservoirs, ponds, agricultural ponds, aquaculture ponds, and ditches, while wetlands were limited to marshes. To align with national standards, this study consolidated waterbody and wetland categories based on morphology, requiring further segmentation to resolve classification conflicts. Through remote sensing and field surveys, we identified 13 wetland types in Lishui: four natural wetland types and nine artificial wetland types, the technical roadmap is shown in the Figure 2.

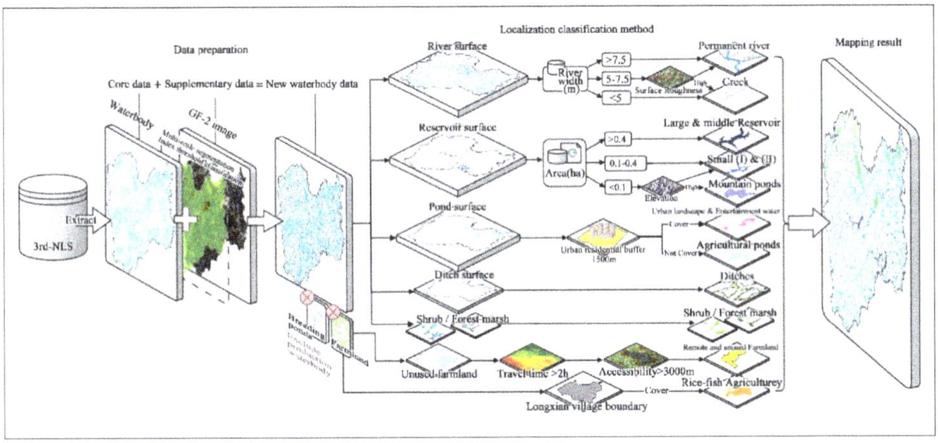

Figure 2. Wetland classification mapping process.

2.4. Function Adjustment by Wetland Type

Due to the diverse types of wetlands and their different functional uses, the monetary evaluation of wetlands was based on the practical connotation of wetland ecosystem services, and the functional quantity and regulation indicators were adjusted according to the range, target, and level of service [9]. We further adjusted the ecosystem service contents provided by different types of wetlands based on ecosystem processes and ecological characteristics (Table 1) and removed some services that are minimally effective or completely replaced by modern technological methods.

Table 1. Service adjustment by wetland type.

	Wetland Type Ecosystem Services		Supply Services	Regulatory Services				Cultural Services
L1 Type	L2 Type	L3 Type	BP	WC	FS	CF	CR	CWT
Natural wetland	River wetland	Permanent river	•	○		•	•	•
		Creek	•			•	•	•
	Marsh wetland	Shrub marsh				•	•	•
		Forest marsh				•	•	•
Artificial wetland	Reservoir	Large and middle	•	•	•	•	•	•
		Small (I)	•	•	•	•	•	•
		Small (II)	•	•	•	•	•	•
		Mountain ponds	•	•	•	•	•	•
	Agricultural pond	Agricultural ponds				•	•	
	Ditch	Ditches				•	•	
	Farmland	Rice–fish agriculture	•			•	•	•
		Remote and unused Farmland				•	•	
	Urban landscape and entertainment water	Urban landscape and entertainment water				•	•	•

Notes: In the table, "•" indicates that the wetland fully provides the respective ecosystem services, while "○" indicates partial provision of the respective ecosystem services.

For functional adjustment, it was based on the characteristics of each wetland type. For ecosystem services related to human activities, the evaluation framework was based on the national standards for wetland definitions, with artificial wetlands primarily referencing the relevant policies and regulations issued by the Water Resources Bureau, which clarified the use and nature of these wetlands. For natural wetlands and micro wetlands that were included, the adjustments were derived from field surveys, during which extensive drone imagery of wetlands was collected, maintaining long-term, multi-temporal, low-altitude digital imagery records of some rivers and streams. In addition, expert consultations provided valuable insights for these adjustments.

2.5. Function Quantity Base Map Optimization

Wetland classification defines the main targets and key functions of waterbody ecosystem services, emphasizing the need to optimize functional accounting in terms of scale, precision, and specificity. Traditional large-scale functional statistics rely on historical data and regional aggregates. In contrast, this study combines multi-source data analysis with optimized scales and specific content to create more accurate valuations for individual patches. Understanding functional quantity, we categorized the three main ecosystem services into natural and social attributes. By integrating geographic and human activity data, spatial statistical analysis was conducted to optimize functional quantity statistics and valuations at the patch scale.

2.5.1. Fishery-Suitable Mapping and Fishery Capacity Base Map

To identify potential fishery-suitable water surfaces for biomass supply services, this study developed a methodology based on fisheries economics while adhering to conservation and land-use regulations. Regulatory documents were reviewed to map restricted fishing areas, including ecological protection zones, municipal water sources, drinking water protection zones, scenic areas, and their buffer zones. The delineation also accounted for forbidden aquaculture zones outlined in the Lishui Aquaculture Waters and Tidal Flats Plan. Artificial fish farms and facility aquaculture sites were excluded, leaving reservoirs, mountain ponds, and rivers—classified as clean waterbodies under wetland classification standards—as the primary fishery-suitable areas.

Lishui's ecological aquaculture model emphasizes community-managed watersheds. To refine suitable areas, restricted zone maps were overlaid with buffer zones around village residential areas, identifying fishery-suitable zones in rivers and streams. In rice–fish symbiotic aquaculture zones, designated as cultural heritage wetland parks, paddy fields were reclassified as wetlands. Differentiation between aquaculture and fishing areas was achieved by applying restrictions and evaluation criteria, excluding aquaculture zones with contractual obligations from fishing areas.

Fishery output from different wetland patches was assessed using a fishery capacity base map (Figure 3a). This map was constructed with a newly designed adjustment model that incorporated a fishery suitability coefficient based on surveys of typical fishery resources [34]. Regional outputs were normalized for comparative purposes, with base data averaged over five years sourced from county-level statistical yearbooks and fishery economic reports. Outputs from aquaculture and fishing were calculated separately due to their distinct characteristics. Additionally, ecological reputation or brand value, reflecting public preference for ecological fishery products [35], was included as a pricing factor [36].

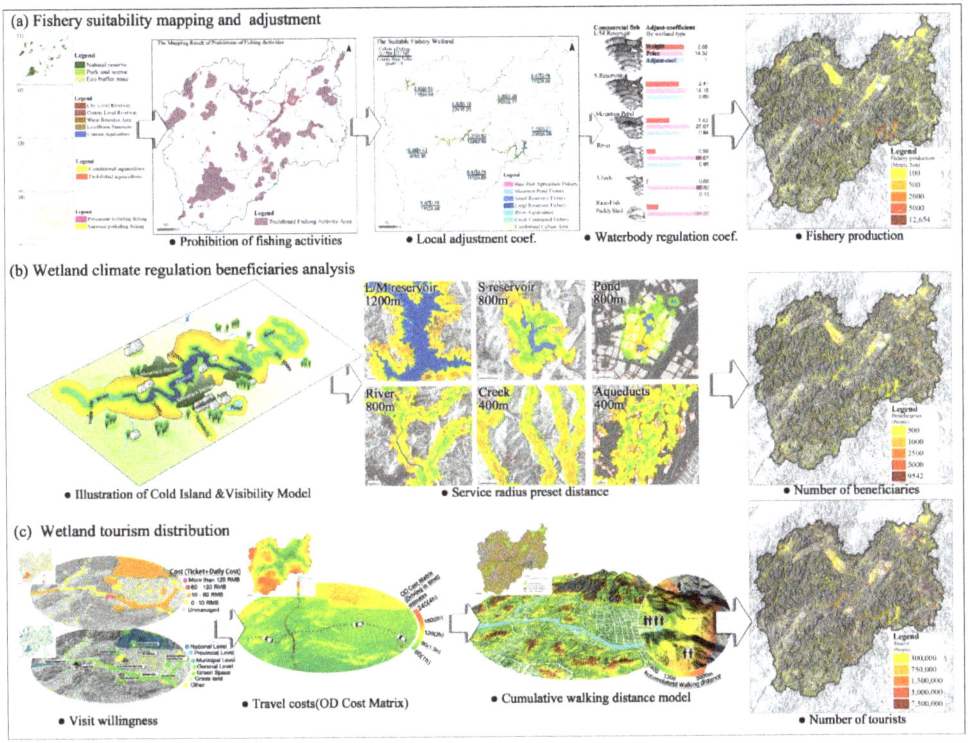

Figure 3. Spatial calculation methods for functional quantities maps based on interpolation optimization. (**a**) Fishery suitability mapping and adjustment. (**b**) Wetland climate regulation beneficiaries analysis and (**c**) wetland tourism distribution.

2.5.2. Wetland Regulatory Services Functional Quantity Base Map

Wetland regulatory services are intrinsically linked to their influence on natural environmental elements, including water conservation, flood control, carbon sequestration, and water purification. The effectiveness of these services is shaped by wetland type and geometric attributes. Larger waterbodies with complex ecosystems exhibit greater self-regulation and resilience, while smaller, fragmented wetlands often provide less efficient services. To improve accuracy in evaluating wetland functions, this study applied correction coefficients based on geometric attributes for different wetland categories, further refining functional quantity estimates through adjustments for average vegetation coverage within newly defined buffer zones.

The social dimension of regulatory services was examined through the cooling effect of wetlands on residential areas during summer. Wetland buffers of 1200 m, 800 m, and 400 m were established based on studies of the water cold island effect [37–39], with adjustments for patch shape and density. A potential beneficiary raster map was constructed using DEM data as a blocking surface(Figure 3b). Population data were sourced from the seventh national census, with interpolation guided by a residential base map derived from 3rd-NLS data, encompassing urban and rural patches. To account for Lishui's urban–rural characteristics, population density was distributed using an area growth optimization index. These distributions were overlaid with the cold island.

2.5.3. Wetland Tourism Population Inversion Model

The cultural services of wetland ecosystems, primarily focused on tourism and wellness, reflect significant social dimensions. Key benchmarks for evaluation included visitor numbers, origins, duration of stay, and consumption patterns. However, city-wide assessments faced challenges due to limited data collection at scenic spots. To address these gaps, a visitor interpolation map was developed for tourism-valued wetlands (see Figure 3c), utilizing five years of cumulative visitor data from over 300 scenic spots across nine counties. Interpolation accounted for spatial links between scenic area entrances and core landscapes, providing a city-wide visitor distribution map.

The interpolated map integrated travel intention thresholds, constructed based on factors such as visit opportunities, travel costs, and access costs, normalized using survey results. Weighting factors, including infrastructure quality, reputation, and unique landscapes, were derived from official documents and online surveys. Exceptional wetlands, such as habitats for the Chinese Merganser and Chinese giant softshell turtle, received higher rankings. Travel and access cost data, collected through questionnaires (324 valid responses), revealed strong preferences for trips under 45 min (92.36%) and daily expenditures below 60 yuan (85.38%). These findings were used to construct a travel cost model incorporating resistance factors from an OD cost matrix.

Wetland accessibility was evaluated using a cumulative walking distance model, estimating distances visitors could travel after reaching core landscapes. Walking distances were categorized into four intervals with associated probabilities: comfortable (<400 m, 100%), moderate (400–1200 m, 50%), fatigued (1200–3000 m, 25%), and extreme (>3000 m, 10%). The model incorporated road types (excluding highways), geomorphology, and land use resistance values. Slope data and land classification from 3rd NLS were included to assess walking difficulty.

2.6. GEP Accounting Standards and Localization Adjustments

The accounting standards for the value of wetland ecological products primarily refer to Technical specification for gross ecosystem product accounting [40]. The categories used in this standard were selected by the National development and reform commission and are mandatory references for this project. Based on this framework, research efforts were made to introduce localized optimizations and implement necessary adjustments in line with the objective realities.

The foundational data for functional quantities were derived from remote sensing quantitative analysis and vectorized results of statistical yearbooks. A refined spatial calculation method was employed to generate the base map of functional quantities. The value calculations for provisioning and regulatory services primarily utilized the residual value method, replacement cost method, and market value method, with coefficient adjustments based on the basic conditions of waterbodies. Cultural services were evaluated mainly using the travel cost method, with accommodation and dining values attributed to wetland-related areas based on the dominance of wetlands in regional tourism. The calculation methods and adjustments are detailed in Table 2 and Figure 4.

Table 2. Gross ecosystem product (GEP) accounting standards and adjustments.

Service	Calculation Formula
BP	$V_p = E_w - E_r - E_a - E_e - E_b$ (1) In Equation (1), V_p: biomass supply value; E_w: value added of biomass products (yuan/a); E_r: employee paid (yuan/a); E_a: depreciation of fixed assets; E_e: net production tax (yuan/a); E_b: normal capital return (yuan/a).
WC	$Q_{wr} = \sum_{i=1}^{n} A_i \times (P_i - R_i - ET_i) \times 10^3$ (2) $V_{wr} = Q_{wr} \times (C_{we} + P_{we} \times D_r)$ (3) In Equation (2), Q_{wr}: wetland ecosystem water conservation capacity (m^3/a); A_i: patch i wetland ecosystem area (km^3); P_i: rainfall (mm/a); R_i: surface runoff (mm/a); ET_i: evapotranspiration (mm/a). In Equation (3): V_{wr}: wetland ecosystem water source conservation value(yuan/a); C_{we}: annual operating cost per unit capacity of reservoir (yuan/(m^3·a)); P_{we}: engineering cost per unit storage capacity of reservoir (yuan/m^3); D_r: annual depreciation rate of reservoirs.
FS	$C_{fm} = C_{rfm} + C_{mfm}$ (4) $V_{fm} = C_{fm} \times (C_{we} + P_{we} \times D_r)$ (5) In Equation (4), C_{fm}: wetland ecosystem flood storage capacity (m^3/a); C_{rfm}: reservoir flood regulation capacity (m^3/a), which is based on based on empirical equations, C_{mfm}. In Equation (5), V_{fm}: wetland ecosystem flood regulation and storage value (yuan/a); P_{we} and D_r are the same as in Equation (3).
CF	$Q_{tCO_2} = \sum_{i=1}^{n} M_{CO_2}/M_C \times SCSR_i \times SW_i \times 10^{-2}$ (6) $V_{Cf} = Q_{tCO_2} \times C_{CO_2}$ (7) In Equation (6), Q_{tCO_2}: physical quantity of carbon fixation (t·CO_2/a); M_{CO_2}/M_C: equals 44/12, the coefficient of conversion from C to CO_2; $SCSR_i$: carbon fixation rate of type i wetland ecosystem (g·C/(m^2·a)); SW_i: type i wetland area. In Equation (7), V_{Cf}: carbon fixation value (yuan/a); C_{CO_2}: carbon dioxide price (yuan/t·CO_2).
CR	$E_{we} = E_{wt} \times \rho_w \times q \times 10^3/(3\,600 \times r)$ (8) $V_{cr} = E_{we} \times P_e$ (9) In Equation (8): E_{we}: energy consumption of evapotranspiration (kW·h/a); E_{wt}:evapotranspiration during open air conditioning cooling period $(m)^3$/a); ρ_w: density of water (g/cm^3); q: volatile latent heat, which is the heat required to evaporate 1 g of water (J/g); r: air conditioning energy efficiency ratio. In Equation (9), V_{cr}: climate regulation value of wetland ecosystems; P_e: local consumption electricity price (yuan/kW·h).
TH	$N_t = \sum_{i=1}^{n} N_{ti}$ (10) $V_{th} = \sum_{i=1}^{n} N_{ti} \times TC_i$ (11) In Equation (10), N_t: total number of wetland natural landscape tourists; N_{ti}: the number of tourists to the patch i wetland natural scenic area (person · time/a). In Equation (11), V_{th}: tourism and health value of wetland ecosystem (yuan/a); TC_i: the average travel cost of tourists to wetland patch i (yuan/(person · time).

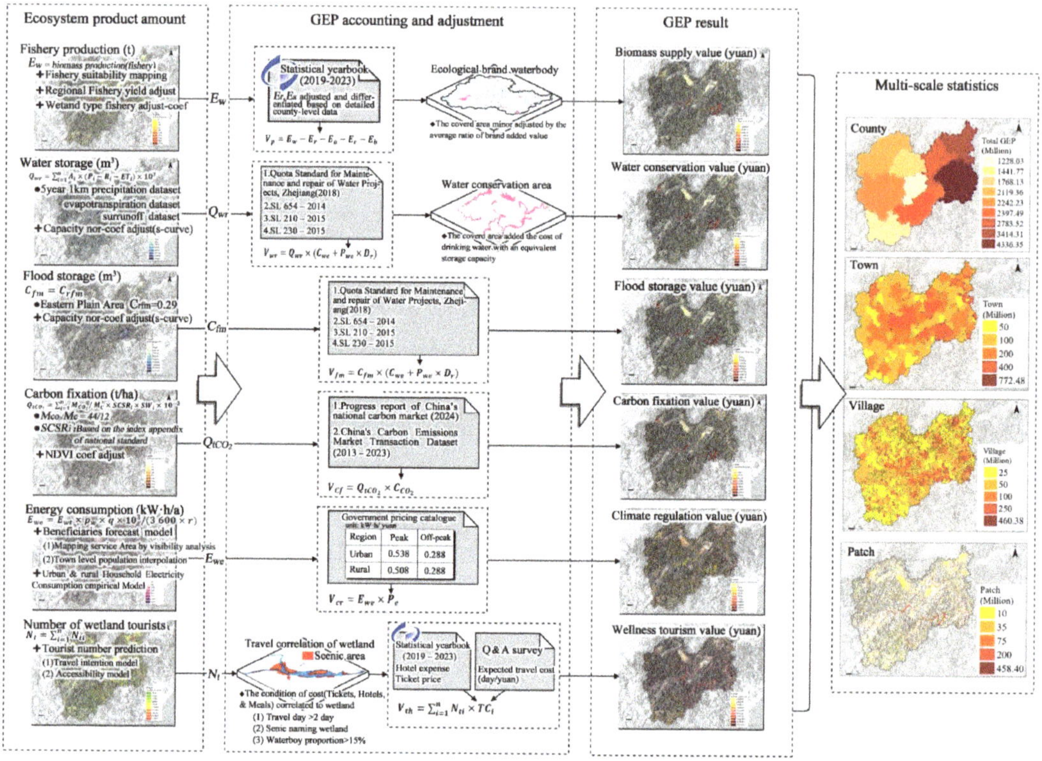

Figure 4. GEP accounting process: In the ecosystem product amout part, the "·" symbol in the figure indicates data calculations based on coefficients or models specified in the standard, while the "+" symbol denotes the spatial calculations or adjustment coefficients added for optimizing functional quantities in the research design.

3. Results

3.1. Wetland Classification Mapping

Wetland classification followed national standards, regulations, and the latest laws and was optimized by combining remote sensing digital products and spatial location analysis for the secondary segmentation of the 3rd NLS. The 3rd NLS data ensured the accuracy of basic waterbody boundaries.

According to the wetland classification map (Figure 5), the total wetland area in Lishui was 40,967.2 ha, with natural wetlands covering 21,221.7 ha (51.80%) and artificial wetlands covering 19,745.5 ha (48.20%). Natural wetlands accounted for more than half of Lishui's wetlands, representing the ecological essence of wetland welfare. Within natural wetlands, river wetlands served as the largest type, covering 18,330.1 ha (86.37%), with a smaller proportion of rocky streams but densely distributed in the city. Artificial wetlands, resulting from human modification or creation, were mostly found in suburban towns and primarily used for water resources, agriculture, forestry, fishing, and domestic water supply. Among artificial wetlands, reservoir wetlands significantly helped to increase the overall proportion, with many townships comprising more than half of their area as reservoir wetlands. As a strong ecological city in an agricultural country, Lishui has numerous agricultural ponds and canals used for irrigation, widely distributed across the city and especially concentrated in the two main plains.

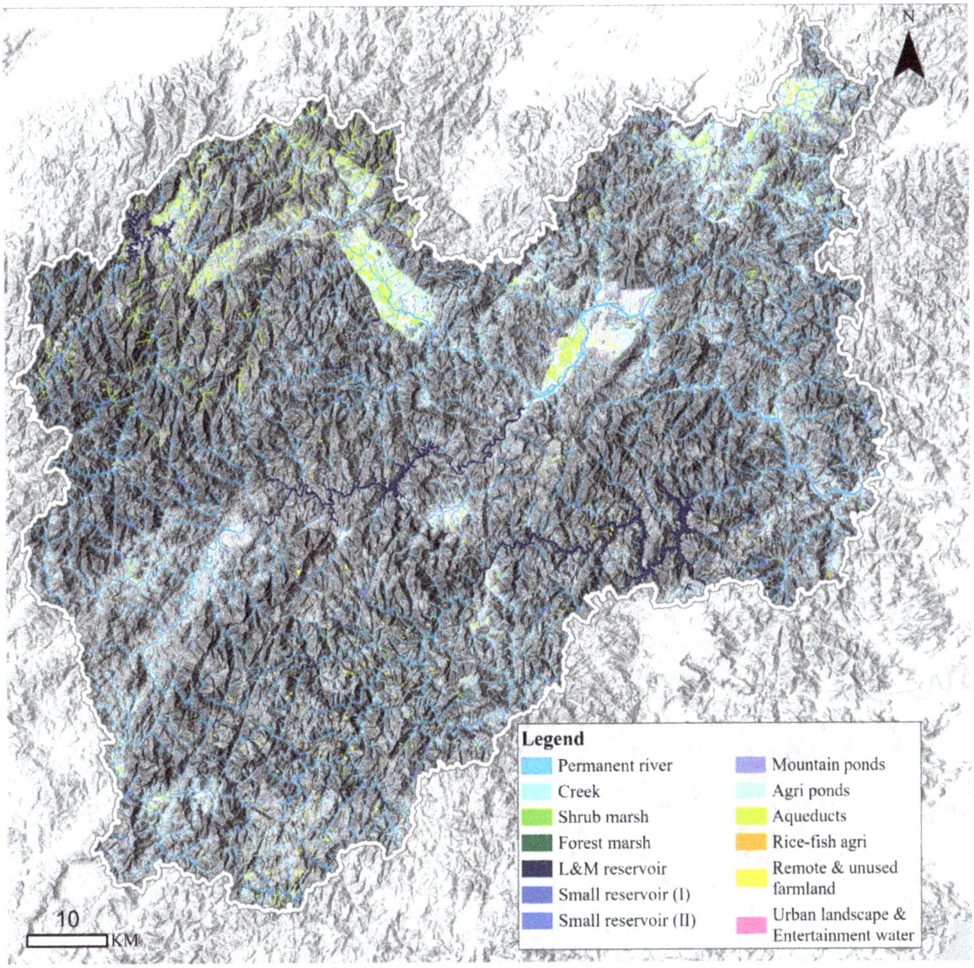

Figure 5. Lishui wetland classification map.

Overall, the distribution of wetland waterbodies at different scales shows significant variations (Figure 6). There are notable differences in the wetland areas and types between counties, towns, and villages, reflecting the complexity and diversity of wetland ecosystems across different administrative divisions. These differences may also be related to the geographical conditions, ecological management practices, and economic development approaches of each region. The reclassified wetland waterbodies were assigned geographic attribute information, including the administrative affiliation, area, and corresponding functional quantities, which could be further used for wetland product value accounting and multi-category wetland management.

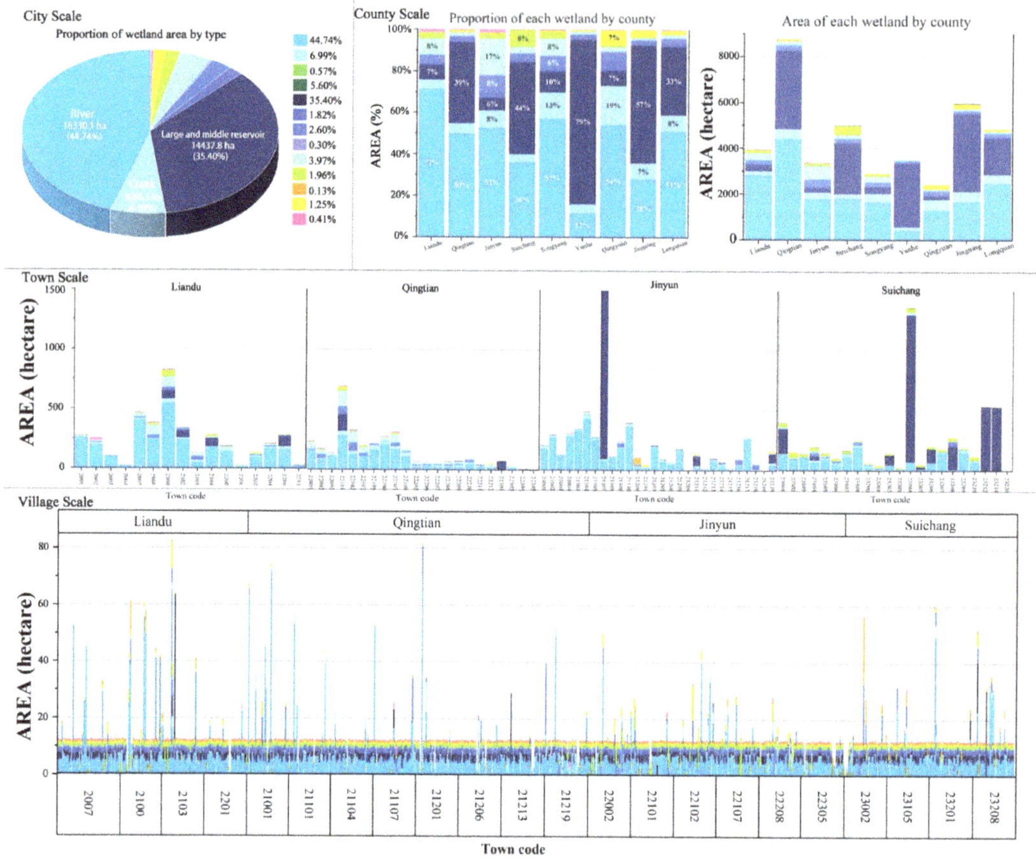

Figure 6. Multi-scale wetland waterbody area statistics.

3.1.1. Multi-Scale GEP Accounting Results and Visualization

According to the calculations result (Figure 7), the total potential GEP value of Lishui's wetlands was approximately 19.121 billion RMB, comprising 865.42 million RMB from supply services, 4471.93 million RMB from regulatory services, and 16,393.84 million RMB from cultural tourism services. Cultural services accounted for the dominant share (over 74.46%), highlighting the critical role of tourism and recreation in Lishui's wetland ecosystem value. At the county level, Qingtian County ranked first with a total value of 3.767 billion RMB, demonstrating strong contributions across all service categories and establishing itself as a model for wetland resource development. In contrast, significant value fluctuations in some counties, coupled with a lack of clear advantages, suggest potential inefficiencies in resource utilization and planning.

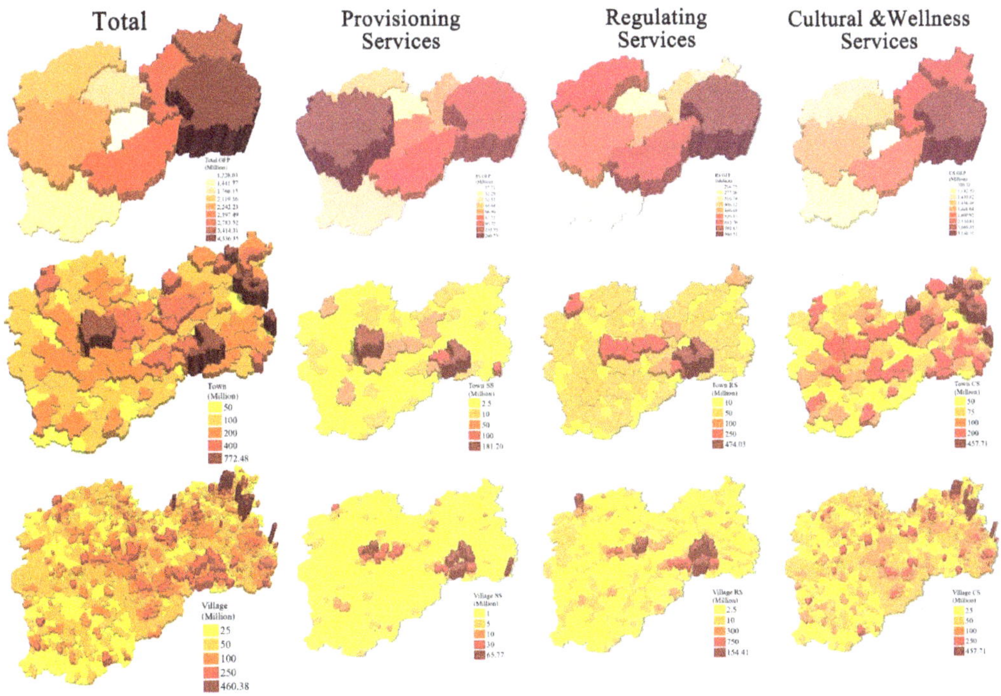

Figure 7. Gross ecosystem product result in multi scale.

Compared to the city and county scales, township-scale analysis revealed a reduction in the number of wetland types and increasing differentiation in the area and quantity. Additionally, the accounting and visualization results at the township scale highlight that highly concentrated high-value areas often contribute disproportionately to the overall totals at broader scales, while low-value townships, which are masked as "high-value" in city- or county-level statistics, are more widely distributed at this finer scale. This reflects the imbalance and strong differentiation of regional wetland GEP values.

At the village scale, the region was further divided into over 2000 administrative units, with the number of wetland types becoming even more reduced and showing greater variation in local water environments and economic differences. Accounting and visualization results at the village scale largely continued the spatial distribution patterns observed at the county level. However, due to the influence of wetland classification and the administrative attribution of waterbodies, the value units were assigned with greater precision. This refinement also provided clearer insights into localized resource utilization and conservation opportunities, enabling more targeted guidance for grassroots planning and projects.

3.1.2. Influence of Classification on Wetland Contributions

The classified wetland GEP results demonstrate continuity and consistency with traditional single-waterbody statistical methods in total values. As shown in Tables 3 and 4, the total GEP of Lishui wetlands under the classified approach aligns closely with traditional statistics, with minor variations observed, such as a −0.77% change in supply services and a −6.03% change in regulatory services. These findings confirm that the classified method maintains overall coherence while enhancing data precision.

Table 3. Wetland area and water patch index analysis.

Twon	Wetland Area Waterbody (ha)	Classified (ha)	±Δ (%)	Water Patch Index NC	NP	PLAND Type	(%)	OD Matrix (Hour)	Wetland Support Tourist Number (M/per)	Beneficiary (Household)
LS	41,285.18	40,967.2	−0.77	12	20,102	River	44.74	103	1422	320,747
S1_XD	156.92	140.46	−10.45	6	150	River	72.21	82.43	49.69	1589
S2_MZ	138.15	139.11	0.64	8	155	River	45.68	112.25	8.13	1691
S3_YC	139.99	139.47	−0.32	5	29	L&m Reservoir	58.95	111.66	5.54	1192
S4_BX	136.56	140.97	12.01	6	64	River	85.31	123.30	3.07	254
S5_BJ	139.40	139.30	−0.01	6	45	River	79.94	99.97	5.56	1385

Table 4. Wetland ecosystem services functional quantities analysis.

Twon	Supply Services Waterbody (Million)	Classified (Million)	±Δ (%)	Regulatory Services Waterbody (Million)	Classified (Million)	±Δ	Cultural Services Waterbody (Million)	Classified (Million)	±Δ
LS	880.59	865.42	−1.72	4759.16	4471.93	−6.03	28,280.00	16,393.84	−42.03
S1_XD	0.78	0.12	−84.61	12.64	11.25	−10.99	-	457.71	-
S2_MZ	0.65	0.26	−60	16.05	15.13	−5.73	-	97.76	-
S3_YC	4.28	1.68	−60.75	17.32	16.00	−7.62	-	50.42	-
S4_BX	0.46	0.02	−95.65	12.07	10.93	−9.44	-	55.46	-
S5_BJ	0.15	0.07	−53.33	12.46	10.92	−12.36	-	48.12	-

The classified approach also introduces greater local specificity, as evidenced by differences across S1–S5, five townships with similar wetland areas. For instance, cultural services in towns BX (S4) and BJ (S5) showed significant reductions compared to others, primarily due to adjustments in wetland types and their associated ecosystem services. Regulatory services followed a similar trend, with notable differences such as −12.36 million RMB in S5 and −16.05 million RMB in S2, reflecting the spatial heterogeneity of wetland functions under the classified system.

Additionally, the classified wetland method facilitates finer-scale analyses by integrating macro-to-micro evaluations. It enables more precise tourism value estimations by incorporating factors such as travel intention and access resistance. This refined approach bridges broader planning with localized assessments, offering a more detailed and accurate representation of regional wetland GEP values.

Compared to the township scale, village-level wetlands are more "public-oriented" and practical waterbodies, serving as direct sites for water resource planning and landscape projects. By aligning wetland services with local needs, classified GEP accounting provides a clearer reflection of village-level wetland characteristics and offers valuable insights for planning and design decisions. As presented in Table 5, four pairs of villages were selected based on two criteria: significant differences in wetland contribution rates (Z-scores) and high similarity in wetland areas (Figure 8). The results indicate that cultural services are the dominant contributor to the total GEP, revealing a significant disparity between cultural services and other ecosystem services. This dominance is primarily attributed to the "Tourist number" variable, as cumulative tourist consumption substantially impacts the total GEP, even under low individual expenditure scenarios. Consequently, regulatory services are often overshadowed by cultural services, yet they play a critical ecological role that is frequently undervalued. For instance, in the P3 group, while P3-1 recorded a higher total GEP, P3-2 exhibited stronger regulatory services, highlighting the significant contribution of regulatory services in villages with limited tourism development. Similar patterns were observed in the P1, P2, and P4 groups, where regulatory service contribution rates between paired villages were relatively close, further emphasizing their importance even when they did not dominate the total GEP.

Table 5. Comparative analysis of village pairs selected by Z-score.

Village Pair	Total GEP (Million)	Wetland Area (%)	Tot Avg. Con (Yuan/m^2)	SS Avg. Con (Yuan/m^2)	RS Avg. Con (Yuan/m^2)	CS Avg. Con (Yuan/m^2)	PLAND Type (%)	Tourist Number (M/per)	Beneficiary (Household)
P1_1	68.79	5.22 (2.65)	1319.03	0.388	9.886	1308.76	S reservoir (50.98)	1.14	287
P1_2	8.12	5.22 (2.61)	155.68	0.018	7.88	147.78	Agri pond (59.33)	0.22	437
P2_1	439.09	17.53 (5.15)	2504.83	0	7.67	2497.16	River (80.75)	7.35	170
P2_2	25.40	17.57 (2.35)	144.51	0.024	7.73	136.76	River (93.82)	0.40	148
P3_1	419.94	24.10 (5.70)	1742.66	0.002	8.06	1734.60	River (81.62)	6.97	207
P3_2	19.48	24.11 (28.70)	80.81	0	14.00	66.81	L&m reservoir (99.93)	0.48	4
P4_1	409.92	37.10 (3.92)	1104.94	0.003	7.99	1096.95	Rive (74.25)	6.78	301
P4_2	38.16	37.12 (4.60)	102.78	0.005	7.44	95.31	Rive (93.71%)	0.59	115

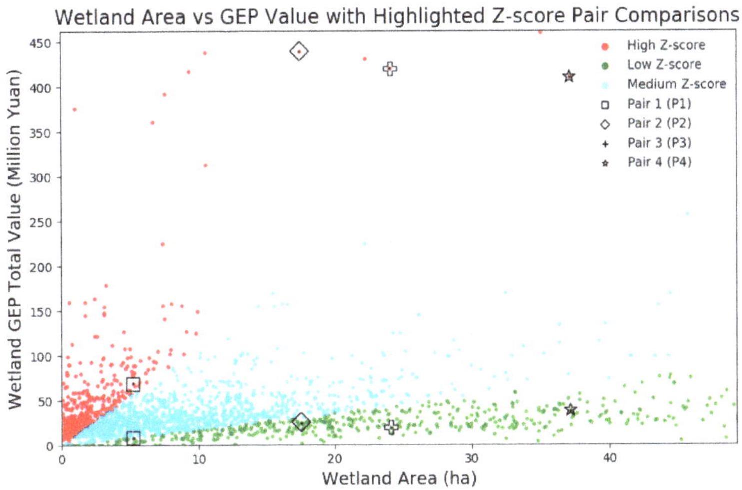

Figure 8. Wetland area vs. GEP value with Z-score selections.

To achieve a more balanced and comprehensive assessment, it is necessary to evaluate wetlands based on a combination of the contribution rates of both regulatory and cultural services.

3.1.3. Strategic Evaluation Framework for Village-Level Wetlands

To better utilize the small-scale GEP accounting results from both macro-level planning and practical development perspectives, this study addresses the imbalance caused by the overemphasis on cultural services in value assessments. A preliminary planning strategy classification method was developed to assist in quickly identifying development and conservation strategies for village-level wetlands. This method is based on two key indicators: wetland contribution clustering and the proportion of wetland area to the total village area.

The clustering analysis classified village-level wetlands into nine categories based on normalized Regulating Service Contribution (RScon) and Cultural Service Contribution (CScon) (Figure 9). These nine categories highlight the differences in ecological and cultural contributions among village wetlands and provide actionable insights for decision-makers in evaluating wetland functions. The wetland area proportion indicator is designed to measure whether a village is highly dependent on water resources and wetland-related economic benefits. Both indicators are weighted equally at 0.5. For more detailed information, please refer to Tables 6 and 7. The results are illustrated in Figure 10.

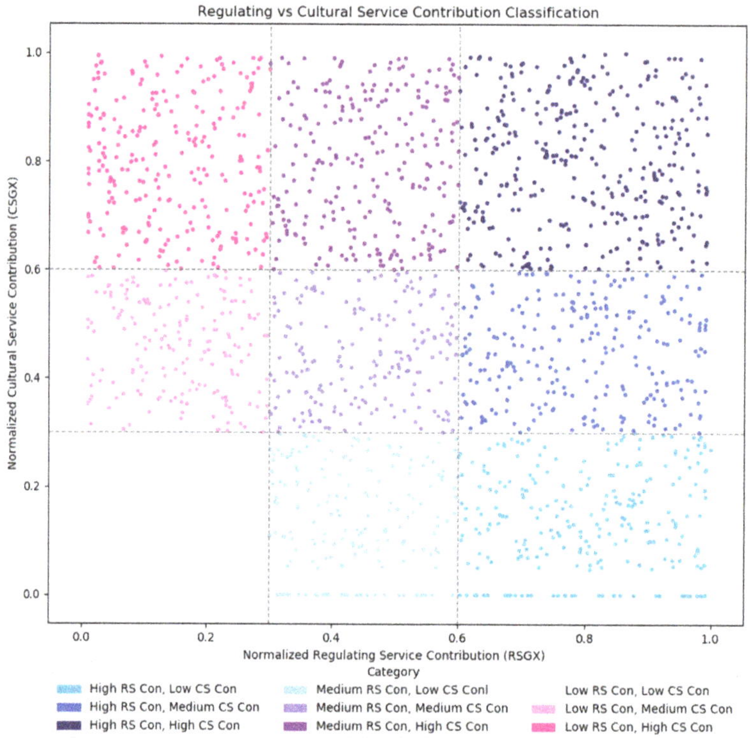

Figure 9. Cluster analysis of regulatory vs. cultural service contributions.

Table 6. Evaluation index system for village-level wetland development strategy.

Indicator	Weight	Value		Grade
W_{con}: Clustering of Wetland Contribution	0.5	RS Con High-	CS Con High	100
			CS Con Med	80
			CS Con Low	70
		RS Con Med-	CS Con High	60
			CS Con Med	60
			CS Con Low	50
		RS Con Low-	CS Con High	50
			CS Con Med	30
			CS Con Low	10
W_{aper} Proportion of Wetland Area to Village Area	0.5	≥20%		100
		5–20%		60
		0.1–5%		30

Table 7. Evaluation index system for village-level wetland development strategy.

Type	Evaluation Score (S)	Development Strategy
A	80–100	Focus on developing CS (cultural services) as the primary goal, with RS (regulatory services) as a secondary priority for protection.
B	65–79	Prioritize the development of CS (cultural services) as the primary goal, with RS (regulatory services) as a complementary enhancement.
C	45–64	Prioritize the development of RS (regulatory services), with localized/minor enhancement of CS (cultural services).
D	20–44	Focus on developing RS (regulatory services).

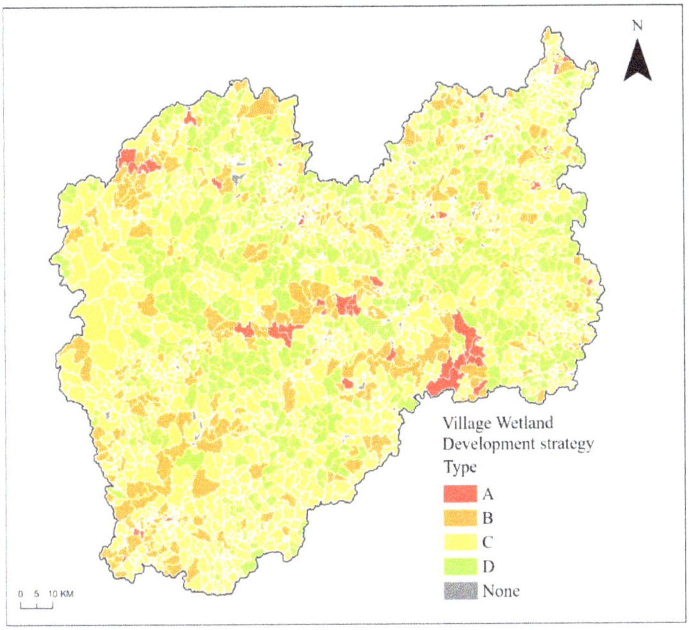

Figure 10. Village-level wetland development strategy map.

4. Discussion

4.1. Impacts of Scale and Resolution Changes in GEP Valuation

Transitioning to finer spatial scales and higher resolution has significantly advanced GEP accounting by enabling more precise integration of ecological values into local planning and development strategies [6,41]. Unlike traditional methods that treat ecosystems as broad economic indicators, fine-scale GEP accounting captures unique wetland characteristics and regional variations, providing more actionable data for urban planning, water resource management, and conservation efforts. However, this refinement introduces challenges, particularly in classifying transition zones and allocating values at smaller administrative levels.

Accurate classification of wetland boundaries is crucial for maintaining ecological continuity and preserving their full ecosystem value. However, current delineation practices often disrupt this continuity, particularly for shallow water zones and biologically diverse transitional areas. Official surveys typically define natural wetland boundaries based on water levels and artificial wetlands according to design plans. Yet, critical ecological buffers in transitional zones are frequently misclassified as forests, grasslands, or other non-wetland types [42,43]. Such misclassification undervalues wetland functions and negatively impacts ecosystem service assessments [44]. In this study, vegetation indices from buffers were incorporated into ecosystem service calculations to address the undervaluation of transitional zones. While this approach showed potential, further research is needed to develop more robust accounting methods to supplement the functional assessment of these areas.

Challenges in population interpolation and service valuation become more pronounced at lower administrative levels, complicating accurate assessments of ecosystem services. Wetlands spanning multiple jurisdictions or exhibiting linear shapes often face difficulties in proportionally allocating population data due to overlapping administrative boundaries [45,46]. Similarly, for smaller wetlands, independent interpolation of population data frequently results in repeated or inflated estimates, further distorting service valuation accuracy. To address these issues, this study aggregated population data at higher administrative levels, applying township-scale maximum population density ranges to improve consistency and reduce duplication [47,48].

4.2. Exploring the Deeper Cultural Service Value of Wetlands

Cultural services play a dominant role in determining wetland GEP, reflecting their substantial social and economic significance [49,50]. However, their prominence can sometimes overshadow other critical services, such as regulatory services, leading to imbalances in wetland valuation and development planning. Addressing this imbalance requires a more nuanced assessment framework.

In this study, the travel cost method was adapted to evaluate cultural services in fragmented wetland patches. While effective for natural scenic wetlands with established data, its adaptation involved interpolating population data based on transportation costs and walkability indices. This approach often fell short in capturing the recreational and wellness functions of rural wetlands, where shoreline accessibility is a key factor [51,52]. Field surveys indicated that many rural wetlands, though less suitable for structured recreational activities, still attract significant leisure tourism, generating substantial expenditures on outdoor and food-related activities. These contributions are often overlooked in current accounting systems, revealing the need for a more inclusive evaluation framework [53,54].

Emerging methods, such as EEG-based studies of landscape emotions, offer innovative ways to quantify public responses to wetland landscapes [55]. However, their experimental nature limits their immediate application for large-scale assessments [56]. Practical tools such as the SolVES model, particularly when integrated with Maxent, provide valuable insights into recreational and social values, enabling the identification of high-value areas and refining travel expenditure estimates [57,58]. Despite these advancements, collecting detailed social survey data for wetlands across a municipality remains a significant challenge.

4.3. Enhancing Wetland GEP Models for Localized and Dynamic Planning

In the preliminary GEP strategy model established in this study, evaluation rules were developed to guide development strategies for village-level wetlands by balancing ecological and cultural functions. Regulatory services, as foundational indicators of natural benefits and ecological health, are prioritized to support cultural tourism. In critical situations, targeted restoration efforts are recommended to improve ecological conditions. The model also takes into account the economic dependence of villages on wetlands, incorporating a wetland proportion score to adjust cultural service priorities. Thus, regions with weaker regulatory services are advised to focus on ecological restoration, while areas with higher cultural service contributions require controlled development to avoid resource overexploitation.

While the scoring-based strategy model provides a useful framework for initial evaluations, it has inherent limitations when dealing with the complex uncertainties that arise from the dynamic interactions between wetland ecosystems and human activities. The fluctuating nature of wetland environments, combined with the unpredictable behavior of humans, makes traditional scoring approaches insufficiently adaptable and precise. To address these challenges, it is necessary for wetland GEP models to integrate advanced optimization frameworks—such as probabilistic and fuzzy methods—to enhance their resilience and provide more effective support for planning and adaptive management [59].

These advanced methods are capable of capturing both natural variability and anthropogenic uncertainties [60], thereby balancing ecological conservation and economic objectives while integrating stakeholder preferences. By optimizing performance in areas such as resource allocation and risk mitigation, these methods improve the model's ability to handle complex scenarios such as urbanization, climate change, and precipitation variability. For instance, they enable better land-use optimization [61], enhance food and water security [62], and support sustainable ecosystem planning [63]. The integration of these advanced methodologies allows wetland GEP models to effectively address the unpredictability of human activities and the complexity of natural systems, thereby significantly improving their applicability in dynamic regulation and long-term management. This ultimately provides more robust and flexible support for localized and regional planning efforts.

5. Conclusions

This study developed a refined wetland classification framework and fine-scale GEP accounting methods tailored for localized wetland ecosystem management. By incorporating the Ramsar Convention guidelines and national standards, the research effectively delineated wetland functions while ensuring the framework's adaptability to high-precision spatial data. Functional calculations were optimized for various wetland types, addressing human-related activities such as fisheries, climate regulation, and tourism, and localized valuation methods were applied to enhance objectivity and accuracy. A village-scale decision-support model was proposed, emphasizing the balance between regulatory and cultural services to guide sustainable wetland management and development.

The study produced several key findings that enhance the understanding and application of wetland GEP accounting:

- Developed a fine-grained wetland classification framework based on a nationally adapted international standard, effectively defining wetland functions.
- Produced high-resolution GEP results at multiple scales, enabling comparisons of regional wetland value and development.
- Achieved total GEP values consistent with those of traditional methods, ensuring continuity while filling gaps at medium and small scales to reflect local characteristics.
- Highlighted the dominance of cultural services in total GEP, underscoring the need to ensure fairness in decisions impacted by service data disparities.
- Proposed a village-scale wetland decision model, balancing regulatory and cultural services, with a decision-support map for wetland management and development.

This study identified several limitations that should be addressed in future research. First, interpolation models heavily rely on statistical and empirical data, which limits their precision, particularly in evaluating cultural services such as visitor-related impacts. Second, the economic valuation framework is constrained by standardized national guidelines, requiring adjustments to better reflect local conditions. Finally, the lack of a dynamic analysis component means the study does not fully account for temporal variations and uncertainties inherent in wetland ecosystems, leaving room for improvement in addressing fluctuating environmental conditions and human influences.

To address these challenges, future research should focus on three priorities. First, it should enhance data accuracy through collaborations with planning and survey agencies, the adoption of real-time monitoring systems, and the use of advanced digital tools to reduce reliance on interpolation. Second, it should incorporate dynamic models to capture seasonal and annual variations in ecosystem functions, improving the adaptability and accuracy of GEP assessments. Third, it should refine decision-support frameworks to address practical needs in wetland management and urban planning while integrating diverse economic resources to better handle external uncertainties and dynamic changes.

Author Contributions: Conceptualization, Z.Z. and K.W.; methodology, Z.Z. and K.W.; software, Z.Z. and S.Z.; validation, Z.Z., K.W. and S.Z.; investigation, Z.Z. and K.W.; data curation, K.W. and Z.Z.; writing—original draft preparation, Z.Z. and S.Z.; writing—review and editing, K.W., Z.W. and W.C.; visualization, Z.Z.; supervision, Z.Z.; project administration, Z.Z.; funding acquisition, Z.Z. and S.Z. All authors have read and agreed to the published version of the manuscript.

Funding: This work was supported by Research Projects of the China (Lishui) Two Mountains Institute, found by the Lishui city development and reform commission [grant numbers FGLS202216]; The public welfare technology application research program, project of lishui, China [grant numbers 2024GYX04].

Data Availability Statement: The data that support the findings of this study are available from Lishui Natural Resources and Planning Bureau. Restrictions apply to the availability of these data, which were used under license for this study. Data are available with the permission of Lishui Natural Resources and Planning Bureau.

Conflicts of Interest: The authors declare no conflict of interest.

References

1. Morris, M.; Chew, C.; Reager, J.T.; Shah, R.; Zuffada, C. A novel approach to monitoring wetland dynamics using CYGNSS: Everglades case study. *Remote Sens. Environ.* **2019**, *233*, 111417. [CrossRef]
2. McCarthy, M.J.; Radabaugh, K.R.; Moyer, R.P.; Muller-Karger, F.E. Enabling efficient, large-scale high-spatial resolution wetland mapping using satellites. *Remote Sens. Environ.* **2018**, *208*, 189–201. [CrossRef]
3. Davidson, N.C. How much wetland has the world lost? Long-term and recent trends in global wetland area. *Mar. Freshw. Res.* **2014**, *65*, 934–941. [CrossRef]
4. Ouyang, Z.; Zhu, C.; Yang, G.; Xu, W.; Zheng, H.; Zhang, Y.; Xiao, Y. Gross ecosystem product: Concept framework and case study. *Acta Ecol. Sin.* **2013**, *33*, 6747–6761. [CrossRef]
5. Huang, Z.; Bai, Y.; Ali, M.; Fang, Z. "Two Mountains concept" leading the green transformation of China's economic society. *J. Environ. Manag.* **2024**, *359*, 120960. [CrossRef]
6. Song, C.; Ouyang, Z. Theoretical Connotation and Application Practice of Gross Ecosystem Product (GEP). *Frontiers* **2023**, *18*, 92–95. [CrossRef]
7. Yang, Q.; Liu, G.; Casazza, M.; Hao, Y.; Giannetti, B.F. Emergy-based accounting method for aquatic ecosystem services valuation: A case of China. *J. Clean. Prod.* **2019**, *230*, 55–68. [CrossRef]
8. Chen, H. At least two accounting systems for Gross Ecosystem Product (GEP) are needed. *J. Environ. Manag.* **2024**, *370*, 122429. [CrossRef]
9. Gao, Y.; Cui, L.; Wang, F.; Li, W.; Lei, Y.; Sun, B. Evaluation of wetland ecosystem services based on big data. *Water Resour. Hydropower Eng.* **2017**, *48*, 1–9+23. [CrossRef]
10. Long, X.; Lin, H.; An, X.; Chen, S.; Qi, S.; Zhang, M. Evaluation and analysis of ecosystem service value based on land use/cover change in Dongting Lake wetland. *Ecol. Indic.* **2022**, *136*, 108619. [CrossRef]
11. Liu, Y.; Jiang, Y.; Yang, C. Land use dynamics and ecosystem service valuation in the Sanmenxia Reservoir wetland of the Yellow River. *Sci. Rep.* **2024**, *14*, 23594. [CrossRef] [PubMed]
12. Lu, D.; Chang, J. Examining human disturbances and inundation dynamics in China's marsh wetlands by using time series remote sensing data. *Sci. Total Environ.* **2023**, *863*, 160961. [CrossRef] [PubMed]
13. Aguilera, M.A.; González, M.G. Urban infrastructure expansion and artificial light pollution degrade coastal ecosystems, increasing natural-to-urban structural connectivity. *Landsc. Urban Plan.* **2023**, *229*, 104609. [CrossRef]
14. Dar, S.A.; Dar, J.A. Linking carbon storage with land use dynamics in a coastal Ramsar wetland. *Sci. Total Environ.* **2024**, *932*, 173078. [CrossRef]
15. Zhang, S.; Tian, J.; Lu, X.; Tian, Q. Temporal and spatial dynamics distribution of organic carbon content of surface soil in coastal wetlands of Yancheng, China from 2000 to 2022 based on Landsat images. *Catena* **2023**, *223*, 106961. [CrossRef]
16. Pattison-Williams, J.K.; Pomeroy, J.W.; Badiou, P.; Gabor, S. Wetlands, flood control and ecosystem services in the Smith Creek Drainage Basin: A case study in Saskatchewan, Canada. *Ecol. Econ.* **2018**, *147*, 36–47. [CrossRef]
17. Gupta, R.; Chembolu, V.; Marjoribanks, T.I.; Dutta, S. Assessing the efficacy of hydro-ecological based wetland management approach for flood resilience of a large river catchment. *J. Hydrol.* **2024**, *641*, 131761. [CrossRef]
18. Aryal, K.; Ojha, B.R.; Maraseni, T. Perceived importance and economic valuation of ecosystem services in Ghodaghodi wetland of Nepal. *Land Use Policy* **2021**, *106*, 105450. [CrossRef]
19. Badamfirooz, J.; Mousazadeh, R.; Sarkheil, H. A proposed framework for economic valuation and assessment of damages cost to national wetlands ecosystem services using the benefit-transfer approach. *Environ. Chall.* **2021**, *5*, 100303. [CrossRef]
20. Bo, X.; Mi, W.; Xu, H.; Dong, J. Estimating of ecological service value for different wetland types based on multi-source data fusion in Ningxia Plain. *J. Zhejiang Univ.* **2016**, *42*, 228–244. [CrossRef]

21. Huang, X.; He, J.; Zhang, Q.; Wu, Z.; Wu, Y. Evaluating wetland ecosystem services value and dominant functions: Insights from the Pearl River Delta. *J. Environ. Manag.* **2024**, *371*, 123069. [CrossRef] [PubMed]
22. Xie, C.; Zeng, Y.; Hao, X.; Ning, Z.; Xie, T. Asymmetric impacts of natural and anthropogenic factors on wetland landscape evolution in Fenhe River Basin, China. *Watershed Ecol. Environ.* **2024**, *6*, 176–186. [CrossRef]
23. Yan, J.; Zhu, J.; Zhao, S.; Su, F. Coastal wetland degradation and ecosystem service value change in the Yellow River Delta, China. *Glob. Ecol. Conserv.* **2023**, *44*, e02501. [CrossRef]
24. Xia, S.; Xue, Z.; Dong, S.; Wu, H.; Yu, X.; Hao, Z. Identification and scoring of conservation gaps in wetlands of China's coastal provinces: Implications for extending protected areas. *J. Environ. Manag.* **2024**, *358*, 120865. [CrossRef]
25. Wang, W.; Xu, J.; Luan, X.; Zhang, Z. Wetland ecosystem service values in Beijing significantly increased from 1984 to 2020: Trend changes, type evolution, and driving factor. *Ecol. Indic.* **2024**, *166*, 112235. [CrossRef]
26. Dang, K.B.; Phan, T.T.H.; Nguyen, T.T.; Pham, T.P.N.; Nguyen, M.H.; Hoang, T.T.H. Economic valuation of wetland ecosystem services in northeastern part of Vietnam. *Knowl. Manag. Aquat. Ecosyst.* **2022**, *423*, 12. [CrossRef]
27. Rooney, R.C.; Royall, O.; Robinson, D.T.; Cobbaert, D.; Trites-Russell, M.; Wilson, M. Evaluating the development and use of a rapid wetland assessment tool (ABWRET-A) in policy implementation in Alberta, Canada. *Environ. Sci. Policy* **2022**, *136*, 575–587. [CrossRef]
28. Lishui Statistical Bureau. *Lishui Statistical Yearbook*; China Statistics Press: Beijing, China, 2019–2023.
29. National Bureau of Statistics of China. *China Population Census Data by Township*; China Statistics Press: Beijing, China, 2020.
30. *GB/T 24708-2009*; General Rules for Wetland Resource Survey. Standards Press of China: Beijing, China, 2009.
31. Standing Committee of the National People's Congress. Wetland Protection Law of the People's Republic of China. Adopted on December 24, 2021, effective June 1; 2022. Available online: https://www.mee.gov.cn/ywgz/fgbz/fl/202112/t20211227_965347.shtml (accessed on 27 December 2021).
32. *GB/T 21010-2017*; Classification of Wetlands. Standards Press of China: Beijing, China, 2017.
33. Yuan, J.; Shi, L.; Tang, X. A Preliminary Analysis of Three Mainstream Wetland Definitions in Wetland Conservation and Management in China. *Wetl. Sci.* **2022**, *20*, 607–612. [CrossRef]
34. Yuan, J.; Lian, Q.; Wang, K.; Yao, Z.; Lu, J.; Zhang, A.; Mi, G. Seasonal variations of fish community structure in Lishui section of Oujiang River main stream. *Chin. J. Ecol.* **2010**, *29*, 1585–1590.
35. Paul, J.; Modi, A.; Patel, J. Predicting green product consumption using theory of planned behavior and reasoned action. *J. Retail. Consum. Serv.* **2016**, *29*, 123–134. [CrossRef]
36. Zhou, Q.; Wu, K.; Yao, L.; Chen, R.; Liu, S.; Xing, H.; Nie, L.; Wu, Z. Bio-ecological remediation of freshwater aquaculture environments: A systematic review and bibliometric analysis. *Water Biol. Secur.* **2023**, *3*, 100229. [CrossRef]
37. Ji, P.; Wang, Y.; Zhu, C.; Sheng, Y. Effects of Air Temperature and Relative Humidity of Small and Medium-sized Lakes and Reservoir in Daqing City during Daytime in Summer. *Wetl. Sci.* **2017**, *15*, 665–669. [CrossRef]
38. Cai, Z.; Han, G.; Chen, M. Do water bodies play an important role in the relationship between urban form and land surface temperature? *Sustain. Cities Soc.* **2018**, *39*, 487–498. [CrossRef]
39. Cai, Y.; Wu, Z.; Chen, Y.; Wu, L.; Pan, W. Investigate the difference of Cooling effect between water Bodies and green spaces: The study of Fuzhou, China. *Water* **2022**, *14*, 1471. [CrossRef]
40. National Development and Reform Commission. *Technical Specification for Gross Ecosystem Product Accounting*; People's Publishing House: Beijing, China, 2022.
41. Kovács, E.; Kelemen, E.; Kalóczkai, Á.; Margóczi, K.; Pataki, G.; Gébert, J.; Málovics, G.; Balázs, B.; Roboz, Á.; Krasznai Kovács, E.; et al. Understanding the links between ecosystem service trade-offs and conflicts in protected areas. *Ecosyst. Serv.* **2015**, *12*, 117–127. [CrossRef]
42. Haukos, D.A.; Johnson, L.A.; Smith, L.M.; McMurry, S.T. Effectiveness of vegetation buffers surrounding playa wetlands at contaminant and sediment amelioration. *J. Environ. Manag.* **2016**, *181*, 552–562. [CrossRef]
43. Feng, W.; Santonja, M.; Bragazza, L.; Buttler, A. Shift in plant-soil interactions along a lakeshore hydrological gradient. *Sci. Total Environ.* **2020**, *742*, 140254. [CrossRef]
44. Antala, M.; Juszczak, R.; van der Tol, C.; Rastogi, A. Impact of climate change-induced alterations in peatland vegetation phenology and composition on carbon balance. *Sci. Total Environ.* **2022**, *827*, 154294. [CrossRef]
45. Bangwayo-Skeete, P.F.; Skeete, R.W. Can Google data improve the forecasting performance of tourist arrivals? Mixed-data sampling approach. *Tour. Manag.* **2015**, *46*, 454–464. [CrossRef]
46. Li, J.; Li, J.; Yuan, Y.; Li, G. Spatiotemporal distribution characteristics and mechanism analysis of urban population density: A case of Xi'an, Shaanxi, China. *Cities* **2019**, *86*, 62–70. [CrossRef]
47. Millward, H.; Spinney, J. Time use, travel behavior, and the rural–urban continuum: Results from the Halifax STAR project. *J. Transp. Geogr.* **2011**, *19*, 51–58. [CrossRef]
48. Li, D.; Xu, D.; Zhou, Y.; Lv, L.; Chen, X. Sustainable rural development through slow tourism images: A case study of Gaochun International Cittàslow in China. *J. Destin. Mark. Manag.* **2024**, *32*, 100903. [CrossRef]
49. Chaikumbung, M.; Doucouliagos, H.; Scarborough, H. Institutions, culture, and wetland values. *Ecol. Econ.* **2019**, *157*, 195–204. [CrossRef]
50. Csurgó, B.; Smith, M.K. The value of cultural ecosystem services in a rural landscape context. *J. Rural. Stud.* **2021**, *86*, 76–86. [CrossRef]

51. Rice, W.L.; Park, S. Big data spatial analysis of campers' landscape preferences: Examining demand for amenities. *J. Environ. Manag.* **2021**, *292*, 112773. [CrossRef]
52. Phillips, K.E.; Rice, W. A Scoping Literature Review of Fairness and Equity Engagement in US River Recreation Allocation Research. *Int. J. Wilderness* **2023**, *29*, 108–122. [CrossRef]
53. Xiang, K.; Cao, Y.; Qiao, G.; Zhang, H. Mechanisms of communitas experience generation in glampers: An interactive ritual perspective. *J. Hosp. Tour. Manag.* **2023**, *55*, 355–367. [CrossRef]
54. Koppen, G.; Sang, Å.O.; Tveit, M.S. Managing the potential for outdoor recreation: Adequate mapping and measuring of accessibility to urban recreational landscapes. *Urban For. Urban Green.* **2014**, *13*, 71–83. [CrossRef]
55. Zhu, H.; Yang, F.; Bao, Z.; Nan, X. A study on the impact of Visible Green Index and vegetation structures on brain wave change in residential landscape. *Urban For. Urban Green.* **2021**, *64*, 127299. [CrossRef]
56. Kerebel, A.; Gélinas, N.; Déry, S.; Voigt, B.; Munson, A. Landscape aesthetic modelling using Bayesian networks: Conceptual framework and participatory indicator weighting. *Landsc. Urban Plan.* **2019**, *185*, 258–271. [CrossRef]
57. Guan, D.; Ran, B.; Zhou, L.; Jin, C.; Yu, X. Assessing and transferring social value of ecosystem services in wetland parks based on SolVES model. *Ecol. Indic.* **2023**, *157*, 111300. [CrossRef]
58. Shi, X.; Zhao, X.; Pu, J.; Gu, Z.; Zhao, Q.; Feng, Y.; Zhou, S. Creating a monetization-SolVES model to visualize the cultural ecosystem services for promoting landscape conservation. *J. Nat. Conserv.* **2024**, *77*, 126521. [CrossRef]
59. Jiang, B.; Wong, C.P.; Cui, L.; Ouyang, Z. Wetland economic valuation approaches and prospects in China. *Chin. Geogr. Sci.* **2016**, *26*, 143–154. [CrossRef]
60. Zeng, X.; Li, T.; Chen, C.; Si, Z.; Huang, G.; Guo, P.; Zhuang, X. A hybrid land-water-environment model for identification of ecological effect and risk under uncertain meteorological precipitation in an agroforestry ecosystem. *Sci. Total Environ.* **2018**, *633*, 1613–1628. [CrossRef]
61. Zeng, X.T.; Huang, G.H.; Yang, X.L.; Wang, X.; Fu, H.; Li, Y.P.; Li, Z. A developed fuzzy-stochastic optimization for coordinating human activity and eco-environmental protection in a regional wetland ecosystem under uncertainties. *Ecol. Eng.* **2016**, *97*, 207–230. [CrossRef]
62. Zeng, X.T.; Zhao, J.Y.; Yang, X.L.; Wang, X.; Xu, C.W.; Cui, L.; Zhou, Y. A land-indicator-based optimization model with trading mechanism in wetland ecosystem under uncertainty. *Ecol. Indic.* **2017**, *74*, 479–499. [CrossRef]
63. Zeng, X.; Zhao, J.; Wang, D.; Kong, X.; Zhu, Y.; Liu, Z.; Dai, W.; Huang, G. Scenario analysis of a sustainable water-food nexus optimization with consideration of population-economy regulation in Beijing-Tianjin-Hebei region. *J. Clean. Prod.* **2019**, *228*, 927–940. [CrossRef]

water

Article

The Hydro-Economic Modeling of Low-Flow Events on the Middle Elbe: Assessing Socio-Economic Impacts on River Navigation

Lukas Folkens *, Daniel Bachmann, Udo Satzinger and Petra Schneider

Department of Water, Environment, Construction and Safety, Magdeburg-Stendal University of Applied Sciences, 39114 Magdeburg, Germany; daniel.bachmann@h2.de (D.B.); udo.satzinger@h2.de (U.S.); petra.schneider@h2.de (P.S.)

* Correspondence: lukas.folkens@h2.de; Tel.: +49-3931-886-4650

Abstract: Low-flow events cause socio-economic impacts in various sectors. However, there are few hydro-economic models to quantify these. This article presents a hydro-economic modeling approach to determine the direct economic damage of low flows to freight and tourist navigation on free-flowing rivers. This includes the description of the required hydrological and economic input variables, a presentation of the calculation approach and the development of the damage functions. Damage and replacement costs were calculated for the study area of the middle Elbe in order to test the model and show how low-flow events affect freight and tourist navigation. Our results indicate that considerable economic losses occur not only during low flows, but also when the reference water levels for navigation are only slightly exceeded over a long period of time. It was also shown that certain river sections are more vulnerable to low-flow events and therefore cause higher costs. The model represents an analytical tool that considers both economic and hydrological aspects. As a part of a holistic risk assessment, it can help decision-makers to understand the interactions between water and the economy and to develop strategies that promote sustainability in water resource management.

Keywords: low-flow risk management (LFRM); hydro-economic low-flow model; hydrological drought; middle Elbe; low-flow damage costs

1. Introduction

The consecutive European summer droughts of recent years represent a historical anomaly [1–3]. Many European rivers reached new hydrological negative extremes in terms of duration, discharge and water levels during this period [4]. In view of climatic changes, low-flow events in Europe are expected to continue to become more frequent in the future [5,6]. As a manifestation of a hydrological drought, low-flow periods reduce the surface water level. A distinction must be made between temporary water shortages caused by hydrological droughts and structural stress conditions, which are referred to as water scarcity [7]. If a hydrological drought affects socio-economic systems, it is referred to as socio-economic drought [8]. As rivers appear as both natural and social systems, they can also be understood as socio-ecohydrological systems [9].

The economic impacts of drought events in Europe are generally discussed extensively in the literature (e.g., [10–12]). For instance, Folkens et al. (2023) [13] have summarized the socio-economic consequences of low-flow events in a review paper. They discuss the associated effects on tourism and recreation, energy production and industry, water suppliers and households, government units, aquatic production, agriculture and forestry, as well as navigation. In the next step, the identified impacts are translated into damage models. For navigation, they state that it is necessary to relate the water level as a reference to associated costs, where lower water levels correlate with higher operating costs for individual entities [13]. However, there are few hydro-economic models that can be used to determine damage costs caused by low-flow events. The main objective of this article is therefore to describe the key elements of such a hydro-economic model, with a focus on freight and tourist navigation. In particular, the correlation between hydrological and economic parameters is clarified in order to show how a changed flow regime in free-flowing rivers affects the cost structure for navigation. The model was calibrated and tested for the middle Elbe.

As transportation routes, rivers provide an ecosystem service [14] of great economic importance, particularly for the cost-effective and sustainable transportation [15,16] of bulk, hazardous and heavy goods and also containers. Thus, one barge with a loading capacity of 1500 tons replaces 15 jumbo rail hoppers or 58 trucks [17]. Focusing on Germany, the network of inland waterways has a length of around 7300 km, 70 percent of which are of international importance according to the European classification system for inland waterways. Inland navigation transports around 230 million tons of goods per year on Germany's rivers and canals [18]. The economic use is contrasted by the considerable impact of inland navigation on biodiversity, as highlighted by Sexton et al. (2024) [19] for European rivers. However, these could not be considered in the study, as the focus is primarily limited to the economic and not the ecological effects of low-flow events.

The development of hydro-economic models to calculate damage costs is important because low-flow events have resulted in enormous social costs in the past, as studies have shown. Koetse and Rietvald (2009) [20], for example, calculated a loss of around EUR 91 million for Rhine shipping in the drought year 2003. Another study published in 2020 estimated economic losses totaling EUR 2.7 billion for inland navigation and industry in Germany and the Netherlands during the 2018 low-flow period [21]. Using water level data over a period of almost 20 years and relating these to freight prices, Jonkeren et al. (2007) [22] estimated the average annual welfare loss due to low water levels on the Rhine at around EUR 28 million. There are further studies for navigation on the Rhine, and the consequences for the Danube navigation were also examined by combining economic factors such as carrying capacity and freight prices with hydrological factors such as water levels [23–25]. Using the example of the Meuse catchment area, Sinaba et al. (2013) [26] investigated the economic damage of low-flow events on inland navigation, as well as on the sectors of energy, agriculture and water supply. The Meuse is a regulated watercourse that is significantly influenced by weirs. The report therefore emphasizes, for example, that a safe minimum water level can be ensured and that no problems arise for navigation due to insufficient water depths. For this reason, the damage assessment refers more to the locking process, which excludes transferability to free-flowing rivers such as the middle Elbe. The approach presented focuses on free-flowing rivers and thus closes a gap in previous research, which has often concentrated on regulated waterways. Moreover, the studies cited focus primarily on the evaluation of historical data for the assessment of low-flow damage, whereas a model-based approach is presented here that combines a hydrodynamic river model with economic input variables. Although historical discharge data can also be used for this purpose, this approach makes it possible to calculate how a change in discharge will affect navigability and how the adjustment of shipping fleets will impact transport figures. In contrast to the studies presented on damage costs on the Rhine, this study not only refers to the water levels of a reference gauge (for the Rhine it is usually the Kaub gauge), but also includes every cross-section of the entire catchment area of the middle Elbe. This allows a comparison of the hydrological and economic results for each river section, which is unique in this form for German navigation in general and for the middle Elbe in particular. No study has yet been carried out for the Elbe to estimate the economic damage to navigation. In the Netherlands, however, the National Water Model [27] already uses the Dutch inland transport model BIVAS, which calculates the annual transport costs based on a daily time series of water levels [28]. The model approach described in this article is partially inspired by this, but has a reduced degree of complexity, a different economic valuation approach and a dedicated focus on free-flowing rivers.

The basic approach to developing a conceptual damage model for low flows is comparable to that for floods, but there are also substantial differences. Damage assessment in the event of flooding starts with the determination of damage to destroyed infrastructure [29], while the focus of damage assessment in the event of low flows is primarily on the damage to ecosystem services. From an economic perspective, freshwater from rivers is a scarce resource in terms of both quality and quantity, and various players are competing for its use. At the same time, it is a public good since it is potentially freely accessible to everyone and can be used by several users at the same time. Accordingly, it is subject to the "tragedy of the commons", which means that it will be overexploited sooner or later due to the absence of, or inadequate, regulation [30]. This emphasizes the need for a holistic low-flow risk management (LFRM) approach that includes not only hydrological and ecological components but also economic components. For the hydro-economic model, the required hydrological and economic input variables are described and the calculation process and the damage parameters are presented. The general structure, basic assumptions and functionality of the model are also discussed. As part of the DryRivers research project, which is developing an LFRM approach called LoFloDes [31,32], the model is an analytical tool that considers both economic and hydrological aspects. It can help decision-makers to understand the interactions between water and the economy and to develop strategies that promote sustainability in water resource management.

2. Materials and Methods

2.1. General Approach

Key factors that influence navigation on waterways are, on the one hand, the draught of the vessel T and, on the other, the depth of the fairway h_f. The most important variable is the water supply in the catchment area of the inland waterways. When water levels are low, cargo ships and passenger vessels alike cannot operate at their maximum capacity, leading to increased costs. The model approach therefore consists of linking hydrological and economic input variables, as shown in the scheme in Figure 1.

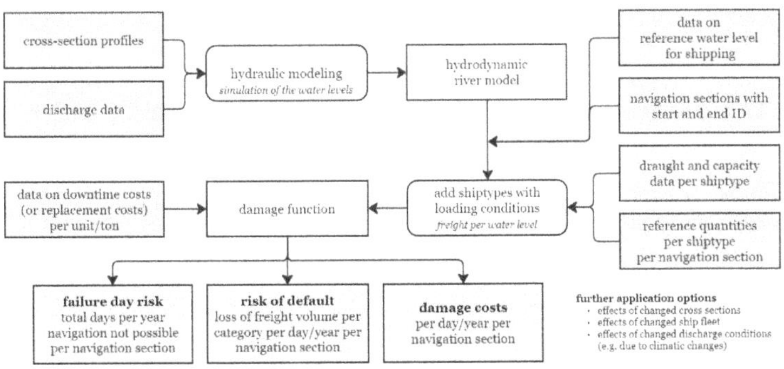

Figure 1. Hydro-economic modeling approach to assess low-flow impacts on river navigation.

Reference data on navigation are added to the river model, which is generated from the cross-sections (c) and discharge data. Furthermore, start and end points can be defined for subdivided river sections (sec), from which the section length L_{sec} can also be calculated. The hydrodynamic calculation provides the water levels h_c (m) per cross-section and allows statements to be made about whether the reference low water levels per cross-section $h_{r,c}$ (m) for navigation according to

$$h_c - h_{r,c} > 0, \tag{1}$$

$$h_c - h_{r,c} < 0, \tag{2}$$

are exceeded (1) or not (2), whereby the most limiting cross-section is representative for the entire river section: $h_{c,min,sec}$ (m). The damage function is controlled based on the calculated difference from $h_{c,min,sec}$ by assigning utilization states u_s (%) per ship type s, with $u_{0,s}$ representing a utilization of 0 percent and $u_{1,s}$ a utilization of 100 percent. This generates a gradual calculation of different loading conditions according to $h_{c,min,sec}$, which are stored by reference freight (or passenger) quantities $q_{s,sec,pot}$ (e.g., t/d). The multiplication of u_s and $q_{s,sec,pot}$ results in $q_{s,sec,state}$ (e.g., t/d), according to the following equation:

$$u_s \times q_{s,sec,pot} = q_{s,sec,state}. \tag{3}$$

By calculating the lost freight volume, the reduction in freight is determined on a daily basis: $q_{s,sec,state}$ (e.g., t/d). The calculated lost freight is multiplied by a damage value d specified in the damage function for economic quantification, resulting in $D_{sec,i}$:

$$(q_{s,sec,pot} - q_{s,sec,state}) \times d = D_{sec,i}. \tag{4}$$

Finally, the annual loss amount $D_{sec,year}$ is calculated.

The damage value d can be expressed on the one hand by downtime costs d_d (e.g., EUR/t) and on the other hand by replacement costs d_r (e.g., EUR/t), as explained in Section 2.2. The general approach is limited to free-flowing rivers and can only be applied wherever discharge and data on the reference water level for navigation $h_{r,c}$, as well as traffic figures, are known. Therefore, the accuracy of the model is highly dependent on the quality and availability of hydrological and economic data. As these data are available for all German inland waterways, the approach described can be applied accordingly to these waterways. As a result, it provides the following parameters, ordered by the requirements of available data, with the lowest requirements first and the highest requirements last:

- Failure day risk according to Equation (2) = total days per year with a utilization rate of zero percent (hydrological characteristic value) (d/a);
- Risk of default as units not transported per day or per year per navigation section (e.g., t/a);
- Damage costs $D_{d,sec,year}$ or replacement costs $D_{r,sec,year}$ per year (EUR/a).

The model can be used to analyze both a current and a future state as well as measures for a free-flowing river. For example, the influence of a change in the cross profiles, e.g., due to a deepening of the fairway, on the downtime days per year can be calculated. Furthermore, the low-flow capability of different ship types can be tested to show how the downtimes develop with a changed fleet. Different discharge scenarios can also be calculated, considering various climate projections, to determine the effects of climatic changes on transportation conditions.

2.2. Downtime and Replacement Costs

As mentioned, the damage value d can be expressed by downtime costs d_d (e.g., EUR/t) or alternatively by replacement costs d_r (e.g., EUR/t). Downtime costs d_d of a cargo ship in a low-flow situation can vary significantly depending on various factors such as the ship type, cargo type, operational costs and market conditions. Similar considerations apply to passenger shipping, where direct downtime costs result from the loss of income for the providers of tourist cruises. Here, these are not expressed in tons per year. Rather, the risk can be quantified in lost visitors per year. This in turn can be monetized if the lost revenue per visitor is included. As exact figures for both cargo and passenger navigation depend heavily on these specific factors and are often not publicly available, it is not possible to give a universally valid figure. However, like all the other input variables and functions that are stored, the downtime costs can also be entered individually by the users themselves. Justified assumptions were made for the Elbe, as shown below. If no downtime costs are available, replacement costs d_r can also be calculated in accordance with the replacement cost method [33], e.g., by calculating the costs for alternative modes of transport (truck and rail) per ton and comparing them with those for inland navigation.

In doing so, the focus can be placed on the evaluation of environmental costs. According to the Federal Environment Agency Methodological Convention 3.0 (MC3.0) for assessing environmental costs, the total economic value of an environmental good is made up of use-dependent and use-independent values [34]. Use-independent values, such as the existence or bequest value, are not included in this article, since the focus here is exclusively on the utility value of watercourses for navigation. Individual preferences of actors are to be seen in the transportation of goods or visitors and form the assessment standard for (potential) damage. Both direct and indirect valuation methods are available to assess individual utility losses. A good overview is provided by Navrud (2000) [35], with the methods for revealed preferences (RP) being of relevance in the present context. A basic distinction can be made between costs of unavoided damage, damage mitigation costs and damage avoidance costs [34]. Here, the focus is on the assessment of direct event-based damage costs. There are also fixed costs, such as wages, insurance and administrative costs, which are incurred even when vessels are not operating. However, due to the high level of complexity, these cannot be considered comprehensively in this hydro-economic model approach. The scale of the temporal consideration is limited to the present and the scale of the spatial consideration is limited to the river itself with its immediately adjacent use for navigation. Long-term or even irreversible damages are not included. According to MC3.0, damage is considered irreversible if natural regeneration does not occur within the relevant planning periods for humans (=150 years) and the damage cannot be reversed by technical anthropogenic means [34]. Following on from this, the economic valuation is partly based on the substitutability of goods. This can be expressed through RP and leads to adaptation reactions, such as the use of alternative goods or innovations.

3. Results

3.1. Middle Elbe Catchment and Navigation

The Elbe is one of the largest rivers in Central Europe. Figure 2 shows its course, with the middle section, which is analyzed here, marked in red.

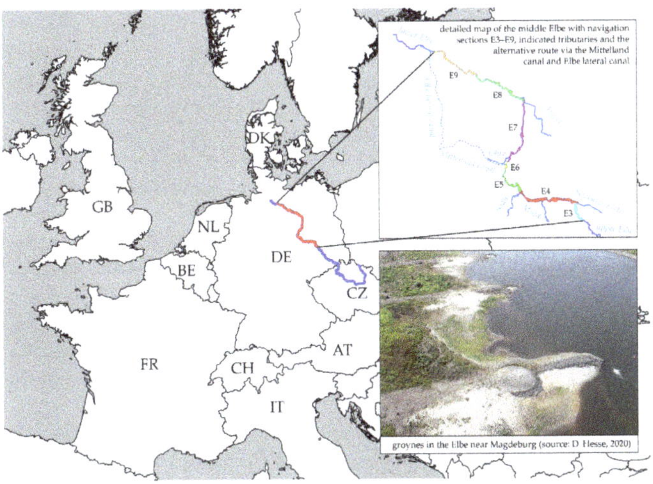

Figure 2. Course of the river Elbe with the study area marked in red and a detailed map with further information on the study area.

The middle Elbe stretches from Riesa, Germany (river kilometer 96.0) to the Geesthacht barrage, Germany (river kilometer 585.9). Apart from the Geesthacht barrage, which limits the tidal flow from the North Sea, there are no barrages in the study area, which is why the Elbe can be characterized here as a free-flowing lowland river. The water flow is therefore subject to natural seasonal fluctuations, e.g., due to precipitation, evaporation rates and snowmelt. There is a humid climate with an average precipitation of 520 mm per year and an average annual temperature of 9.5 degrees Celsius in the reference period between 1981 and 2010 at the Magdeburg monitoring site [36]. Furthermore, the river is affected both qualitatively and quantitatively by anthropogenic factors such as withdrawals and discharges and by the reservoir system in the upper reaches of the Elbe (Czech Republic). The latter causes a low-flow elevation of more than 20 cm for the lower middle Elbe and up to 35 cm for the upper middle Elbe [37].

Around 13.3 million tons of goods were handled on the Elbe federal waterway in 2023 [38]. Furthermore, a study shows that commercial shipping on the Elbe has regional economic effects on a total of 16,400 direct, indirect and induced employees [39]. Even though around 6900 groynes stabilize the inland Elbe (Figure 2) [40], there are significant restrictions for navigation during low flows. In the low-flow year 2018, the Elbe had a navigable depth of less than 1.40 m in some sections on more than 230 days of the year and was therefore impassable for two thirds of the year [41]. In particular, the lower reaches between Dömitz and Hitzacker (river kilometer 508 to 521), located in river section E9, are considered a critical section [42,43]. However, sections E7 to E9 can be bypassed via the artificial waterways of the Mittelland canal and the Elbe lateral canal, as can be seen in the detailed map in Figure 2. The situation on the Elbe illustrates the need for suitable risk management approaches that can help decision-makers to develop well-founded river development plans and action programs.

3.2. Inland Cargo Shipping

For the simulation of h_f, a hydrodynamic 1D river model was created in LoFloDes using cross-section profiles and discharge data from the Elbe and its biggest German tributaries, Schwarze Elster, Mulde, Saale, Ohre and Havel (Figure 2), as a boundary condition. The discharge data were provided by the Federal Institute of Hydrology (BfG) in Germany. A model-based simulation of h_c was then carried out for the period from 2012 to 2020. Data on the reference water levels for navigation $h_{r,c}$, the currently valid equivalent low water level GlW2010, were provided by the Federal Waterways Engineering and Research Institute (BAW) in Germany and assigned to the cross-sections from the hydrodynamic model. The GlW is a statistically determined reference water level that defines the water level at which the target depth of the navigation channel is still guaranteed. For the Elbe, the maintenance target is 1.40 m. A drop in the water level below GlW according to Equation (2) therefore means that the possible draught T, and thus the cargo capacity of the ships is severely restricted. In the model, u_s corresponds to zero, although some ship types can still operate below the GlW, as will be explained in more detail below. From the difference between GlW ($h_{r,c}$) and the current water level h_c, the unloading depth and thus the possible payload is calculated for inland navigation. For a gradual damage calculation, the different ship types with the different loading conditions from $u_{0,s}$ to $u_{1,s}$ (%) must be considered. Motor cargo vessels (mcv) and barges in the size classes up to 1500 tons are primarily relevant for Elbe shipping. Table 1 contains the section length L_{sec} for the river sections E3 to E9 in the study area, and also the ship classes that are most relevant for navigation on the Elbe, analogously to the BAW traffic figures [44], each with the respective draught T and the reference quantity $q_{s,sec,pot10}$ in 2010.

In the model, $q_{s,sec,pot10}$ was assigned accordingly for all route sections in the study area. To calculate the required $h_{f,s}$, a safety margin (so-called "flotation") of approx. 30 cm must be added. Therefore, the required $h_{f,s}$ per ship class is added in brackets in Table 1. If the level falls below this limit, the ships must reduce the cargo volume to reduce T. As h_c decreases, the profitability per ship also declines. A gradual analysis is possible if it is assumed that the maximum unloading depth corresponds to one hundred percent capacity utilization $u_{1,s}$ and an undershoot of GlW corresponds to zero percent capacity utilization $u_{0,s}$. For a motor cargo vessel with a loading capacity of up to 1500 tons, the utilization rate u and the required water level above GlW are shown in Figure 3 as an example.

Table 1. Section length L_{sec} (km) for Elbe sections E3 to E9 and ship classes with average draught T, required fairway depth $h_{f,s}$ [45] and quantities $q_{s,sec,pot10}$ (p.a.) in 2010 (data source: TraVis [1] [44]).

Section	T ($h_{f,s}$) (m)	E3 [2]	E4	E5	E6	E7	E8	E9
L_{sec} (km)	-	29.6	92.1	42.1	11.1	78.9	79.45	66.95
pushed barges [3] < 1500 t	2.89 (3.19)	706	809	991	1043	1163	1360	1372
mcv [4] 1001–1500 t	2.66 (2.96)	292	365	472	402	347	339	339
mcv [4] 901–1000	2.62 (2.92)	59	69	82	48	17	47	47
mcv [4] 651–900	2.55 (2.85)	175	195	219	155	73	66	66
mcv [4] 401–650	2.45 (2.75)	155	186	207	179	258	382	380
mcv [4] < 400	2.35 (2.65)	4	4	4	2	1	1	1

Notes: [1] The sections from TraVis were summarized in E3 to E9 according to the classification from ELWIS [41]. [2] E3 is only partially located in the study area and is therefore only included with 29.6 of a total of 89.2 km. [3] For pushed barges, TraVis does not make a more detailed distinction. All push barges up to a loading capacity of 1500 tons are included here. [4] mcv = motor cargo vessels.

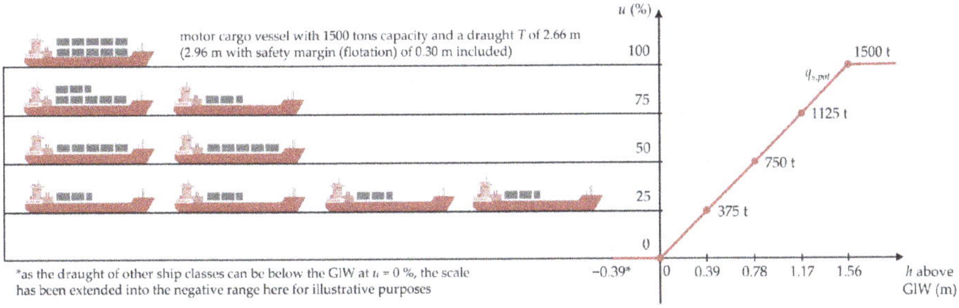

Figure 3. Utilization of a motor cargo ship with a capacity of up to 1500 t at different water levels above GlW.

For the model implementation, the ship classes listed in Table 1 were defined with $q_{s,sec,pot10}$ [44]. Furthermore, the different loading conditions $u_{0.25,s}$, $u_{0.50,s}$, $u_{0.75,s}$ and $u_{1,s}$ were defined for each category, which were a result of the deviation from the GlW (see Figure 3). The values in between were interpolated accordingly. According to Equation (3), $q_{s,sec,state}$ represents these values. The difference between $q_{s,sec,state}$ and $q_{s,sec,pot10}$, in turn, is included in the damage function as a loss of freight volume per day in accordance with Equation (4) by multiplying it with a damage value d. In each case, the most limiting cross-section profile is representative for the entire section ($h_{c,min,sec}$). Table 2 shows the number of days per year on which the GlW was undercut for each section of the Elbe between 2012 and 2020, according to Equation (2), comparing the h_f data from the Electronic Waterway Information Service (ELWIS) of the Federal Waterways and Shipping Administration of Germany (WSV) [41] with the data from the LoFloDes 1D river model.

The model is particularly accurate for the low-flow years 2018 to 2020. Apart from that, there are occasional deviations of up to 49 days (E9, 2014). The deviations can be explained by the fact that the model was calibrated specifically for extreme low-flow events. Adjustments, especially to the roughness coefficient, lead to very accurate results during low-flow events, but for medium water levels, there are larger deviations due to the changed flow and friction conditions (e.g., influence of groynes). At medium low-flow conditions, the water level is underestimated.

As figures on d_d are not available for the Elbe, approximate values from the literature, obtained with the help of artificial intelligence (ChatGPT), were assumed. In their study, Jonkeren et al. (2007) [22] calculated an average price of EUR 8.50 per ton for the river Rhine. ChatGPT gives a rough estimate of EUR 100 to 300 per ton per day in damage costs for cargo ships with load capacities between 400 and 1500 tons. The scientific interpretation of the information provided by ChatGPT is set out in the discussion section.

Table 2. Days with fairway depths below the reference water level GlW, classified by Elbe sections (data source: ELWIS [41]) [1].

Elbe Section	2012			2013			2014			2015			2016			2017			2018			2019			2020			Ø		
	ELWIS	Model	Deviation	ELWIS	Model	Deviation	ELWIS	Model	Deviation	ELWIS	Model	Deviation	ELWIS	Model	Deviation	ELWIS	Model	Deviation	ELWIS	Model	Deviation	ELWIS	Model	Deviation	ELWIS	Model	Deviation	ELWIS	Model	Deviation
E3	12	0	12	10	0	10	37	16	21	130	125	5	32	33	1	52	59	7	186	179	7	126	117	9	55	46	9	71	64	7
E4	66	114	38	16	17	1	116	154	38	178	181	3	98	107	9	147	149	2	235	232	3	229	219	10	208	202	6	144	153	9
E5	4	14	10	0	0	0	21	25	4	119	138	19	37	49	12	45	64	19	188	189	1	164	157	7	99	98	1	75	82	6
E6	0	0	0	0	0	0	0	0	0	48	66	18	20	19	1	1	3	2	171	161	10	98	99	1	14	23	9	39	41	2
E7 [2]	8	35	27	2	0	2	16	47	31	133	160	27	48	61	13	74	95	21	214	213	1	178	171	7	119	150	31	88	104	16
E8 [2]	18	54	36	3	5	2	51	58	7	149	169	20	68	81	13	57	52	5	219	222	3	200	210	10	189	198	9	106	117	11
E9 [2]	65	97	32	13	16	3	47	96	49	162	175	13	95	102	7	52	83	31	233	233	0	230	239	9	222	229	7	124	141	17
Max	66	114	38	36	17	10	116	154	49	178	181	27	98	107	13	147	149	31	235	233	10	230	239	10	222	229	31	144	153	17
$\|Ø - Max_n\|$	78			108			28			34			46			3			91			86			78					

Notes: [1] Gaps in the data records (e.g., due to excessively high or low water levels) were corrected using a standardized procedure. [2] Sections E7, E8 and E9 can be bypassed via the artificial waterways of the Elbe lateral canal and Mittelland canal, as illustrated in Figure 2.

As explained above, replacement costs d_r can also be calculated by calculating the costs for alternative modes of transport. Corresponding environmental cost rates for different modes of transport in Germany can be found in MC3.1 [46], with 2.15 EUR-cents per ton-kilometer for inland cargo shipping and 2.97 EUR-cents per ton-kilometer for truck (28–40 t). Based on the deviation (0.82 EUR-cents per ton-kilometer), the environmental costs per kilometer can be determined.

Several scenarios using different d were calculated for testing purposes. The costs calculated by the model are included in the Supplementary Material in Table S1 and are explained below. Firstly, the reference transport volumes $q_{s,sec,pot10}$ from 2010 obtained via TraVis [44] were applied for each section of the catchment area. In addition, different cost rates were used, namely an estimated damage cost d_d per ton of EUR 8.50 [22], EUR 200 (mean value of the ChatGPT estimate) and a substitution cost d_r of EUR 0.0082 per ton per kilometer. The model uses the transport volumes $q_{s,sec,pot10}$ to calculate the transport volume $q_{s,sec,state}$ for the individual years according to Equation (3) and then, using Equation (4), the damage costs $D_{d,sec,year}$ or replacement costs $D_{r,sec,year}$ per section per year are calculated. Figure 4 shows $D_{d,sec,year}$ calculated with the reference transport volumes of 2010, with onediagram per year.

Two columns per section are shown, corresponding to the two estimated cost rates d_d. The columns show the annual costs $D_{d,sec,year}$ resulting from (4), with d_d equal to 200 EUR/t in light blue and d_d equal to 8.50 EUR/t in black. Analogously, the primary axis applies to the former and the secondary axis to the latter. Firstly, it is striking that sections E8 and E9 have the highest values of all the years. This can be attributed to the hydrological conditions. Section E9, for example, is one of the critical areas for shipping, as mentioned above [42,43]. However, sections E7 to E9 can be bypassed via the Mittelland canal and the Elbe lateral canal. Nevertheless, it would be misleading to exclude them from the overall assessment, as they are part of the BAW's traffic forecast and thus part of the Federal Transport Infrastructure Plan (BVWP) 2030 [44]. This forms the basis for planning new construction and replacement investments in the federal waterway network. All section values must therefore be included in the average value accordingly. This is shown in the form of the dashed lines and provides an approximation of the total costs. As a ship usually passes through several sections and is therefore statistically recorded multiple times, the sections cannot be summed up to make a statement about the total damage. For this reason, an average value was calculated for the entire area. It is also noticeable that the average damage values are relatively close together over the years, except for 2013. In 2013, the Elbe had high water levels and even an extreme flood [47]. This can also be seen from the figures in Table 2. The modeled damage costs for low flows are therefore lower than in the other years. In contrast, the highest damage was calculated for the low-flow years 2018, 2019 and 2020. These are closely followed by 2015 and also

2014 which, according to Table 2, do not initially appear to be classic low-flow years. This can be explained by the fact that a high number of days with water levels just above GlW can sometimes lead to greater damage than low-flow peaks. This aspect is addressed in more detail in the discussion section.

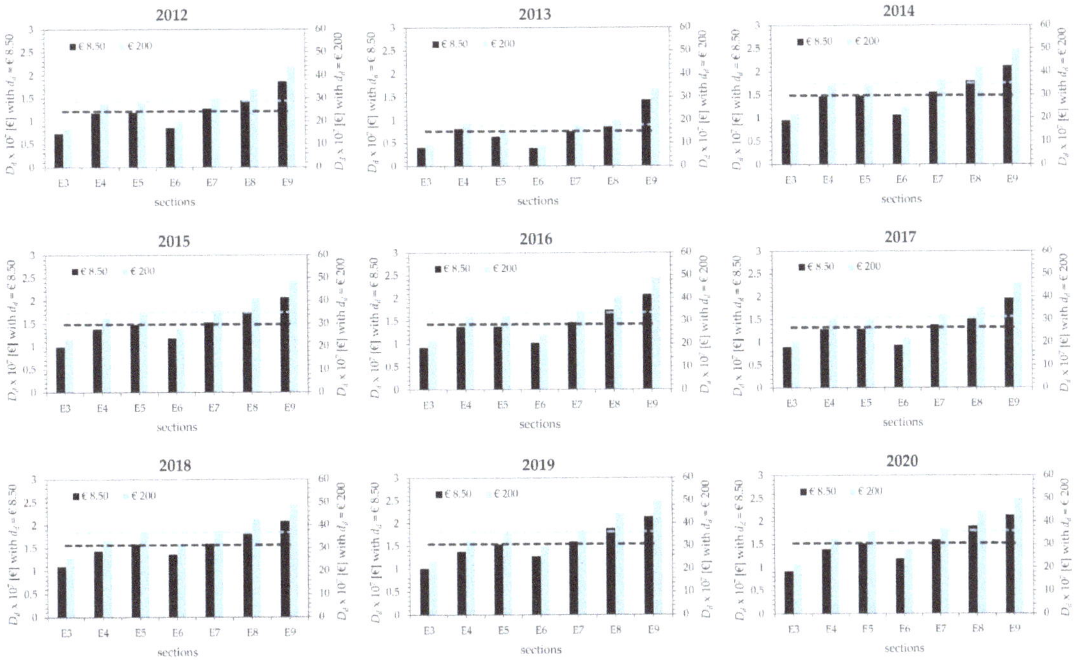

Figure 4. Damage costs $D_{d,sec,year}$ (10 million EUR/a) for cargo shipping in Elbe sections E3 to E9 for the years 2012 to 2020 calculated with the transport volumes of 2010.

Furthermore, it is striking that the overall scale, especially for a d_d of EUR 200, appears very high. For example, the model calculates an average loss amount across all sections of EUR 369 million for 2018. For a d_d of EUR 8.50 per ton, this results in almost EUR 16 million, which seems more realistic overall. The relationship to the dimensions from other studies is also addressed in the discussion section in more detail.

The evaluation of the replacement costs D_r has a special aspect compared to the previous analysis, namely that the cost rate d_r of EUR 0.0082 per ton is to be applied per kilometer. The environmental damage caused by transporting the quantity of freight by truck rather than by ship is calculated. A replacement route is assumed that corresponds to the length of the respective river section L_{sec}. Figure 5 shows $D_{r,sec,year}$, with one diagram per year.

As L_{sec} varies greatly for the individual sections (see Table 1), there are minor changes in relation to Figure 4. The shortest sections E6 (L_{sec} = 11.1 km) and E3 (L_{sec} = 29.6 km) incur the lowest costs, and E4, the longest section (L_{sec} = 92.1 km), incurs higher costs compared to the previous analysis. This can also be explained by the fact that the hydrological conditions in sections E3 and E6 are the best overall (see Table 2). Furthermore, E8 and E9 continue to have the highest costs, although the route length is significantly less than that of E4. The reasons for the differences between the years are the same as in the previous analysis. Here, too, 2013 has the lowest values and all other years are close together. The highest average value is also in 2018, at EUR 905 thousand. This value therefore provides an indication of the additional environmental costs incurred for alternative transportation by truck in 2018. Overall, it can be stated that if the lengths of the replacement routes were set to be the same for all sections (e.g., 100 km), there would be a 1:1 correlation with Figure 4, which illustrates the influence of the route length on the cost structure.

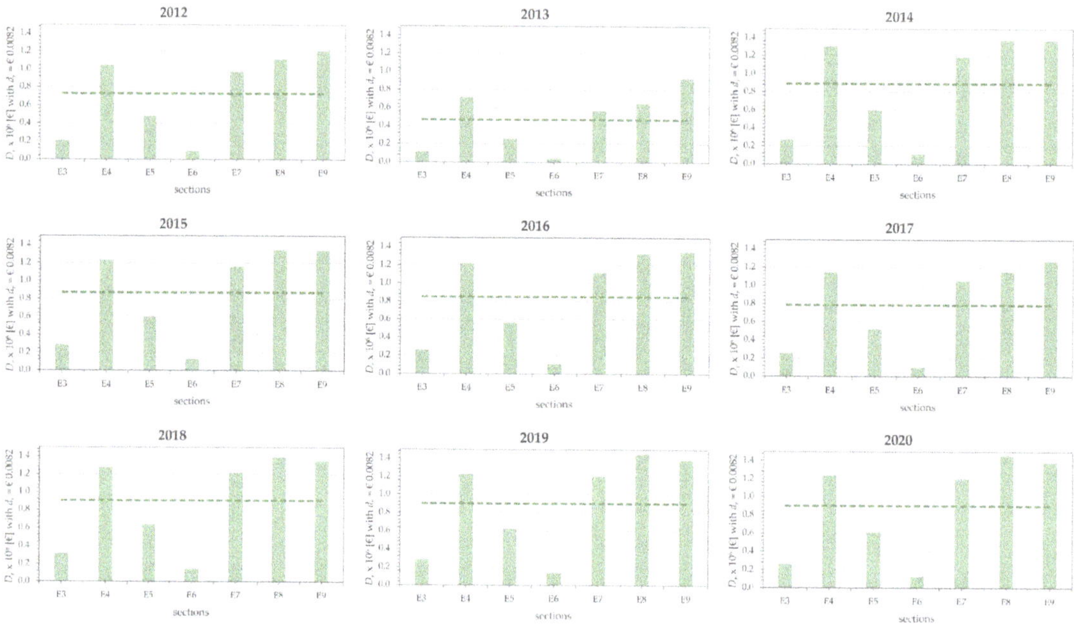

Figure 5. Replacement costs $D_{r,sec,year}$ (million EUR/a) for cargo shipping in Elbe sections E3 to E9 for the years 2012 to 2020 calculated with the transport volumes of 2010.

3.3. Tourist Shipping

The downtime costs d_d for the leisure and recreation sector extend to many subsectors, such as tourist shipping, the water sports and rental industry, gastronomy and accommodation, as well as local recreation. For tourist shipping, the hydro-economic assessment approach described in Section 2 can be adopted. As they have a shallower draught ($T \approx 0.90$ m), passenger ships can generally still navigate at fairway depths h_f of 1.20 m. A corresponding ship type has been stored in the model. However, in contrast to freight ships, no section-related quantities $q_{s,sec,pot}$ are available for the middle Elbe, but only data recorded for the Magdeburg city section counting point. Table 3 shows the passenger ships and sport boats recorded in the period from 2012 to 2020, which are included in the WSV's traffic reports [48].

Table 3. Touristic and leisure shipping on the Elbe (Magdeburg city section) from 2012 to 2020 (data source: WSV's traffic reports [48]).

	2012	2013	2014	2015	2016	2017	2018	2019	2020 [1]	Ø 2012–2020
Passenger ships	1396	1527	1610	1303	1514	1454	757	840	892	1255
Sport boats	2871	2673	3089	3421	3321	4024	4248	4151	2422	3358

Note: [1] Figures only partially recorded.

Direct downtime costs result from the loss of income for the providers of tourist cruises. Here, these are not expressed in tons per year. Rather, the damage can be expressed in lost visitors per year. This in turn can be monetized if the lost revenue per visitor is included. To test the model, a type III inland passenger vessel was used, as is frequently used on the Elbe. As described above, ships of this type usually have a draught T of 0.90 m when empty. Including flotation water, the channel depth h_f must therefore be at least 1.20 m. If such a vessel at full capacity (e.g., 150 visitors) has a draught T of 1.10 m [49,50] and therefore requires a fairway h_f of 1.40 m, a gradual consideration can be made analogous to Figure 3, with negative values for h above GlW. The average value of 1.255 ships was assumed as the transport volume $q_{s,pot}$ for every section for the calculation according to Equations (3) and (4), as no section-related quantities were available. However, default costs d_d had to be defined for this, which can again be adjusted as required. The model was calculated with a d_d of EUR 50 per passenger, consisting of EUR 25 in ticket costs and EUR 25 in catering costs. This led to the following results (Figure 6).

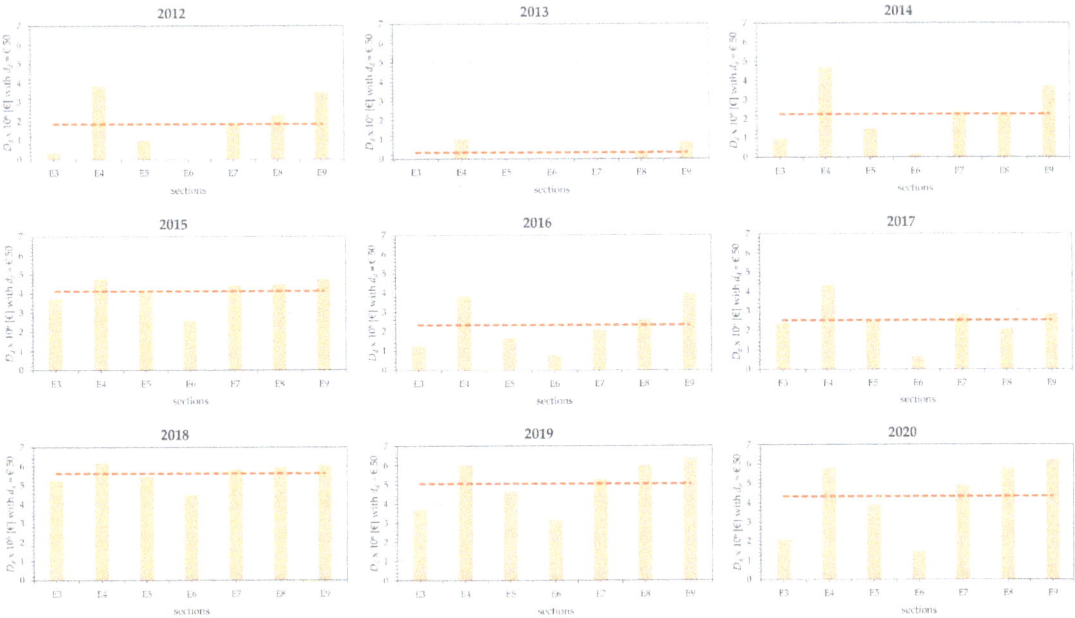

Figure 6. Damage costs $D_{d,sec,year}$ (million EUR/a) for passenger shipping in Elbe sections E3 to E9 for the years 2012 to 2020, calculated with the reference quantity $q_{s,pot}$ of 1.255 ships/a.

Figure 6 differs greatly from both previous analyses. This is mainly because damage occurs only at lower water levels due to the shallower draught T of the passenger vessels. For example, since the fairway depth h_f of 1.40 m was not exceeded on any day in 2013 in sections E3 and E6 according to the modeled data (Table 2), no damage occurred. In total, a loss $D_{d,year}$ of EUR 348 thousand was calculated for the average of all sections for 2013. Overall, the influence of the shallower draughts results in the extreme low-flow years (particularly 2015, 2018, 2019 and 2020) being more significant than the others. The year with the highest average total loss was 2018, with a calculated loss $D_{d,year}$ of EUR 5.6 million. When comparing the individual sections, it is noticeable that once again sections E7 to E9, and also E4 in particular, stand out.

The consequences of low-flow events also potentially mean restrictions on water sports activities. However, as can be seen in Table 3, the highest number of sport boats in the long-term period were counted on the Magdeburg city section in the low-flow years of 2018 and 2019. Only incomplete data are available for 2020. It can be assumed that there will be little or no low-flow consequences on the middle Elbe due to the shallower draughts. This therefore also applies to the rental industry (canoes, kayaks, sailing boats, stand-up paddles, etc.). Due to the low socio-economic significance, parameterization was not carried out. There are further negative impacts in the fifteen areas approved for waterskiing and four areas approved for personal watercraft on the middle Elbe [51]. However, damage costs cannot be quantified due to a lack of data.

4. Discussion

The hydro-economic model represents a component that can be used to derive generalized and validated damage functions. It combines hydrological and economic input variables. Considering Table 2, the benefit of this approach becomes clear. The figures on the undercutting of the GlW would suggest that the years 2015, 2018, 2019 and 2020 are particularly prominent in the damage calculation. However, considering Figure 4, 2014 in particular shows that a high level of damage can also occur even if the GlW undercutting is relatively low. If the GlW is slightly exceeded for a large part of the year, this may have a greater impact than the low-flow peaks with a period of GlW undershoots, where the rest of the year has solid water levels. Figure 7 can be used to underline this.

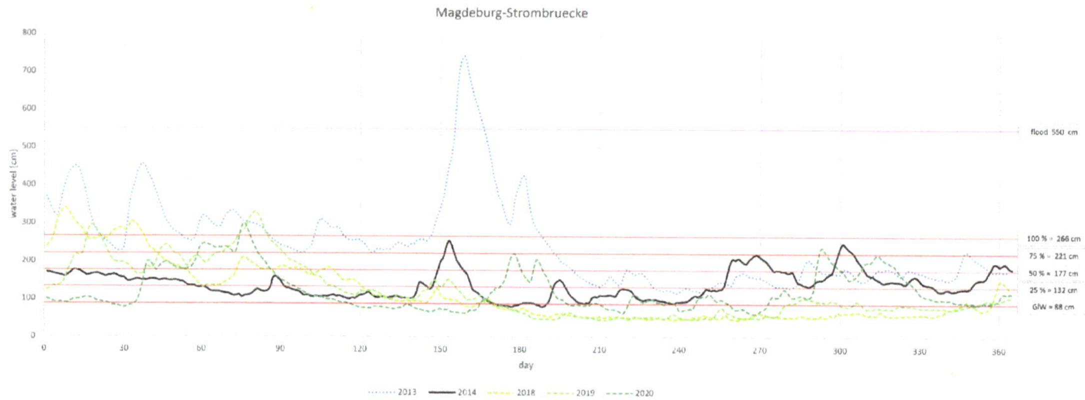

Figure 7. Modeled water level hydrographs for the years 2013, 2014, 2018, 2019 and 2020 for the Magdeburg-Strombruecke gauge with load conditions for a motor cargo vessel with a maximum carrying capacity of 1500 tons.

Looking at 2018 and 2019, the second half of the year in particular determined the low-flow period. At the beginning of the year, in contrast, there were high water levels, where a capacity utilization of 100 percent $u_{1,s}$ was even achieved at times. In 2014, on the other hand, capacity utilization u_s was low almost all year round, which also led to high damage costs overall. A capacity utilization of 100 percent $u_{1,s}$ was not achieved throughout the course of the year. With one brief exception, this also applies to 2020. Overall, 2014 and 2020 are comparable, with more favorable conditions for navigation in 2020 at the beginning of the year, but there were several GlW undershoots during the rest of the year. In addition, 2013 was illustrated, which has a flood peak but has almost optimal navigation conditions, especially in the first half of the year. As the model is primarily limited to the economic assessment of low-flow events, the economic impact of floods on navigation is not adequately considered here.

Uncertainties apply to both the hydrodynamic and the damage model. For example, the fairway depths calculated in the model depend directly on the GlW data provided. As described, GlW2010 is currently used for the Elbe. However, as the discharge conditions and the riverbed are changeable, the GlW value must be checked at regular intervals and adjusted by the responsible authorities (WSV) if necessary. As already briefly discussed above, the deviations in Table 2 could also be partly due to this. It should also be noted that the GlW by definition describes a statistically determined low water level that is undercut on a long-term average of 20 ice-free days per year [52]. Furthermore, the data basis for the draughts of the ship categories is from 2008 [45]. The draughts T may have changed due to technological developments. However, since all ship types can be customized as required, both with the stored draughts T and the assigned reference quantities $q_{s,pot}$, newer data can be added. The relevance of this is reflected here in the example of passenger transportation, where damage occurs at lower water levels due to shallower draughts. Another source of uncertainty is the cost rate assumptions d_d and d_r (e.g., [53]), which can also be adjusted by potential users. It is also important to mention here that the elasticity of the cost rates has not yet been considered. Further research is needed here. In comparison with other studies [20–22], it is noticeable that the values appear disproportionately high when using d_d from ChatGPT. ChatGPT states that it partly considers profitability analyses from shipping companies and insurance companies as well as scientific studies, but it is not clear exactly how the range of EUR 100 to 300 is calculated. Rather, it results from a large number of included data sets and a wide range of influencing factors that have an impact on downtime costs. The figures thus include not only the goods not transported, but also the costs for the crew, insurance, administration and port fees, as well as contractual penalties. However, assuming the cost rate d_d of EUR 8.50 per ton from Jonkeren et al. (2007), the results are quite realistic in comparison. Koetse and Rietvald (2009) [20–22], for example, calculated a loss of around EUR 91 million for Rhine shipping in the drought year 2003. In comparison, the hydro-economic model for the middle Elbe calculates costs of EUR 15.7 million for the low-flow year 2018, which reflects the differences in the importance and size of the two waterways well. The results also appear realistic in relation to the results of Streng et al. (2020) [21] and Jonkeren et al. (2007) [22]. Another point of discussion is that the standard assumption in the hydro-economic model is that there is full capacity utilization of the ships, with the deviation determining a loss. A full capacity utilization does not correspond to reality, which is why Jonkeren et al. (2007) [22], for example, include a mean load factor. To show the dependence of the results on the assumptions, sensitivity calculations could be carried out in further studies, whereby it must be defined which sensitivities are to be tested. Furthermore, the parameters developed so far need to be further validated and tested in other river basins and with other boundary conditions. For example, projected BAW traffic figures for 2030 $q_{s,sec,pot30}$ [44], as well as yearly traffic figures from the WSV's traffic reports [48], are also available and can be included in the model.

From a holistic point of view, further parameters for low-flow impact assessment can be examined. Folkens et al. (2023) [13] have identified a variety of low-flow impacts and possible parameters. One example, with relevance for the Elbe, is surface water abstraction. Further damage costs result from potential downtime costs for the accommodation, camping and catering industry. Overnight stays can be used as a key figure for RP. It can be said that there are at least 150 accommodation and catering businesses in the immediate area of the middle Elbe [54]. There are also at least 19 camping operations [55]. Indirect costs can be seen, for example, in the replacement costs that must be incurred to travel to more distant recreational areas. How such effects can be transferred to a hydro-economic model is the subject of future research. Furthermore, the model must be embedded in a holistic risk approach. In traditional risk assessment, the expected value of the damage is calculated by multiplying the amount of damage by the probability of occurrence. This step is essential for developing the LFRM approach [30].

5. Conclusions

In view of climatic changes and the projected increase in low-flow events in the northern hemisphere, the need for risk management strategies is increasing. Reduced surface water runoff has a variety of consequences for ecology, society and the economy. A hydro-economic model for the calculation of damage costs for low-flow events in free-flowing rivers can help to collect, analyze and use information in order to better understand the impact on the environment, the economy and society. It has been shown that the approach is suitable for quantifying the economic damage to navigation. For the middle Elbe, a total loss $D_{d,2012–2020}$ of EUR 152 million for navigation was calculated, summing up all the damage costs D_d for passenger navigation and cargo shipping (with a d_d of EUR 8.50 per ton) in the period from 2012 to 2020. In the annual analysis, 2018 has the highest total damage costs for freight shipping (EUR 15.7 million, with a d_d of EUR 8.50 per ton) and tourist shipping (EUR 5.6 million), followed by 2019 and 2020. However, significant economic losses do not only occur during low flows, but also when the reference water levels for navigation are only slightly exceeded over a longer period of time, as the year 2014 illustrates. Here, the damage costs for freight shipping amount to EUR 14.9 million (with a d_d of EUR 8.50 per ton). When comparing the river sections, it is noticeable that section E9 has the highest values in most analyses, which underlines its classification as a critical section for navigation. E3 and E6, on the other hand, have the best hydrological conditions and therefore the lowest damage costs.

As an analytical tool and part of a holistic risk assessment, the model can help decision-makers to understand the interactions between water and the economy and develop strategies that promote sustainability in water resource management. Here, it is not crucial that the calculated damage is correct in absolute terms, but different states can be brought into reference with each other in the form of a relative change. A major strength of the approach is its hydrological resolution, as river sections rather than separate gauges can be analyzed and compared based on multiple cross-sectional profiles. Based on this, well-founded decisions can be made on maintenance measures for individual or several river sections. In addition, the approach can be adopted by authorities, scientists or economic players as required, for example, by adjusting the ship types, utilization states or cost rates. However, the tool is only to be understood as a fragment of a holistic LFRM approach, which includes hydrological, ecological and economic components. Ecological components, such as the continuity of fish populations or the conditions for macrozoobenthos, must be considered just as much as economic factors, such as abstraction and discharges, hydropower generation or the use of watercourses for tourism. This is discussed in more detail in the DPSIR study by Folkens et al. (2023) [13]. From a strictly economic point of view, shipping is of great importance due to its economic significance. As described, the network of inland waterways in Germany has a length of around 7300 km, of which only 490 km (middle Elbe) were included in this study. As data on discharge, the reference water level for navigation GlW and traffic figures are available for all German inland waterways, the method can be applied accordingly as a nationwide approach by the authorities (WSV and BAW). It can also be used internationally if the appropriate data are available. As an analytical tool, it could be used to calculate the influence of a change in the cross profiles, e.g., due to a deepening of the fairway, on the downtime days, as well as downtime and replacement costs per year. Furthermore, new ship types can be applied to show how the downtime costs develop with a changed fleet of ships that requires less draught. Different discharge scenarios can also be calculated in the model, considering various climate projections to determine the effects on transportation conditions. It thus provides the scientific community with a multitude of use cases and further development options. In addition, there are also applications for the economy, for example, for the profitability calculations of shipping companies or the location planning of multinational corporations.

Supplementary Materials: The following supporting information can be downloaded at https://www.mdpi.com/article/10.3390/w16233497/s1: Table S1: Calculated costs for E3 to E9 at different cost rates.

Author Contributions: Conceptualization, L.F.; methodology, L.F., D.B. and U.S.; software, U.S., D.B. and L.F.; validation, L.F. and U.S.; formal analysis, L.F. and U.S.; investigation, L.F.; writing—original draft preparation, L.F.; writing—review and editing, L.F., U.S., P.S. and D.B.; visualization, L.F. and U.S.; supervision, D.B. and P.S.; project administration, D.B.; funding acquisition, D.B. All authors have read and agreed to the published version of the manuscript.

Funding: This research was conducted as part of the DryRivers project, which was funded within the WaX—Water Extreme Events grant from the Federal Ministry of Education and Research (BMBF) (FKZ 02WEE1628A). The APC was funded through DryRivers project funds.

Data Availability Statement: The data used in this study, except for the discharge data of the Elbe, are available upon reasonable request. Similarly, the software (LOFLODES: https://github.com/dabachma/LoFloDes, version 0.1, accessed on 31 November 2024) and Python scripts used are also available. Publicly available data have been referenced in the text.

Acknowledgments: Our gratitude goes to Daniel Hesse (Department of Water, Environment, Construction and Safety, Magdeburg-Stendal University of Applied Sciences) for providing the aerial photo of the Elbe groynes (Figure 2). We would also like to thank the employees of the Federal Waterways Engineering and Research Institute (BAW) for their time and expertise during discussions on the research approach.

Conflicts of Interest: The authors declare no conflicts of interest.

Nomenclature

Parameter	Formula Symbol	Unit
draught of the vessel	T	m
depth of the fairway	h_f	m
cross-section	c	-
river section	sec	-
section length	L_{sec}	km
water level per cross-section	h_c	m
reference low water levels per cross-section	$h_{r,c}$	m
limiting cross-section of the river section	$h_{c,min,sec}$	m
ship type	s	-
utilization state per ship type	u_s	%
reference freight (or passenger) quantities	$q_{s,sec,pot}$	e.g., t/d
calculated freight (or passenger) quantities	$q_{s,sec,state}$	e.g., t/d
damage cost rate	d	e.g., EUR/t
downtime cost rate	d_d	e.g., EUR/t
replacement cost rate	d_r	e.g., EUR/t
damage per river section per day	$D_{sec,i}$	EUR/d
annual loss amount per river section	$D_{sec,year}$	EUR/a
damage costs per year	$D_{d,sec,year}$	EUR/a
replacement costs per year	$D_{r,sec,year}$	EUR/a

References

1. Hari, V.; Rakovec, O.; Markonis, Y.; Hanel, M.; Kumar, R. Increased future occurrences of the exceptional 2018–2019 Central European drought under global warming. *Sci. Rep.* **2020**, *10*, 12207. [CrossRef] [PubMed]
2. Vogel, M.M.; Zscheischler, J.; Wartenburger, R.; Dee, D.; Seneviratne, S.I. Concurrent 2018 Hot Extremes Across Northern Hemisphere Due to Human-Induced Climate Change. *Earth's Future* **2019**, *7*, 692–703. [CrossRef] [PubMed]
3. Van der Wiel, K.; Batelaan, T.J.; Wanders, N. Large increases of multi-year droughts in north-western Europe in a warmer climate. *Clim. Dyn.* **2023**, *60*, 1781–1800. [CrossRef]
4. Piniewski, M.; Eini, M.R.; Chattopadhyay, S.; Okruszko, T.; Kundzewicz, Z.W. Is there a coherence in observed and projected changes in riverine low flow indices across Central Europe? *Earth-Sci. Rev.* **2022**, *233*, 104187. [CrossRef]
5. Marx, A.; Kumar, R.; Thober, S.; Rakovec, O.; Wanders, N.; Zink, M.; Wood, E.F.; Pan, M.; Sheffield, J.; Samaniego, L. Climate change alters low flows in Europe under global warming of 1.5, 2, and 3 °C. *Hydrol. Earth Syst. Sci.* **2018**, *22*, 1017–1032. [CrossRef]
6. Spinoni, J.; Vogt, J.V.; Naumann, G.; Barbosa, P.; Dosio, A. Will drought events become more frequent and severe in Europe? *Int. J. Climatol.* **2017**, *38*, 1718–1736. [CrossRef]
7. Tsakiris, G. Proactive Planning Against Droughts. *Procedia Eng.* **2016**, *162*, 15–24. [CrossRef]
8. Wilhite, D.A.; Glantz, M.H. Understanding the Drought Phenomenon: The Role of Definitions. *Water Int.* **1985**, *10*, 111–120. [CrossRef]
9. Hein, T.; Hauer, C.; Schmid, M.; Stöglehner, G.; Stumpp, C.; Ertl, T.; Graf, W.; Habersack, H.; Haidvogl, G.; Hood-Novotny, R.; et al. The coupled socio-ecohydrological evolution of river systems: Towards an integrative perspective of river systems in the 21st century. *Sci. Total Environ.* **2021**, *801*, 149619. [CrossRef]
10. Naumann, G.; Cammalleri, C.; Mentaschi, L.; Feyen, L. Increased economic drought impacts in Europe with anthropogenic warming. *Nat. Clim. Change* **2021**, *11*, 485–491. [CrossRef]

11. Conradt, T.; Engelhardt, H.; Menz, C.; Vicente-Serrano, S.M.; Alvarez Farizo, B.; Peña-Angulo, D.; Domínguez-Castro, F.; Eklundh, L.; Jin, H.; Boincean, B.; et al. Cross-sectoral impacts of the 2018–2019 Central European drought and climate resilience in the German part of the Elbe River basin. *Reg. Environ. Change* **2023**, *23*, 32. [CrossRef] [PubMed]
12. Klages, S.; Heidecke, C.; Osterburg, B. The Impact of Agricultural Production and Policy on Water Quality during the Dry Year 2018, a Case Study from Germany. *Water* **2020**, *12*, 1519. [CrossRef]
13. Folkens, L.; Bachmann, D.; Schneider, P. Driving Forces and Socio-Economic Impacts of Low-Flow Events in Central Europe: A Literature Review Using DPSIR Criteria. *Sustainability* **2023**, *15*, 10692. [CrossRef]
14. MEA. Ecosystems and Human Well-Being. A Framework for Assessment. *Millennium Ecosystem Assessment*. Available online: https://www.millenniumassessment.org/en/Framework.html (accessed on 6 September 2024).
15. Rohács, J.; Simongáti, G. The role of inland waterway navigation in a sustainable transport system. *Transport* **2007**, *22*, 148–153. [CrossRef]
16. Sys, C.; van de Voorde, E.; Vanelslander, T.; van Hassel, E. Pathways for a sustainable future inland water transport: A case study for the European inland navigation sector. *Case Stud. Transp. Policy* **2020**, *8*, 686–699. [CrossRef]
17. US Army Corps of Engineers. Inland Waterway Navigation–Value to the Nation. Available online: https://www.mvp.usace.army.mil/Portals/57/docs/Navigation/InlandWaterways-Value.pdf (accessed on 11 September 2024).
18. BDB. The Waterway System. Available online: https://www.binnenschiff.de/system-wasserstrasse/wasserstrasse/ (accessed on 6 September 2024). (In German)
19. Sexton, A.N.; Beisel, J.-N.; Staentzel, C.; Wolter, C.; Tales, E.; Belliard, J.; Buijse, A.D.; Martínez Fernández, V.; Wantzen, K.M.; Jähnig, S.C.; et al. Inland navigation and land use interact to impact European freshwater biodiversity. *Nat. Ecol. Evol.* **2024**, *8*, 1098–1108. [CrossRef]
20. Koetse, M.J.; Rietveld, P. The impact of climate change and weather on transport: An overview of empirical findings. *Transp. Res. Part D Transp. Environ.* **2009**, *14*, 205–221. [CrossRef]
21. Streng, M.; van Saase, N.; Kuipers, B. Economische Impact Laagwater-Een Analyse van de Effecten van Laagwater op de Binnenvaartsector en de Nederlandse en Duitse Economie. Final Report; Erasmus Centre for Urban, Port and Transport Economics: Rotterdam, The Netherlands, 2020. Available online: https://mcusercontent.com/9a6d55ece9db05ec49eeb87e0/files/c1fe06ba-31ef-42f1-91df-bf5760d84b8a/Erasmus_UPT_Eindrapport_Economische_impact_laagwater.pdf (accessed on 9 February 2023). (In Dutch)
22. Jonkeren, O.; Rietveld, P.; van Ommeren, J. Climate Change and Inland Waterway Transport: Welfare Effects of Low Water Levels on the river Rhine. *J. Transp. Econ. Policy* **2007**, *41*, 387–411.
23. Ademmer, M.; Jannsen, N.; Meuchelböck, S. Extreme Weather Events and Economic Activity: The Case of Low Water Levels on the Rhine River. *Ger. Econ. Rev.* **2023**, *24*, 121–144. [CrossRef]
24. Beuthe, M.; Jourquin, B.; Urbain, N.; Lingemann, I.; Ubbels, B. Climate change impacts on transport on the Rhine and Danube: A multimodal approach. *Transp. Res. Part D Transp. Environ.* **2014**, *27*, 6–11. [CrossRef]
25. Scholten, A.; Rothstein, B. *Navigation on the Danube-Limitations by Low Water Levels and Their Impacts*; EUR 28374 EN; Publications Office of the European Union: Luxembourg, 2017.
26. Sinaba, B.; Bauwens, A.; Boeckx, L.; Deckers, P.; Degré, A.; De Keizer, O.; Döring, R.; Drogue, G.; Fournier, M.; Hissel, F.; et al. *Quantification of the Impacts of Future Low Flows on the Economy in the Transnational Meuse Basin*; AMICE Action 7 Report; EPAMA: Charleville-Mézières, France, 2013.
27. Mens, M.; Minnema, B.; Overmars, K.; van den Hurk, B. Dilemmas in developing models for long-term drought risk management: The case of the National Water Model of the Netherlands. *Environ. Modell. Softw.* **2021**, *143*, 105100. [CrossRef]
28. Mens, M.J.P.; van Rhee, G.; Schasfoort, F.; Kielen, N. Integrated drought risk assessment to support adaptive policymaking in the Netherlands. *Nat. Hazards Earth Syst. Sci.* **2022**, *22*, 1763–1776. [CrossRef]
29. Meyer, V.; Messner, F. *National Flood Damage Evaluation Methods: A Review of Applied Methods in England, The Netherlands, the Czech Republik and Germany*; UFZ Discussion Paper No. 21/2005; UFZ: Leipzig, Germany, 2005.
30. Ostrom, E. Tragedy of the Commons. In *The New Palgrave Dictionary of Economics*, 2nd ed.; Durlauf, S.N., Blume, L.E., Eds.; Palgrave Macmillan: New York, NY, USA, 2008; pp. 6716–6719. Available online: https://hdl.handle.net/10535/5887 (accessed on 16 February 2023).
31. Satzinger, U.; Bachmann, D. Conceptual approach for a holistic low-flow risk analysis. *Hydrol. Process.* **2024**, *38*, e15217. [CrossRef]
32. LoFloDes. 2023. Available online: https://promaides.myjetbrains.com/youtrack/articles/LFD-A-1/General (accessed on 30 April 2024).
33. Geisendorf, S.; Gronemann, S.; Hampicke, U. *The Importance of Natural Assets and Biodiversity for a Sustainable Economy*; Erich Schmidt Verlag: Berlin, Germany, 1999. (In German)
34. Bünger, B.; Matthey, A. *Methodological Convention 3.0 for the Assessment of Environmental Costs: Methodological Principles*; German Federal Environment Agency: Dessau-Roßlau, Germany, 2018. (In German)
35. Navrud, S. Valuation Techniques and Benefit Transfer Methods: Strengths, Weaknesses and Policy Utility. In *Valuing Rural Amenities*; OECD: Paris, France, 2000; pp. 15–40.
36. DWD. Climate on-site data for Magdeburg. Available online: https://www.dwd.de/EN/weather/weather_climate_local/saxony-anhalt/magdeburg/_node.html (accessed on 4 September 2024).

37. ICPER. *Hydrological Evaluation of the 2018 Low Water Situation in the Elbe Catchment Area*; ICPER: Magdeburg, Germany, 2022. Available online: https://www.ikse-mkol.org/fileadmin/media/user_upload/D/06_Publikationen/02a_Niedrigwasser/2022_IKSE-NW-2018.pdf (accessed on 5 September 2024). (In German)
38. Statista Research Department. Freight Handling by German Inland Navigation in the Elbe Region from 2005 to 2023. Available online: https://de.statista.com/statistik/daten/studie/419656/umfrage/deutsche-binnenschifffahrt-gueterumschlag-im-elbegebiet/ (accessed on 6 September 2024). (In German).
39. HTC. *Economic Importance of Commercial Navigation on the Elbe (Elbe Navigation Study)*; Final Report; HTC: Hamburg, Germany, 2015. Available online: https://www.hamburg.de/contentblob/6547366/4036c418cab0a7c70c87db3b89ded29f/data/elbschifffahrtsstudie-2016.pdf (accessed on 6 September 2024). (In German)
40. WSV. The Elbe. Available online: https://www.gdws.wsv.bund.de/DE/wasserstrassen/01_bundeswasserstrassen/07_Elbe-Oder/Elbe.html?nn=1214418 (accessed on 6 September 2024). (In German).
41. WSV. Electronic Waterway Information Service (ELWIS): Fairway and Immersion Depths Between the Elbe and Oder Rivers. Available online: https://www.elwis.de/DE/dynamisch/Ft/Start (accessed on 11 January 2024).
42. Flörke, M.F.; Wimmer, F.; Laaser, C.; Vidaurre, R.; Trolzsch, J.; Dworak, T.; Stein, U.; Marinova, N.; Jaspers, F.; Ludwig, F.; et al. *Climate Adaption—Modelling Water Scenarios and Sectoral Impacts*; Final report ClimWatAdapt Project; Center for Environmental Systems Research: Kassel, Germany, 2011.
43. GKE. Elbe Residual Section. Available online: https://www.gesamtkonzept-elbe.de/Webs/Projektseite/GkElbe2020/DE/Projekte/Reststrecke/Reststrecke-node.html (accessed on 6 September 2024). (In German)
44. BAW. Transport Quantity Visualization. Available online: https://travis.baw.de/ (accessed on 14 August 2024).
45. PLANCO. Current European inland waterway fleet. In *Benefit-Cost Analysis for the Expansion of the Hanover-Linden Branch Canal for Large, Motorized Cargo Ships*; Final Report; Planco: Essen, Germany, 2008; pp. 19–27.
46. Matthey, A.; Bünger, B. *Methodological Convention 3.1 for the Assessment of Environmental Costs: Cost Rates*; German Federal Environment Agency: Dessau-Roßlau, Germany, 2020. (In German)
47. Merz, B.; Elmer, F.; Kunz, M.; Mühr, B.; Schröter, K.; Uhlemann-Elmer, S. The extreme flood in June 2013 in Germany. *La Houille Blanche* **2014**, *1*, 5–10. [CrossRef]
48. WSV. Publications of the WSV: Traffic Reports. Available online: https://www.gdws.wsv.bund.de/webcode/4317470 (accessed on 22 January 2024). (In German)
49. Dobratz, S. 2024: MS Berlin-Technical Specifications. Available online: http://schifffahrt-schwerin.de/flotte/06-ms-berlin.html (accessed on 2 September 2024). (In German)
50. Puls, H. 2024: White Fleet Magdeburg–Charter Tours. Available online: https://www.weisseflotte-magdeburg.de/Charterfahrten (accessed on 2 September 2024). (In German)
51. WSV. Water Sports on Federal Waterways between the Elbe and Oder Rivers. Available online: https://www.gdws.wsv.bund.de/SharedDocs/Downloads/DE/Publikationen/_GDWS/Schifffahrt/Sportschifffahrt_Ost.pdf;jsessionid=614F8CC3E7C42F3F714E7DC773458640.live21323?__blob=publicationFile&v=20 (accessed on 9 April 2024). (In German)
52. Muilerman, G.-J.; Maierbrugger, G.; Arnbrecht, H.; de Schepper, K.; Turf, S.; van Liere, R.; Quispel, M. *Good Navigation Status*; European Commission: Brussels, Belgium, 2018. Available online: https://op.europa.eu/publication-detail/-/publication/7980f36c-3eca-11e8-b5fe-01aa75ed71a1 (accessed on 5 September 2024).
53. Bieler, C.; Sutter, D. External Costs of Transportation in Germany. Final Report: Zurich, Switzerland, 2019. Available online: https://www.infras.ch/media/filer_public/b0/c9/b0c9923c-199c-4642-a235-9e2440f0046a/190822_externe_kosten_verkehr_2017.pdf (accessed on 3 September 2024). (In German)
54. Elbe Cycle Route Central Coordination Office (2024): Your Gastronomy Along the Elberadweg. Available online: https://www.elbe-cycle-route.com/gastronomy-search/ (accessed on 2 September 2024).
55. Blaues Band. The Elbe kilometer route from Torgau to Wittenberge. Available online: https://www.blaues-band.de/elbe/elbe-kilometrierung.php (accessed on 2 September 2024). (In German)

water

MDPI

Article

Valuation of Ecosystem Services of Fluvial Beaches in the Southeastern Peruvian Amazon

Gabriel Alarcon-Aguirre [1,2,3,4,*], Yesenia Del Águila Romero [2], Mauro Vela-Dafonseca [1,3], Percy Amílcar Zevallos Pollito [1,3], Liset Rodriguez Achata [3,4,5], Dalmiro Ramos Enciso [6], Jorge Cardozo Soarez [1], Jorge Luís Diaz Revoredo [7], Rembrandt Canahuire-Robles [1,3] and Jorge Garate-Quispe [1,3,4,8,*]

1 Departamento Académico de Ingeniería Forestal y Medio Ambiente, Facultad de Ingeniería, Universidad Nacional Amazónica de Madre de Dios, Puerto Maldonado 17001, Peru; mvela@unamad.edu.pe (M.V.-D.); pazpolli@unamad.edu.pe (P.A.Z.P.); jorgec@unamad.edu.pe (J.C.S.); rcanahuire@unamad.edu.pe (R.C.-R.)
2 Centro de Teledetección para el Estudio y Gestión de los Recursos Naturales (CETEGERN), Facultad de Ingeniería, Universidad Nacional Amazónica de Madre de Dios, Puerto Maldonado 17001, Peru; yedaro07@hotmail.com
3 Research Group: Earth Sciences & Dynamics of Ecology and Landscape, Universidad Nacional Amazónica de Madre de Dios, Puerto Maldonado 17001, Peru; lrodriguez@unamad.edu.pe
4 Research Group: Ecology & Restoration of Tropical Ecosystems, Universidad Nacional Amazónica de Madre de Dios, Puerto Maldonado 17001, Peru
5 Departamento Académico de Ciencias Básicas, Facultad de Ingeniería, Universidad Nacional Amazónica de Madre de Dios, Puerto Maldonado 17001, Peru
6 Departamento Académico de Sistemas e Informática, Facultad de Ingeniería, Universidad Nacional Amazónica de Madre de Dios, Puerto Maldonado 17001, Peru; dramos@unamad.edu.pe
7 Departamento Académico de Derecho y Ciencias Políticas, Facultad de Educación, Universidad Nacional Amazónica de Madre de Dios, Puerto Maldonado 17001, Peru; jdiaz@unamad.edu.pe
8 Department of Evolutionary Biology, Ecology and Environmental Sciences, Faculty of Biology, University of Barcelona, 08028 Barcelona, Spain
* Correspondence: galarcon@unamad.edu.pe or galarcona@hotmail.com (G.A.-A.); jgarate@unamad.edu.pe or garate.qjs@gmail.com (J.G.-Q.)

Abstract: Riverine beaches in the Amazon are valuable ecosystems for local populations, providing areas for recreation and classic beach activities. However, these ecosystems are subject to multiple pressures. The study presents the results of the willingness to pay (WTP) of 518 respondents at two beaches (Hawaii and Bora Bora) in the Peruvian Amazon (Puerto Maldonado, Madre de Dios). Over 58% of respondents indicated that they would use DAP to maintain beach ecosystem services (BES) beyond recreational use. The amount of payment was an average WTP value of USD 1.41/person/visit for Hawaii and USD 1.34/person/visit for Bora Bora. While factors related to environmental perception had a decisive influence, WTP at beaches was independent of economic factors such as income. The results can support decision-makers with quantitative data on social preferences regarding beach improvement policies in the southeastern Peruvian Amazon.

Keywords: Amazon beaches; conservation; contingent valuation method; hypothetical scenario; logit model; willingness to pay

1. Introduction

The importance of ecosystem services has evolved to become a fundamental aspect of wilderness management [1,2]. The Amazon's freshwater ecosystems, from wetlands to lakes, lagoons, swamps, rivers, estuaries, and streams, among others, have in common the presence of a permanent or temporary body of water. These ecosystems cover an area of approximately one million square kilometers and play an essential role in climate regulation, nutrient transport, water quality, biodiversity support, recreation, and food production, benefiting local, regional, and global communities [1,2]. Compared to other ecosystems, the biodiversity of these freshwater systems is disproportionately high, but the surface area of these systems is less than 1% of the planet [1]. The frequent proximity of freshwater ecosystems to human population centers has made these areas attractive for visitation. However, the impact of activities in these areas is intense [1,3,4].

Freshwater biodiversity is affected not only in the Amazon ecosystem but globally, due to a number of factors that threaten its continuity. The reasons for the decline of freshwater biodiversity are many, but the most important threats are habitat degradation, pollution, alteration of water flows and extraction, overfishing, and the introduction of exotic species; factors that will be exacerbated by the effects of climate change. All of these human-induced actions are not permanent and will eventually affect human well-being. This is due to the intimate link between human livelihoods and freshwater biodiversity as a basic service; water-related services that support the health, livelihoods, and well-being of people, taking into account the needs of Indigenous and local communities, as well as people in situations of poverty and vulnerability [1,5].

In particular, coastal and inland beaches are under severe pressure as components of freshwater ecosystems; they are viewed as ecosystems that offer advantages that are directly related to tourism, aesthetics, and recreation [1,6]. Beaches provide a range of ecosystem services that benefit society and are essential for human use. This is because beaches are strongly influenced by and interact physically and biologically with freshwater systems [1,6]. This means that sandy beach systems play an important role in the global land–freshwater interface [1,7]. When discussing impacts on the dynamic ecosystems of freshwater beaches and their associated goods and services, it is important to consider the potential impacts on adjacent habitats, both physical and ecological [1,7].

Over the years, economic valuation techniques have focused on people's preferences in real markets. However, for natural resources and environmental goods (such as scenic and recreational beauty), there was no defined market to determine consumer preferences and willingness to pay [1,7]. Contingent valuation research conducted in aquatic ecosystems in Latin America and the Amazon focused on obtaining income for recreational values and environmental services, social benefits, and public policy implementation. Similarly, consumer economic behavior is measured by the responses obtained for the range of prices set, as well as the variation in willingness to pay for socioeconomic and environmental variables in the surveys [1,7]. This direct valuation process facilitates the identification of the preferences expressed by current or potential visitors, as well as the evaluation of the maximum willingness to pay (WTP) to prevent the degradation of environmental quality in the Amazonian aquatic ecosystems [1,7].

Recognizing the value of beach ecosystem services and how they may be affected, studies have been carried out to determine how bathers value these ecosystems [4]. This refers to willingness to pay (WTP) studies, as they facilitate the identification of environmental preferences and are often used in public environmental projects [1,8]. In order to provide relevant information on possible solutions to the progressive degradation of beach ecosystems, these studies used the contingent valuation method to estimate the WTP for the beach ecosystem service. WTP can be calculated using revealed preferences [1,9], which determine WTP by dividing individual payments to consume a resource or by analyzing stated preferences (economic value through a hypothetical market) and asking respondents to report their WTP directly [1,9–11].

Many studies analyze differences in spatial heterogeneity using the Contingent Valuation Method (CVM) [1,12] as well as directly identifying ideal market scenarios through field studies to assess visitor satisfaction and improve ecosystem services [1,11,12]. Despite its widespread use, the contingent valuation method has some limitations, such as the deviation from the starting point, which presents a hypothetical scenario and does not ensure that respondents really answer the following questions [13]. In general terms, several methodological caveats have been identified. However, experts in the field have noted that the results of properly conducted processes approximate reality [11].

Despite the favorable context for the use of VCMs in the valuation of ecological services, studies on freshwater or inland beaches are scarce, as most of them refer to coastal or marine areas, such as water treatment plants [1,14–16], for beach restoration [1,17], and its application in tourism services [1,16,18].

The economic, recreational, aesthetic, and cultural aspects of beaches make them a desirable resource [1,19], but human activities are always putting pressure on them. This is the case of the freshwater beaches of the Peruvian Amazon, where there are several problems related to water pollution [20] and the quality of sand and silt on beaches [21–24]. There is no history of studies on WTP in freshwater beach ecosystems in the southern Peruvian Amazon, but there are private beaches that charge for access and maintenance services, without any methodological basis for estimation. Therefore, here we present an alternative view by investigating the WTP of visitors for ecosystem services in two free access river beaches (Bora Bora and Hawaii) in the city of Puerto Maldonado, Tambopata, Madre de Dios–Peru. We address the following research questions: (1) What are the descriptive characteristics of the river beaches? (2) Which socio-economic variables influence the WTP for the ecosystem services of the river beaches? (3) What is the WTP for the ecosystem services of the river beaches using the Contingent Valuation Method (CVM)? (4) What is the average value of the WTP for the ecosystem services of the river beaches?

2. Materials and Methods

2.1. Study Area

In the southeast of the Peruvian Amazon lies the department of Madre de Dios. It borders Puno to the south, Cusco to the west, and Ucayali to the north, and internationally with Brazil and Bolivia. It has an area of about 85,000 km^2 and a population of about 141,000 inhabitants [25].

The study areas were the river beaches of Bora Bora and Hawaii, located on the outskirts of the city of Puerto Maldonado, which has an area of 16.61 km^2 and a population of 85,024 inhabitants [25]. Puerto Maldonado lies between the Madre de Dios and Tambopata rivers. It is geographically located between the coordinates 12°38′49″–12°32′56″ south latitude and 69°11′40″–69°13′40″ west longitude, with an average altitude of 201 m above sea level [25].

The climate is hot and humid, the hottest months being August and September, with annual rainfall of more than 2000 mm and an average temperature of 26°. The dry season is from June to August, with the heaviest rainfall from October to April. The surazo or friaje is caused by cold polar winds from the south, with temperatures dropping to an average of 8 °C for several days [25–27].

Bora Bora Beach is located on the left bank of the Madre de Dios River, in the area of El Triunfo, 3.5 km from the center of the city of Puerto Maldonado (Figure 1). The access road is terrestrial and the entrance to the beach is free and has a nice view of the Continental Bridge. Hawaii Beach is located on the right bank of the Tambopata River, in front of the Tambopata Port in Puerto Maldonado, 2.2 km from the center of the city of Puerto Maldonado. Access is by boat, usually on Saturdays and Sundays throughout the day. On these beaches, you can enjoy beautiful landscapes at sunset. These beaches were chosen because they are places that the population can access without payment restrictions. Evaluations to determine how much visitors are willing to pay for services at Bora Bora and Hawaii beaches in Puerto Maldonado were conducted in 2021.

2.2. Beach Characterization

Seasonal visits were made to river beaches during the months of June through August, according to [1] and adapted by [28]. A technical inspection was carried out in the study area to establish a baseline since there is little scientific and official information about the two beaches. In this field inspection, the characteristics of the beaches were described in detail. For this purpose, information was collected on the generalities, uses, and activities of the beach, its environmental characteristics, the pollution present, the services and facilities available, and the use of the space [1].

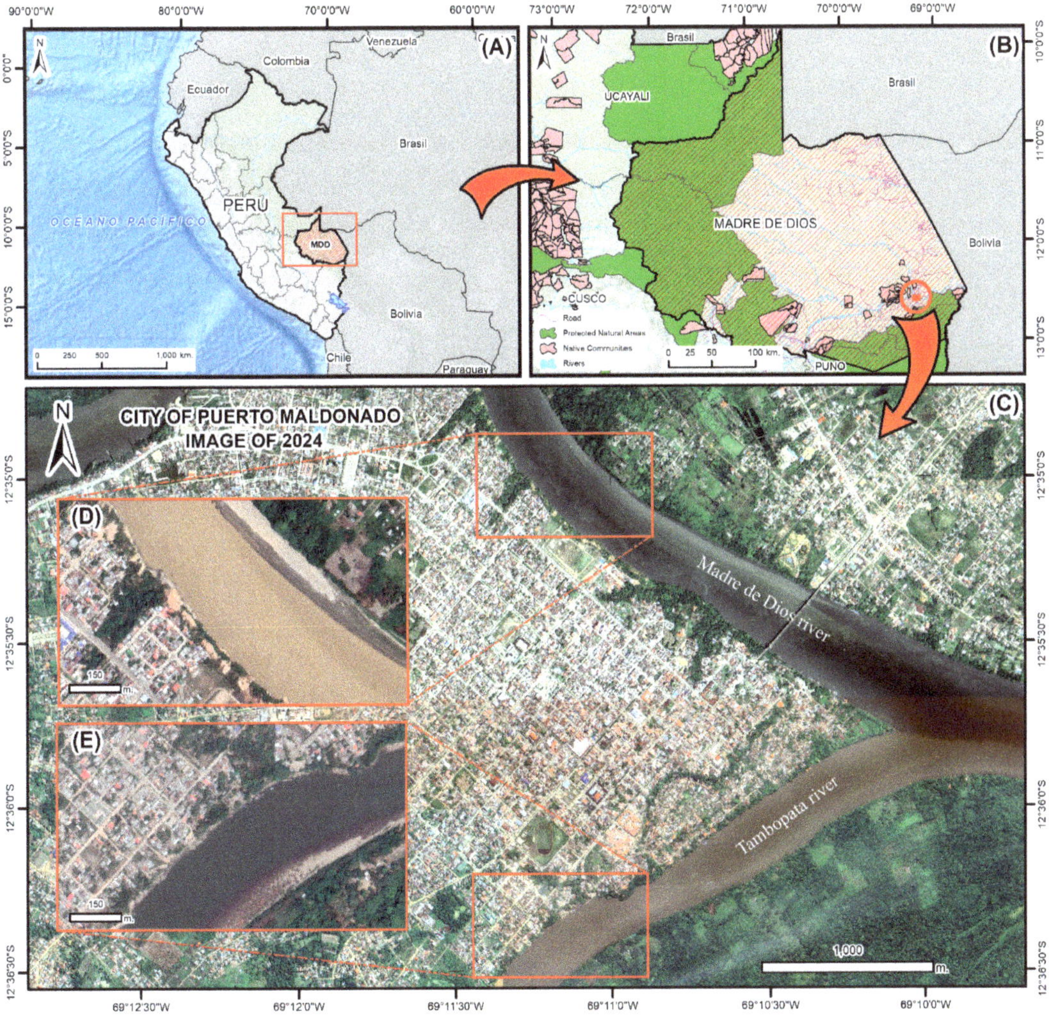

Figure 1. Study area location, related to Peru (**A**), Madre de Dios (**B**), and the city of Puerto Maldonado (**C**); Bora Bora beach (**D**) and Hawaii beach (**E**).

2.3. Contingent Valuation and Willingness to Pay

The study proposes the use of the Contingent Valuation Method (CVM), which determines the monetary value of a good or service without a market [1,29–34].

WTP was projected by means of a question to accept or not (simple bounded dichotomous format) a random amount for the maintenance of beach ecosystem services [29–33,35]. The surveys simulated the hypothetical scenario that the resident will face while making a decision on whether or not to purchase a certain good in the market: "The river beaches of Bora Bora and Hawaii, surrounding the city of Puerto Maldonado, provide adequate conditions of quality of use and permanent maintenance of ecosystem services by the competent authority that guarantee the safety of visitors".

To reduce the hypothetical bias, it was considered that the construction of the hypothetical market should accurately reflect the ecosystem service of river beaches. To this end, all support was provided to clearly define and explain the environmental good or service, as well as the specific characteristics of the change in BES. Also, they were provided with the mechanism or method of collection (WTP) in the form of public services managed by local governments [1,34,36].

Based on previous DAP studies [1,34,36], a survey was designed to determine the willingness to pay of visitors to the two selected river beaches. Structure of the survey questionnaire for the contingent valuation (CV) study [1,34,36], was structured in three pieces for the current study: the first section collected socioeconomic data from visitors, including standard questions about gender, age, occupation, education level, monthly income, frequency of visits, interest in ecology and environmental issues, satisfaction, and the time cost of beach access. Second, it included Beach Ecosystem Services (BES), including the importance of BES and preservation of BES for future generations; and finally, questions related to WTP, hypothetical prices obtained in the pilot survey (15% of respondents in the final sample), considered open-ended questions to visitors by WTP. The hypothetical or starting price values with the highest frequencies were assigned to the final survey for Hawaii (USD 0.26, USD 0.79, USD 1.32, and USD 1.84) and Bora Bora (USD 0.26, USD 0.79, and USD 1.32), where the surveys were distributed with specifications of the maximum amount to be paid. The survey has been validated by experts [10,11,37,38].

Specific questions concerning beach usage were posed to the BES, including how frequently people visit the beaches each month, what their primary activities are, and how satisfied they are with the beaches.

Following the experience of beach ecosystem valuation [4], respondents were given an explanation of the many types of ecosystem services and examples of each type. In this case, the following topics were covered: (i) the importance of each BES category; and (ii) the respondents' desire to conserve BES. The criteria ranged from not very interested to very interested, and high, medium, and low values for preserving BES for future generations were formed to classify the importance of BES (provisioning, regulating, supporting, and cultural).

"Would you be willing to pay for the preservation of the ecological services of the beach?" was the proposed WTP. An open-ended survey was used to determine WTP values for payments per visit, and a final survey was used to determine payment ranges. Socioeconomic criteria for the WTP analysis of BES maintenance were discovered through the survey. In this regard, the CVM has been used extensively around the world to determine user WTP for maintaining the benefits associated with river beaches [1,13,29,34,36,39,40].

A total of 518 surveys (Bora Bora (190 visitors surveyed) and Hawaii (328 visitors surveyed)) were conducted, with a margin of error of approximately 5% and a confidence level of 95%. Based on the hypothetical prices obtained, a simple random probability sample was taken, where everyone had an equal chance of participating and being selected for the study. For this purpose, visitors who were 18 years of age or older and able to pay were considered. In the case of Bora Bora beach, according to visitors and local residents, an average of 1600 visitors/month is estimated. In the case of Hawaii beach, 9600 visitors/month.

2.4. Statistical Analysis

Data were extracted and compiled from a comprehensive questionnaire administered between June and August 2021. For the statistical data analysis, descriptive and inferential techniques, as well as the Chi-square test, were used. Additionally, a binary logistic regression (logit, Equation (1)) model was employed to identify the various factors that may have a significant impact on visitors' WTP (Willingness to Pay) for the beaches. All statistical analysis were made using STATA software (version 18).

$$Pi = P(Z_i \leq X_i\beta = F(X_i\beta) = \frac{e^{X_i\beta}}{1 + e^{X_i\beta}} \quad (1)$$

where Pi = it is the probability that the dependent variable equals one, so β is the change in the probability that $P = 1$ is associated with a unit change in x_i, holding the other explanatory variables constant.

The likelihood function was expressed as follows:

$$\text{Log L} = \sum_{i}^{n} Y_i(X_i\,\beta) - \sum_{i}^{n} \log\left(1 + e^{X_i\beta}\right) \quad (2)$$

To determine the marginal effects of changes in the regressor variables on the conditional probability, models based on the derivatives of the probability with respect to a given explanatory variable were used (Equations (3) and (4)).

$$\frac{\partial Pi}{\partial xij} \equiv \frac{\partial}{\partial xij} P\left(yi = \frac{1}{xi}\right) = \beta_j \cdot f(x_j\beta_j) \quad (3)$$

where $f(z)$ is the corresponding density function (Equation (4)).

$$\frac{\partial Pi}{\partial xij} = \frac{\partial}{\partial xij} P\left(yi = \frac{1}{xi}\right) = \beta_j \cdot \frac{e^{X_i\beta}}{\left(1 + e^{X_i\beta}\right)^2} \quad (4)$$

The following equation was used to calculate the marginal effects for the mean value of the explanatory variables (Equation (5)).

$$n^{-1} \sum_{i=1}^{n} f(x_j\beta_j)\beta \; f(\overline{x}_j\beta_j)\beta \quad (5)$$

Taking into account previous studies such as [1,41], binary regression analysis was used to explain how socioeconomic variables influenced participants' willingness-to-pay responses to yes/no questions (dichotomous outcome).

Three models were evaluated according to the level of significance of the socioeconomic variables, total, 10% and 5%. It was decided to use a model with a 10% significance level (0.10) to include more variables. In the Hawaii study, the variables hypothetical price (hp), interest in environmental issues (ica), and frequency of visits (fv) were included. In the Bora Bora study, the variables hypothetical price (hp) and time cost to access the beach (ctaevu) were used.

The following equation was used to determine the probability of answering yes for WTP for the maintenance of beach ecosystem services [42–46] (Equation (6)).

$$Prob(yes) = \beta_0 - \beta_1(WTP) + \sum \beta_i Z_i \quad (6)$$

where *Prob*(*yes*) is the parametric method for estimating *WTP* using logit regression; where the dependent variable is beachgoers who say "yes" to paying or "no" to paying the bid level.

The WTP for the maintenance of beach ecosystem services in this type of model was:

$$WTP = \frac{\hat{\beta}_0 \Sigma_2^n \hat{\beta}_i Z_i}{\hat{\beta}_1} \quad (7)$$

The parametric estimation of the minimum *WTP* was carried out using the logit model, which mathematical representation of the probability (P_k) of accepting a payment for the maintenance of beach ecosystem services is as follows:

$$P_k = E\left(Y = \frac{1}{X_k}\right) = \frac{1}{1 + e^{-(\hat{\beta}_0 + \hat{\beta}_1 X_1 + \ldots + \hat{\beta}_k X_k)}} \quad (8)$$

where, $Y = 1$ if the answer is affirmative (yes) and $Y = 0$ if the answer is negative (no), with respect to the willingness to accept a minimum compensation, and X_k represents the set of socioeconomic and cultural variables characteristic of the survey.

The criteria used to evaluate the variables were as follows: Sex (male, female); Age (18–35, 36–55, >55); Level of education (no education, primary school, high school or bachelor's degree); Interest in environmental issues (low, medium, high); Income (<252.63 USD, 252.89 USD to 526.32 USD, 526.58 USD to 921.05 USD, 921.32 USD to 1315.79 USD, >1315.79 USD); Frequency of visits (biannual, monthly, bi-weekly, weekly); Satisfaction (very dissatisfied, dissatisfied, satisfied, very satisfied); Access time (60 min, 30–60 min, 15–30 min).

To ensure the validity of the results, a variance inflation factor (VIF) was used to control for multicollinearity. Hawaii beach reported VIF values for the variables; income with 1.32, education level with 1.23, frequency of visits with 1.13, gender with 1.11, satisfaction with 1.08, age with 1.07, interest in environmental issues with 1.07, time of access to the beach with 1.06, and hypothetical price with 1.05. For Bora Bora beach, it was income with 1.71, education level with 1.142, frequency of visits with 1.24, gender with 1.34, satisfaction with 1.05, age with 1.12, interest in environmental issues with 1.10, time of access to the beach with 1.04, and hypothetical price with 1.11. In each case, they have a low correlation and do not need to be tested [47].

3. Results

3.1. River Beach Characterization

The beaches of Hawaii and Bora Bora cover approximately 5.37 ha and 6.38 ha, respectively; both, however, lack infrastructure and services. During the visits, we observed pollution, especially litter and waste on the beach, with no specific regulation, except for sewage. However, the environmental characteristics are still acceptable for recreational use (Table 1). Despite the abandonment and lack of regulation by the competent authority, it is necessary that the authority develops beach conservation plans through immediate public policies to avoid the deterioration of ecosystem services due to seasonal pollution.

Table 1. Beach characterization.

Beach Characterization		Hawaii	Bora Bora
Infrastructure and services	Beach access	Limited access	Good access
	Road conditions	Good access	Good access
	Type of transport	Private	Private
	Parking areas	Absence	Presence (not zoned)
	Public toilets	Absence	Absence
	Waste bins	Absence	Absence
	Lifeguard	Absence	Absence
	Control and monitoring	Absence	Absence
	Beach activities	Enjoy sunbathing and swimming	Enjoy sunbathing and swimming
	Recreational and sports equipment (sports grounds)	Absence	Absence
	Trading	Presence (Unorganized)	Presence (Unorganized)
	Motor vehicles on the beach	Absence	Absence
	Equipment (umbrellas, chairs)	Presence	Presence
	Signage–Public information	Absence	Absence

Table 1. *Cont.*

Beach Characterization		Hawaii	Bora Bora
Contamination	Odors	Seasonal Only	Seasonal Only
	Waste	Seasonal Only	Seasonal Only
	Waste piles	Seasonal Only	Seasonal Only
	Discharges or discharges to the river (Wastewater/domestic)	Absence	Absence
Environmental characteristics	Beach area	>100 m	>100 m
	Beach shape	Straight	Straight
	Beach width	>100 m	>100 m
	Beach particles	Sand	Sand
	Sand color	Gray	Gray
	Sand grain type	Medium sand	Medium sand
	Type of swell	Waters with currents	Waters with currents
	Mouths	Absence	Absence
	Turbidity	Clear	Clear

On the other hand, it is important to mention that the influx of visitors to private beaches is mainly due to the adequate environmental conditions they offer for recreation and rest. In this context of use and challenges related to infrastructure and services, pollution, as well as the conditions of free access to river beaches, present similarities with other regions worldwide; therefore, the presence of the minimum environmental conditions that offer recreational enjoyment and rest perceived by visitors are sufficient for their access, as researchers have found in different areas of the world [17,39,41,48–51].

3.2. Visitor/Bather Perception

According to the data obtained, the sampled population is local, which is common in the river beaches of the Peruvian Amazon. According to surveys of locals and visitors to the beaches, it is estimated that Bora Bora has an average of 1600 visitors/month during the dry season, while Hawaii has 9600 visitors/month.

The results showed that the highest percentage of respondents at the beaches studied were women between the ages of 18 and 35. The main educational level of visitors to Hawaii and Bora Bora was primary school, with 50% and 59%, respectively. Interest in environmental issues was generally high. The majority of visitors were employed, with salaries ranging from USD 252.81 to USD 526.32. Bora Bora had visitors with the highest and lowest purchasing power; 1.1% of respondents reported incomes above USD 1315.79, while 28.1% of respondents reported incomes between USD 0 and USD 252.63 (Table 2).

Table 2. Descriptive metrics of socioeconomic characteristics affecting river beach ecosystem services.

Beach	Sex	Age	Education Level	Interest in Environmental Issues	Income	Frequency of Visits	Satisfaction	Access Time	Hypothetical Price
				Hawaii (n = 328)					
Category	Woman	18–35	Primary	High	252.89 US$ to 526.32 US$	Semi-annual	Satisfied	60 min	0.26 US$
Frequency	178	146	164	217	204	161	178	317	66
Percentage	27.8%	44.51%	50%	66.16%	62.20%	49.08%	54.27%	96.64%	20.12%
				Bora Bora (n = 190)					
Category	Woman	18–35	Primary	High	<252.63 US$	Semi-annual	Satisfied	60 min	0.26 US$
Frequency	130	111	112	101	103	112	126	180	45
Percentage	68.4%	58.4%	59.0%	53.2%	54.2%	59.0%	66.3%	94.7%	39.8%

Notes: Variables: Sex (female and male); Age (18 to 35, 36 to 55, and >55); Level of education (no education, primary school, high school or bachelor's degree); Interest in environmental issues (low, medium, high); Income (<252.63 USD, 252.89 USD to 526.32 USD, 526.58 USD to 921.05 USD, 921.32 USD to 1315.79 USD, >1315.79 USD); Frequency of visits (biannual, monthly, bi-weekly, weekly); Satisfaction (very dissatisfied, dissatisfied, satisfied, very satisfied); Access time (15 to 30 min, 30 to 60 min and 60 min).

Most visitors visit the beaches on a monthly and semi-annual basis, primarily for recreational reasons. Visitors report varying degrees of satisfaction with beach use, with Hawaii reporting the highest satisfaction (54%) compared to Bora Bora (32%) (Table 2).

Regarding the entry price (hp) obtained in the pilot survey and used in the final survey, in both beaches; Hawaii (USD 0.26, USD 0.79, USD 1.32, and USD 1.84) and Bora Bora (USD 0.26, USD 0.79, and USD 1.32) opted for the lowest price (S/1.00), with a positive response of 20.1% and 39.5%, respectively. This confirms the economic theory of consumption in terms of tastes and preferences.

Cultural services were the most important (77%), followed by provisioning services (77%), support services (76%), and regulatory services (74%). It should be noted that the services ranked as most important differed between the two beaches. In Hawaii, support and cultural services were most important, while in Bora Bora, cultural and regulatory services were most important. At the level of importance for their maintenance, Hawaii and Bora Bora presented mostly medium values (interested) of BES, with priority given to support services for Hawaii and cultural services for Bora Bora.

3.3. *Willingness to Pay for River Beach Ecosystem Services*

Before proceeding with the econometric analysis, we verified that the hp variable met the assumptions of the dichotomous logit model using the contingent valuation method (CVM). In our case, the coefficient β of hp for both beaches was negative.

The logit model considered ($p < 0.10$) of the willingness to pay (WTP) for ecosystem services; Hawaii beach presents a logit model coefficient (R^2) of 0.17, while Bora Bora has 0.14, which suggests an adequate model to classify individuals, a situation consistent with the principles of demand. As for the LR $chi^2(3)$ test, it is assumed that the null hypothesis that no variable infers WTP is rejected (LR $chi^2(3)$ =0 for Hawaii and LR $chi^2(2)$ =0 for Bora Bora). Overall, the logistic trend shows that the response rate decreases as the level of the WTP offer increases, which is consistent with demand-side principles.

For the Hawaii beach, hp had a negative impact per unit change as the price increased, so the probability of visitors paying for the ecosystem service decreased by 1.31 times and 7% on WTP. Factors such as frequency of visits (fv) and interest in environmental issues (ica) were positive and significant ($p < 0.05$), suggesting that these factors positively influenced WTP (Table 3). The variable fv contributes 1.34 times to the occurrence of the event, while at the marginal effects level, a higher frequency of visits increases the probability of WTP by 7%. As for ica, it contributes 1.75 times to the occurrence of the event, while at the marginal effects level, a greater interest in environmental issues increases the probability of WTP by 14%.

Table 3. Descriptive metrics of socioeconomic characteristics affecting river beach ecosystem services.

Hawaii Beach Variables	Coefficients	Standard Error	z	*p*-Value	Odds Ratio	Marginal Effect (dy/dx)
hp	−0.27	0.06	−4.85	0.00	0.76	−0.07
fv	0.29	0.14	2.06	0.04	1.34	0.07
ica	0.56	0.24	2.34	0.02	1.75	0.14
_cons	−0.54	0.72	−0.76	0.45		
LR $chi^2(3)$				30.95		
Pseudo R^2				0.17		
Bora Bora Beach Variables	**Coefficients**	**Standard Error**	**z**	***p*-Value**	**Odds Ratio**	**Marginal Effect (dy/dx)**
hp	−0.21	0.09	−2.25	0.02	0.81	−0.05
ctaevu	1.65	0.92	1.79	0.07	5.20	0.39
_cons	−0.70	0.97	−0.72	0.47		
LR $chi^2(2)$				11.30		
Pseudo R^2				0.14		

Notes: Sex (sex), age (age), education level (edu), interest in environmental issues (ica), income (ing), frequency of visits (fv), access time (ctaevu), and hypothetical price (hp).

As for the beach of Bora Bora, hp negatively influences the unit change as the price increases; consequently, the visitor's probability of paying for the ecosystem service decreases by 1.24 times and the willingness to pay by 5%. While ctaevu was positive and significant ($p < 0.05$), indicating that this variable positively influences WTP (Table 3). The variable ctaevu contributes 5.20 times to the occurrence of the event, while at the marginal effects level, a shorter beach access time increases the probability of WTP by 39%.

In both beaches, whose access is free, curiously, the variables income, age, level of education, or sex were not determinant in the WTP. For the inhabitants of the city of Puerto Maldonado, Bora Bora beach is more distant, located on the northeast side of the city, crossing one of the longest bridges in Peru (continental) over the Madre de Dios River, so the cost of time to access the beach is fundamental in the WTP decision for the ecosystem service. In contrast, at Hawaii Beach, located close to the city on the banks of the Tambopata River, visitors are more interested in environmental issues, which is reflected in the frequency of visits for personal or family recreation purposes, which drives the WTP. Visitor demand is reflected in an average of 9600 visits per month at Hawaii Beach and 1600 visits per month at Bora Bora.

The predictive ability of the model based on the final survey data from Hawaii Beach adequately determined the membership of 148 people in group D (WTP) and 88 in group ~D (no WTP). Conversely, 43 people did not accept WTP when they actually did, while 49 people did not accept WTP. The probability of predicting people's WTP for the beach was 77.5%, while the opposite was 35.8%. The overall goodness of fit of the model was 60.06%. Regarding the beach of Bora Bora, the model determined that 85 people belonged to group D (WTP) and 48 to group ~D (no WTP). Conversely, 28 people did not accept the WTP when in fact they did, and 29 people did not accept the WTP. The probability of predicting people's WTP for the beach was 75.2%, while the opposite was 37.7%. The overall goodness of fit of the model is 60%.

Overall, WTP (+) predominated among visitors to the two river beaches, with 58.2% at Hawaii and 59.5% at Bora Bora: Descriptive statistical analysis was conducted by beach to determine the value visitors were willing to pay (Table 4). The analysis revealed an average WTP of USD 1.41/person/visit, slightly higher than Bora Bora beach with a WTP of USD 1.34/person/visit.

Table 4. Estimated WTP payable at each beach (per revenue—USD).

Variable	Observations	Mean	Standard Deviation	Minimum	Maximum
Hawaii Beach					
WTP	328	1.41	0.35	0.58	2.24
Bora Bora Beach					
WTP	190	1.34	0.76	1.17	5.25

4. Discussion

4.1. River Beach Characterization

Information on the contingent valuation of river beaches in the Amazon is scarce compared to coastal beaches or lakes. Several studies have investigated the possible factors influencing the economic valuation of river beaches [5,17,19,28,40,41,52]. The analysis of beaches with different natural characteristics, pollution problems, and services allows us to understand the elements that influence the use and enjoyment of the beach. The results of the study (Table 1) suggest that the two beaches analyzed have similarities and some slight differences. To highlight one aspect, both beaches are long and have low turbidity (clear water). The favorable environmental conditions have a positive impact on activities such as beach soccer, volleyball, swimming, and sunbathing. However, the fact that they are open to the public without government control means that there is often chaos and pollution due to the accumulation of rubbish at the end of the day [53–56].

4.2. Visitor/Bather Perception

The conservation of marine and riverine beaches has been debated to varying degrees in the literature [1,14,41,50,52,57]. The consensus is that, in general, beaches are vulnerable to man-made elements and climate variability [58]. Long-term droughts, floods, water scarcity, decreased soil productivity, agricultural yields, disease outbreaks, invasion of alien species, water levels, decreased mangrove and reed cover, biodiversity status, and water purity are some of the ecological indicators that indicate that the beach ecosystem is in danger. In the case of the Amazon, what is usually mentioned is the progress of deforestation and the increase in activities that threaten the sustainability of natural resources.

The Madre de Dios and Tambopata Rivers are two of the most important watercourses in the Madre de Dios region, essential for the development of forestry, fishing, and agricultural activities. The current situation shows that population pressure, reduced land-use capacity, and contamination of fisheries by agricultural and gold mining activities are forcing the local population to seek other alternatives, accelerating the degradation of the beach ecosystem. This phenomenon is also observed in other areas with freshwater beaches [51,59,60].

Different people expressed different perceptions of WTP for the Hawaii and Bora Bora beaches. These different perceptions were associated with marginal utility derived from the preserved river ecosystem, and the results were manifested in WTP responses and quantities by significant variables ($p < 0.10$).

During the study period, an unfavorable interaction was identified in relation to beach pollution, where visitors exert a negative influence that would lead to ecosystem degradation due to a lack of attention to sustainability in their recreational activities. This attitude indicates a willingness to engage in beach recreation regardless of the environment. These findings are consistent with those of other studies conducted in similar contexts [53–56].

Visitors clearly identified cultural, provisioning, and support services, while regulating services were less recognized by visitors. The identification of BES may have been biased because direct-use provisioning services are crucial to both local economic and cultural elements, particularly tourism. Also, when asked about support services, they were not recognized as precursors of the other services. Consideration should be given to the most appropriate classification system for ecosystem services based on their fitness for purpose. Nevertheless, the research and questionnaire design may have contributed to the bias in the results presented here by approaching the classification of BES from research rather than a practical standpoint. In the present research, four categories were chosen. However, there are sometimes discrepancies in the identification of services, more so in the case of regulatory and support services, which causes confusion among visitors and requires a clear separation between them [2,14,40,60].

4.3. Willingness to Pay for Ecosystem Services of Beaches

Several studies of WTP for the preservation of the natural benefits of beaches have reported that visitors show a positive willingness to pay when the resources they could hypothetically contribute are used to preserve or improve the condition of beaches [1,2,14,18,52,60]. In particular, this study has found that a number of factors influence the presence of WTP (+) on both beaches, as determined by logistic regression analysis.

According to this study, the proposed WTP for the beach in Hawaii is USD 1.41/person/visit, while that of Bora Bora is USD 1.34/person/visit. The estimated willingness to pay for the ecosystem services of Hawaii and Bora Bora beaches guarantees their use and conservation, but there is a slight variation with respect to private beaches, which range from 1.58 USD to 2.63 USD, with the Botafogo, Miranda, and Taricaya beaches standing out.

Data from Hawaii and Bora Bora beaches showed that 58.2% and 59.5% of respondents, respectively, were willing to pay because, as in previous research, they believed the hypothetical situation would improve ecological services and benefit future generations [12,14,18,40,52], it was found that WTP (+) is not solely determined by income. Consequently, the logistic regression showed that the responses were influenced by the frequency of visits, interest in environmental issues, and time cost of access to the beach, all of which were mostly related to the secondary and higher education levels.

On the other hand, 41.8% of respondents who answered "no to payment" in Hawaii and 40.5% in Bora Bora are mostly at the same educational level. However, they are constrained by a moderate to low income. Moreover, 19.5% of respondents in Hawaii and 18.4% in Bora Bora said they could not afford it because they believe it is the government's responsibility and because they do not trust the local government structures assigned to manage the funds, attributing this mistrust to high levels of corruption, a common problem in developing countries. On the other hand, 22% in Hawaii and 19.5% in Bora Bora did not do so because of their low income. The reality and analysis are similar to numerous studies conducted in inland water environments, such as lakes and rivers [12,15,18,24,57,61].

4.4. Limitations of the Study

It is important to remember that the contingent valuation approach used in the study could not have fully captured the more complex phases of the BES. This is because the method only allows for the detailed analysis of one scenario, rather than evaluating multiple potential scenarios in terms of environmental trade-offs and WTP. Therefore, it is suggested that a detailed analysis be carried out to address the various related aspects of how environmental change affects WTP, as well as social preferences in terms of the economic valuation of BES.

The quantification of the population of visitors to the beaches of Hawaii and Bora Bora was based on information provided by the locals, as there is currently no local, regional, or national institution that keeps records of visitors to the beaches. Based on this information, a sample was selected to analyze the WTP. On the other hand, many visitors were reluctant to be interviewed, so more time was needed for data collection.

5. Conclusions and Policy Implications

The beaches of Hawaii and Bora Bora, located near the city of Puerto Maldonado, are open to the public. Despite the lack of management by the competent authority, there is a high demand from bathers due to the favorable environmental conditions for recreational activities, despite the lack of infrastructure and basic services.

There was a higher representation of women among the total number of respondents. In the context of improving the quality of use and continuous maintenance of ecosystem services, the most influential socio-economic variables in WTP were identified as frequency of visits and interest in environmental issues in the case of Hawaii, and the cost of access time in the case of Bora Bora.

The average WTP per person per visit was USD 1.41 for Hawaii and USD 1.34 for Bora Bora. Visitor WTP results are lower than for private beaches, but consistent with the local socio-economic reality. However, it is important to analyze the data in monetary terms to ensure the continued provision and maintenance of ecological services.

The implementation of a strong environmental education policy is essential to increase the knowledge and commitment of visitors to river beaches. This education has a number of benefits, including the training of river beach managers, public access to relevant information on important river-related issues, direct community involvement in the management of river beach areas, and the promotion of environmentally sound practices to reduce negative impacts.

Consequently, since interest in environmental issues has emerged as a crucial factor in beaches, it is imperative to address environmental issues such as solid waste management and promote orderly visitation through education and awareness at various levels; initial, primary, secondary, and higher education, authorities, managers, visitors/bathers and tourism operators, in order to achieve greater awareness and ensure the sustainable use of river beaches.

Finally, it is necessary to implement a means of payment that gives confidence to the visitors, through funds managed by public-private institutions, where the value to be paid for the ecosystem service of the river beaches is intended for such purposes and not questioned for acts of corruption.

Author Contributions: Conceptualization, G.A.-A. and Y.D.Á.R.; methodology, G.A.-A., J.L.D.R. and Y.D.Á.R.; software, G.A.-A., L.R.A. and M.V.-D.; validation, G.A.-A., J.C.S., J.L.D.R. and Y.D.Á.R.; formal analysis, G.A.-A. and D.R.E.; investigation, G.A.-A., J.C.S., J.L.D.R., L.R.A. and Y.D.Á.R.; Data curation, G.A.-A., D.R.E. and J.G.-Q.; writing—original draft preparation, G.A.-A.; writing—review and editing, J.G.-Q., J.L.D.R. and P.A.Z.P.; visualization, R.C.-R. and J.G.-Q.; supervision, G.A.-A. and P.A.Z.P. All authors have read and agreed to the published version of the manuscript.

Funding: This research received no external funding.

Data Availability Statement: The raw data supporting the conclusions of this article will be made available by the authors upon request.

Acknowledgments: We thank Franchesca Zamudio Zambrano for her assistance with field data collection. We thank the local people around the Hawaiian and Bora beaches for providing information about visitors to the study area. We also thank Foster Brown for his suggestions and revision of the English version of the manuscript.

Conflicts of Interest: The authors declare no conflicts of interest.

References

1. Enriquez, T.; Botero, C.M.; Cantero, R.; Pertuz, A.; Suarez, A. Willingness to pay for Beach Ecosystem Services: The case study of three Colombian beaches. *Ocean Coast. Manag.* **2018**, *161*, 96–104. [CrossRef]
2. Nahuelhual, L.; Vergara, X.; Kusch, A.; Campos, G.; Droguett, D. Mapping ecosystem services for marine spatial planning: Recreation opportunities in Sub-Antarctic Chile. *Mar. Policy* **2017**, *81*, 211–218. [CrossRef]
3. Mendoza, G.; Martínez, M.L.; Lithgow, D.; Pérez, O.; Simonin, P. Land use change and its effects on the value of ecosystem services along the coast of the Gulf of Mexico. *Ecol. Econ.* **2012**, *82*, 23–32. [CrossRef]
4. Paffett, K.; Stevens, L.E.; Springer, A.E. Chapter 4.5.3—Ecological Assessment and Rehabilitation Prioritization for Improving Springs Ecosystem Stewardship. In *Wetland and Stream Rapid Assessments*; Dorney, J., Savage, R., Tiner, R.W., Adamus, P., Eds.; Academic Press: London, UK, 2018; pp. 475–487.
5. Schuhmann, P.W.; Mahon, R. The valuation of marine ecosystem goods and services in the Caribbean: A literature review and framework for future valuation efforts. *Ecosyst. Serv.* **2015**, *11*, 56–66. [CrossRef]
6. Alcívar, A.A. Propuesta de un Plan de Marketing Turístico para los Humedales Ribereños de la Parroquia Honorato Vásquez. Manabí 2016. Available online: https://repositorio.ug.edu.ec/items/32e434a3-b1a8-4649-8f23-4a36afda67dc (accessed on 10 September 2024).
7. Beck, M.; Reckhardt, A.; Amelsberg, J.; Bartholomä, A.; Brumsack, H.-J.; Cypionka, H.; Dittmar, T.; Engelen, B.; Greskowiak, J.; Hillebrand, H. The drivers of biogeochemistry in beach ecosystems: A cross-shore transect from the dunes to the low-water line. *Mar. Chem.* **2017**, *190*, 35–50. [CrossRef]
8. Risén, E.; Nordström, J.; Malmström, M.E.; Gröndahl, F. Non-market values of algae beach-cast management–Study site Trelleborg, Sweden. *Ocean Coast. Manag.* **2017**, *140*, 59–67. [CrossRef]
9. Christie, M.; Fazey, I.; Cooper, R.; Hyde, T.; Kenter, J.O. An evaluation of monetary and non-monetary techniques for assessing the importance of biodiversity and ecosystem services to people in countries with developing economies. *Ecol. Econ.* **2012**, *83*, 67–78. [CrossRef]
10. Alarcón, G.; Díaz, J.L.; Vela, M.; Quiñonez, J.J.; Zevallos, P.A.; Gutiérrez, J.D. Valor de conservación en bosques de comunidades indígenas: Un estudio de caso en la Amazonia Peruana, San Jacinto y Puerto Arturo. *J. High Andean Res.* **2018**, *20*, 301–314. [CrossRef]
11. Alarcon, G.; Zevallos, P.A.; Quispe, R.; Ramos, D.; Garate-Quispe, J.S. Valor de conservación de un bosque en el sureste de la Amazonia Peruana: El caso de Madre de Dios. *Rev. Ecosistemas* **2020**, *29*, 1947. [CrossRef]
12. Ren, Y.; Lu, L.; Zhang, H.; Chen, H.; Zhu, D. Residents' willingness to pay for ecosystem services and its influencing factors: A study of the Xin'an River basin. *J. Clean. Prod.* **2020**, *268*, 122301. [CrossRef]
13. McFadden, D.; Train, K. *Contingent Valuation of Environmental Goods: A Comprehensive Critique*; Edward Elgar Publishing: Northampton, MA, USA, 2017; p. 336.
14. Beharry, N.; Scarpa, R. Valuing quality changes in Caribbean coastal waters for heterogeneous beach visitors. *Ecol. Econ.* **2010**, *69*, 1124–1139. [CrossRef]
15. Hess, S.; Beharry-Borg, N. Accounting for latent attitudes in willingness-to-pay studies: The case of coastal water quality improvements in Tobago. *Environ. Resour. Econ.* **2012**, *52*, 109–131. [CrossRef]
16. Peng, M.; Oleson, K.L.L. Beach recreationalists' willingness to pay and economic implications of coastal water quality problems in Hawaii. *Ecol. Econ.* **2017**, *136*, 41–52. [CrossRef]

17. Matthews, Y.; Scarpa, R.; Marsh, D. Stability of willingness-to-pay for coastal management: A choice experiment across three time periods. *Ecol. Econ.* **2017**, *138*, 64–73. [CrossRef]
18. Prayaga, P. Estimating the value of beach recreation for locals in the Great Barrier Reef Marine Park, Australia. *Econ. Anal. Policy* **2017**, *53*, 9–18. [CrossRef]
19. Williams, A.T.; Rangel-Buitrago, N.G.; Anfuso, G.; Cervantes, O.; Botero, C.M. Litter impacts on scenery and tourism on the Colombian north Caribbean coast. *Tour. Manag.* **2016**, *55*, 209–224. [CrossRef]
20. Ibana-Lopez, K.; Sihuay-Perales, M.; Garate-Quispe, J.; Araújo-Flores, J.; Herrera-Machaca, M.; Alarcón-Aguirre, G.; Rodriguez-Achata, L. Contaminación de agua superficial de la periferia urbana de Puerto Maldonado, al sureste de la amazonia peruana. *Rev. De Investig. Vet. Del Perú* **2021**, *32*, e20365. [CrossRef]
21. Alarcón, G.; Díaz, J.; Vela, M.; García, M.; Gutiérrez, J. Deforestación en el sureste de la amazonia del Perú entre los años 1999-2013; caso Regional de Madre de Dios (Puerto Maldonado–Inambari). *J. High Andean Res.* **2016**, *18*, 319–330. [CrossRef]
22. Bonotto, D.M.; Wijesiri, B.; Vergotti, M.; da Silveira, E.G.; Goonetilleke, A. Assessing mercury pollution in Amazon River tributaries using a Bayesian Network approach. *Ecotoxicol. Environ. Saf.* **2018**, *166*, 354–358. [CrossRef]
23. Gerolin, C.R.; Pupim, F.N.; Sawakuchi, A.O.; Grohmann, C.H.; Labuto, G.; Semensatto, D. Microplastics in sediments from Amazon rivers, Brazil. *Sci. Total Environ.* **2020**, *749*, 141604. [CrossRef]
24. Velásquez, M.G.; Vega Ruiz, C.M.; Gomringer, R.C.; Pillaca, M.; Thomas, E.; Stewart, P.M.; Gamarra Miranda, L.A.; Dañobeytia, F.R.; Guerrero Barrantes, J.A.; Gushiken, M.C.; et al. Mercury in soils impacted by alluvial gold mining in the Peruvian Amazon. *J. Environ. Manag.* **2021**, *288*, 112364. [CrossRef] [PubMed]
25. INEI, Instituto Nacional de Estadística e Informática del Perú. *Magnitud y Crecimiento Poblacional*; INEI: Lima, Perú, 2017; p. 1521.
26. GOREMAD; IIAP. *Macro Zonificación Ecológica Económica de Madre de Dios*; GOREMAD: Puerto Maldonado, Perú, 2009; p. 208.
27. Perz, S.; Castro, W.; Rojas, R.; Castillo, J.; Chávez, A.; García, M.; Guadalupe, Ó.; Gutiérrez, T.; Hurtado, A.; Mamani, Z.; et al. La Amazonia como un sistema socio-ecológico: Las dinámicas de cambios complejos humanos y ambientales en una frontera trinacional. In *Naturaleza y Sociedad: Perpectivas Socio-Ecológicas Sobre Cambios Globales en América Latina*; Postigo, J., Young, K., Eds.; desco, IEP e INTE-PUCP: Lima, Perú, 2016; p. 444.
28. Federigi, I.; Balestri, E.; Castelli, A.; De Battisti, D.; Maltagliati, F.; Menicagli, V.; Verani, M.; Lardicci, C.; Carducci, A. Beach pollution from marine litter: Analysis with the DPSIR framework (driver, pressure, state, impact, response) in Tuscany, Italy. *Ecol. Indic.* **2022**, *143*, 109395. [CrossRef]
29. Cuccia, T. Contingent valuation. In *Handbook of Cultural Economics*, 3rd ed.; Edward Elgar Publishing: Northampton, MA, USA, 2020; p. 552.
30. Ginsburgh, V. Contingent valuation, willingness to pay, and willingness to accept. In *Economic Ideas You Should Forget*; Springer: Cham, Switzerland, 2017; pp. 65–66.
31. Haab, T.C.; McConnell, K.E. *Valuing Environmental and Natural Resources: The Econometrics of Non-Market Valuation*; Edward Elgar Publishing: Northampton, MA, USA, 2002; p. 352.
32. Hoyos, D.; Mariel, P. Contingent valuation: Past, present and future. *Prague Econ. Pap.* **2010**, *4*, 329–343. [CrossRef]
33. Song, X.; Lv, X.; Li, C. Willingness and motivation of residents to pay for conservation of urban green spaces in Jinan, China. *Acta Ecol. Sin.* **2015**, *35*, 89–94. [CrossRef]
34. Pascual, U.; Muradian, R.; Brander, L.; Gómez-Baggethun, E.; Martín-López, B.; Verma, M.; Armsworth, P.; Christie, M.; Cornelissen, H.; Eppink, F. The economics of valuing ecosystem services and biodiversity. In *The Economics of Ecosystems and Biodiversity: Ecological and Economic Foundations*; Roudledge: London, UK, 2011; pp. 183–256.
35. Mousavi, S.; Akbari, S. Estimated value of forest conservation in Iran: A case study of Fars Province. *Afr. J. Agric. Res.* **2011**, *6*, 6407–6411. [CrossRef]
36. Ferreira, S.; Marques, R.C. Contingent valuation method applied to waste management. *Resour. Conserv. Recycl.* **2015**, *99*, 111–117. [CrossRef]
37. Elangovan, N.; Sundaravel, E. Method of preparing a document for survey instrument validation by experts. *MethodsX* **2021**, *8*, 101326. [CrossRef]
38. Perni, Á.; Barreiro-Hurlé, J.; Martínez-Paz, J.M. Contingent valuation estimates for environmental goods: Validity and reliability. *Ecol. Econ.* **2021**, *189*, 107144. [CrossRef]
39. Venkatachalam, L. The contingent valuation method: A review. *Environ. Impact Assess. Rev.* **2004**, *24*, 89–124. [CrossRef]
40. Zerouali, S.; Yacoubi-Khebiza, M.; El Qorchi, F. Monetary Value Change of Some Provisioning Ecosystem Services of Middle Draa Valley, South of Morocco. In *Climate Change and Its Impact on Ecosystem Services and Biodiversity in Arid and Semi-Arid Zones*; IGI Global: Hershey, PA, USA, 2019; pp. 67–77.
41. Castaño, J.; Newball, R.; Roach, B.; Lau, W.W.Y. Valuing beaches to develop payment for ecosystem services schemes in Colombia's Seaflower marine protected area. *Ecosyst. Serv.* **2015**, *11*, 22–31. [CrossRef]
42. Horowitz, J.L.; Savin, N. Binary response models: Logits, probits and semiparametrics. *J. Econ. Perspect.* **2001**, *15*, 43–56. [CrossRef]
43. Linares, P.; Aguilera, A.; Romero, C. Economía y medio ambiente: Herramientas de valoración ambiental. In *Tratado de Tributación Medioambiental*; Thomson Reuters: Madrid, España, 2008; pp. 1189–1225.
44. McFadden, D.; Train, K. Mixed MNL models for discrete response. *J. Appl. Econom.* **2000**, *15*, 447–470. [CrossRef]

45. Bishop, R.C.; Heberlein, T.A. Measuring values of extramarket goods: Are indirect measures biased? *Am. J. Agric. Econ.* **1979**, *61*, 926–930. [CrossRef]
46. Bishop, R.C.; Heberlein, T.A. *Simulated Markets, Hypothetical Markets, and Travel Cost Analysis: Alternative Methods of Estimating Outdoor Recreation Demand*; Department of Agricultural Economics, University of Wisconsin-Madison: Madison, WI, USA, 1980.
47. Bayman, E.O.; Dexter, F. Multicollinearity in Logistic Regression Models. *Anesth. Analg.* **2021**, *133*, 362–365. [CrossRef]
48. Alves, B.; Rigall-I-Torrent, R.; Ballester, R.; Benavente, J.; Ferreira, Ó. Coastal erosion perception and willingness to pay for beach management (Cadiz, Spain). *J. Coast. Conserv.* **2015**, *19*, 269–280. [CrossRef]
49. Boyle, K.J. Contingent valuation in practice. In *A Primer on Nonmarket Valuation*; Springer: Dordrecht, The Netherlands, 2017; pp. 83–131.
50. Chang, J.-I.; Yoon, S. Assessing the Economic Value of Beach Restoration: Case of Song-do Beach, Korea. *J. Coast. Res.* **2017**, *79*, 6–10. [CrossRef]
51. Dejen, E.; Anteneh, W.; Vijverberg, J. The Decline of the Lake Tana (Ethiopia) Fisheries: Causes and Possible Solutions. *Land Degrad. Dev.* **2017**, *28*, 1842–1851. [CrossRef]
52. Makwinja, R.; Mengistou, S.; Kaunda, E.; Alamirew, T. Willingness to pay for the ecological restoration of an inland freshwater shallow lake: Case of Lake Malombe, Malawi. *Heliyon* **2022**, *8*, e08676. [CrossRef]
53. Pereira, L.C.C.; Pessoa, R.M.C.; Sousa-Felix, R.C.D.; Dias, A.B.B.; Silva, B.R.P.D.; Costa, R.M.D. How sustainable are recreational practices on Brazilian Amazon beaches? *J. Outdoor Recreat. Tour.* **2024**, *45*, 100741. [CrossRef]
54. da Costa, I.D.; Costa, L.L.; da Silva Oliveira, A.; de Carvalho, C.E.V.; Zalmon, I.R. Microplastics in fishes in amazon riverine beaches: Influence of feeding mode and distance to urban settlements. *Sci. Total Environ.* **2023**, *863*, 160934. [CrossRef]
55. Lima, A.K.d.S.; Silva, A.C.; Pereira, L.F.; Bezerra, C.M.; Soares, L.S.; Castro, A.C.L.d.; Marinho, Y.F.; Funo, I.C.d.S.A.; Lourenço, C.B. Anthropogenic litter on the macrotidal sandy beaches of the Amazon region. *Mar. Pollut. Bull.* **2022**, *184*, 114124. [CrossRef] [PubMed]
56. Pereira, L.C.C.; Sousa-Felix, R.C.d.; Costa, R.M.d.; Jimenez, J.A. Challenges of the recreational use of Amazon beaches. *Ocean Coast. Manag.* **2018**, *165*, 52–62. [CrossRef]
57. Henao, E.; Cantera, J.R.; Rzymski, P. Conserving the Amazon River Basin: The case study of the Yahuarcaca Lakes System in Colombia. *Sci. Total Environ.* **2020**, *724*, 138186. [CrossRef] [PubMed]
58. Makwinja, R.; Kaunda, E.; Mengistou, S.; Alamirew, T. Impact of land use/land cover dynamics on ecosystem service value—A case from Lake Malombe, Southern Malawi. *Environ. Monit. Assess.* **2021**, *193*, 492. [CrossRef]
59. Chiotha, S.; Jamu, D.; Nagoli, J.; Likongwe, P.; Chanyenga, T. *Socio-Ecological Resilience to Climate Change in a Fragile Ecosystem: The Case of the Lake Chilwa Basin, Malawi*; Routledge: London, UK, 2018.
60. Nagoli, J.; Mulwafu, W.; Green, E.; Likongwe, P.; Chiwona-Karltun, L. Conflicts over natural resource scarcity in the aquatic ecosystem of the Lake Chilwa. *Environ. Ecol. Res. J.* **2016**, *4*, 207–216. [CrossRef]
61. Polizzi, C.; Simonetto, M.; Barausse, A.; Chaniotou, N.; Känkänen, R.; Keränen, S.; Manzardo, A.; Mustajärvi, K.; Palmeri, L.; Scipioni, A. Is ecosystem restoration worth the effort? The rehabilitation of a Finnish river affects recreational ecosystem services. *Ecosyst. Serv.* **2015**, *14*, 158–169. [CrossRef]

water

MDPI

Article

Willingness-to-Pay for Blue Ecosystem Services of Natural Pools in Sri Lanka: A Discrete Choice Experiment

Menuka Udugama [1], Bader Alhafi Alotaibi [2], Madhushi Navoda [1], Mohamed M. M. Najim [3], Lahiru Udayanga [4,*] and Abou Traore [5]

1 Department of Agribusiness Management, Faculty of Agriculture & Plantation Management, Wayamba University of Sri Lanka, Makadura 60170, Sri Lanka
2 Department of Agricultural Extension and Rural Society, College of Food and Agriculture Sciences, King Saud University, Riyadh 11451, Saudi Arabia
3 Faculty of Agriculture, Sultan Sharif Ali Islamic University (UNISSA), Kampus Sinaut, Km 33, Jln Tutong, Tutong TB1741, Brunei; najim.mujithaba@unissa.edu.bn
4 Department of Biosystems Engineering, Faculty of Agriculture & Plantation Management, Wayamba University of Sri Lanka, Makadura 60170, Sri Lanka
5 Department of Community Sustainability, College of Agriculture and Natural Resources, Michigan State University, 328 Natural Resources Building, East Lansing, MI 48824, USA
* Correspondence: udayanga@wyb.ac.lk

Abstract: Ecosystem services offered by freshwater ecosystems, in the form of natural pools have not been fully realized by the public, which has led to limited attention on the conservation of these pools. This study therefore was conducted to investigate the user preferences for sustainable enhancement of recreational values of natural pools and their immediate environment. A total of 320 local users of natural pools located in Rangala and Nillambe were surveyed as the sample. A Discrete Choice Experiment (DCE) was employed to elicit the preference and user Willingness to Pay (WTP). The Marginal Willingness to Pay (MWTP) for the improvement of recreational values of natural pools was estimated using a conditional logit (CL) model. Outcomes of the WTP disclosed a clear preference hierarchy for various enhancements and contributions. Users were willing to pay Sri Lankan Rupees (LKR) 297.6 to reduce the environmental damage by 50% and LKR 84.4 to raise the community income by 20%. The option to have a higher number of recreational activities was highly valued. Respondents were willing to pay a value of LKR 554.8 per year for the multiple benefits provided by the pool ecosystems. Conclusively, the study suggested that efforts to upgrade these natural pools should prioritise income generation, broadening of recreational activities and environmental conservation, in line with respondents' inclinations.

Keywords: discrete choice experiment; ecosystem services; natural pools; user; willingness-to-pay (WTP)

1. Introduction

Blue ecosystem services refer to the benefits derived from marine and freshwater ecosystems. These services are crucial for human well-being and include a variety of functions provided by aquatic environments such as oceans, rivers, lakes, wetlands, and estuaries. Natural pool ecosystems, often referred to as freshwater pools, are small bodies of standing water found in various terrestrial landscapes. It is a type of pool that uses a natural water purification system to maintain the quality of water [1]. These ecosystems are characterised by their relatively small size, shallow depth, and often isolated nature. Natural pools are typically fed by surface water runoff, groundwater seepage, or precipitation. They may also receive inputs from nearby streams or rivers during periods of high flow [2]. Despite their small size, natural pools can support a diverse array of aquatic and semi-aquatic species, including fish, amphibians, aquatic insects, and various types of vegetation. These ecosystems provide important habitat for both resident and migratory species [3]. Further, natural pools play a key role in nutrient cycling and energy flow within ecosystems [4].

The hydrology of natural pools can vary seasonally and in response to changes in precipitation and temperature. Therefore, these may experience fluctuations in water level, temperature, and dissolved oxygen concentrations, which can influence the distribution and abundance of aquatic species [3]. Natural pools provide a range of important ecological functions and ecosystem services; provisioning, regulating, supporting and cultural such as fish, habitat provision, water storage, groundwater recharge, and flood mitigation and recreation [5]. They also contribute to the overall landscape heterogeneity and biodiversity of terrestrial ecosystems. From a human use perspective, these ecosystems can serve as recreational sites for activities such as swimming, fishing, and wildlife observation [6,7].

Recreation, which refers to an activity of leisure and the refreshment of mind and body, is a broad field of study that encompasses various theoretical and practical aspects. It is considered as a key human activity that shapes individual leisure time behaviours [8]. These recreational activities are essential for maintaining health, physical and social development of people. Engagement in leisure activities, together with recreation, has been linked to weight reduction, improved cardiovascular health, positive mental health outcomes and subjective well-being [9]. Recreation activities can fulfill individual and societal needs, channel excess energy into socially acceptable activities, and promote social interactions [10]. Engagement in outdoor recreation contributes to economic growth, job creation, and increased economic activity [11,12]. Valuing recreational services provided by freshwater ecosystems involves assessing the economic benefits users and visitors derive from activities such as fishing, boating, and swimming. These recreational services are a significant component of the overall value of freshwater ecosystems, influencing both individual well-being and local economies. However, if under studied and mismanaged, unregulated recreational activities could lead to negative environmental externalities such as pollution, habitat destruction, and introduction of invasive species, which deletariously influence these fragile ecosystems [13–15]. Recreation in natural pools can significantly influence water quality and biodiversity, particularly, when there is an increased number of visitations [16,17]. Thus natural pools, as common-pool resources, are often subject to challenges related to exploitation and management due to their open-access nature [18].

Sri Lanka is blessed with 103 rivers that carry water from the central highlands into the western, southern, and eastern coasts [19] resulting in biodiversity-rich natural pools or nature pools, which can offer multiple benefits. Among these uses, recreational benefits are commonly enjoyed by both villagers and visitors from outside of the village. Natural ecosystems in Sri Lanka provide opportunities for tourists to engage in these activities and experience the diverse ecological landscapes. Currently, there seems to be a potential shift towards natural pools as a preferred recreational resource among tourists visiting tropical destinations [20]. Tourism is a major contributor to Sri Lanka's economy, representing over 10% of Gross Domestic Production (GDP) and creating employment opportunities for around 500,000 people [21,22]. Therefore, conservation and restoration of natural pools can be economically advantageous for the recreational industry. However, a strategic and sustainable approach is needed to overcome challenges and capitalise on the potential future trends in the recreational services sector [23,24].

Several activities can be planned and implemented for the purpose of improving recreational activities around freshwater ecosystems. Community involvement in natural pool management can enhance both natural and social systems, leading to improved health and well-being [25]. Engaging communities in such projects can increase environmental consciousness and promote local environmental action [26]. Community-driven approaches to develop water trails and recreational areas can improve health, quality of life, and community engagement. Developing access points, monitoring water quality, managing woody debris, and implementing safety plans for water trails are few key actions that can be taken by the communities to improve recreation around the freshwater ecosystems, as it plays a crucial role in supporting and maintaining watershed functions and conservation [27].

Integrated watershed development models have shown a 28% increase in family incomes in villages located in watersheds, compared to non-watershed villages, with a significant contribution from crop cultivation [28].

Willingness to Pay (WTP) is a concept used to measure the value individuals place on certain goods or services, specifically in the context of enhancing recreational facilities. It is measured using contingent valuation methods and is influenced by factors such as perceived value, income levels, and alternative recreational options. Considering WTP in decision-making processes for enhancing recreational facilities can facilitate resource allocation, evaluate welfare benefits, and support sustainable development [29,30]. Discrete Choice Experiments (DCEs) and Contingent Valuation Approach (CVA) are two of the commonly used methods to assess WTP and estimate individual choice behaviour. Both of these approaches are based on stated preference [31].

In environmental and natural resource literature, various methodologies and approaches have been employed to assess the economic value of freshwater ecosystems in general and particularly to understand how these ecosystems contribute to human well-being and the economy. The majority of these studies centre around benefits such as clean water, biodiversity, flood regulation, and recreational opportunities offered by freshwater ecosystems. A recent study conducted by Sierra et al. has assessed the economic value of key natural benefits of freshwater ecosystems using a market value method considering transfer of benefits and direct uses. Results of this study have revealed that users consider ecotourism and prevention of flooding to be the most important values provided by freshwater ecosystems [32]. Since there are complex relationships in freshwater ecosystem services, the value of these ecosystem services often depends upon other ecosystem services provided [33,34]. A meta-analysis conducted by Brouwer et al. has found that services provided by freshwater ecosystems such as lakes are greatly valued than the values reported for wetlands by the users [35]. A recent study conducted by Ureta et al. has employed economic valuation techniques such as the payment card approach to explore the WTP towards protection of blue water ecosystem services in South Carolina. According to the findings of Ureta et al. people are willing to pay more for improvements that increase recreational activities, such as better fishing, presence of more types of species, and better access to water areas [36]. Therefore, assessment of WTP has assisted to guide the policy makers on prioritisation of river protection programmes in South Carolina [36].

Another study conducted in five Kenyan counties (Migori, Siaya, Busia, Kisumu, and Homa Bay) has evaluated how much the residents are willing to pay for the conservation of the Lake Victoria Ecosystem. The findings of this study have reported that around 40.9% of respondents are willing to contribute approximately Kenyan Shilling (KES) 500 each, resulting in an estimated total annual WTP of KES 616,279,069 [37]. Using a contingent valuation approach, Bueno et al. has attempted to investigate how local communities value efforts to restore water quality in Sampaloc Lake in Philippines, amid urbanisation pressures. The findings have revealed that households around the lake are willing to pay Philippine Peso (PHP) 177.09 per month, totaling PHP 7,102,017 annually, for these improvements [38].

Many studies have evidenced that people are willing to pay for services and contribute towards conservation of freshwater ecosystems, which directly benefit them or improve their quality of life [36,38]. Further, implementing an environmental users fee system to fund restoration of such freshwater ecosystems has been identified as an effective sustainable solution for management of such sensitive ecosystems [38]. However, such attempts require coordinated efforts on elevating environmental education and comprehensive policies to manage freshwater ecosystems [36,38]. Further, WTP for ecosystem services often varies with numerous factors, including socio-economic status, cultural values, awareness of ecosystem benefits, and local environmental conditions [39]. Previous studies have shown that people are more likely to pay for ecosystem services when they understand their importance and when there are clear mechanisms in place to link their payments to tangible outcomes, such as improved environmental quality or increased access to resources [37].

Utilizing nature-based solutions to ecosystem management have been proven to be sustainable and result in positive impacts on the socio-economic conditions of rural communities, including enhanced income distribution [40,41]. Particularly, participatory management programmes tend to lead to positive changes in the lives of marginal communities, while ensuring the sustainable conservation of freshwater ecosystems in different parts of the world [42]. For this, governments should facilitate policy-making, policy-lobbying and provide resources, and establish partnerships to promote integrated blue water ecosystem management [40,42,43]. However, designing such programmes requires an in-depth understanding on the perceptions of resource users and local communities on different values of freshwater ecosystems, along with their willingness to contribute towards such efforts either financially or from labour [44,45]. To the best knowledge of the authors, no studies have valued the confounded multiple benefits of natural pools, particularly the non-market values, applying a DCE in Sri Lanka, which is a developing country. Therefore, this study provides a significant contribution to this knowledge gap in literature from a developing country perspective.

Further, ecosystem services offer opportunities for diversifying livelihoods of local communities, beyond traditional sectors such as agriculture and forestry. Developing natural pool ecosystems as multi-purpose revenue generating entities can lead in to environmental, economic as well as social benefits [44,46]. Existing research on how much local stakeholders are ready to spend for the enhanced enjoyment and services from bettered recreation spots in natural pools of Sri Lanka is sparse. Hence, there is a noticeable demand to create strategies for enduring enhancement of these areas for recreation and their environs. Therefore, this study explores user preferences for improvement of recreational activities of natural pools and elicits user WTP for conservation of natural pools to ensure sustainable development. The insights from this research could support policy-making, enabling the government to refine recreational offerings and sustainably harness the untapped potential of natural pool resources.

2. Materials and Methods

2.1. Study Area

Natural pools located in the Kandy district, specifically in the Nillambe and Rangala areas were considered as the study sites in the current study. The Kandy District (6.93° to 7.50° N and 80.43°) is located in the central highlands of Sri Lanka processing a wide array of natural environmental features. Both Rangala and Nillambe areas are covered with mountain ranges, tea plantations and a diverse array of natural pools (Figure 1), leading these to become major tourist attractions. The local communities in these areas primarily are low-income tea pluckers.

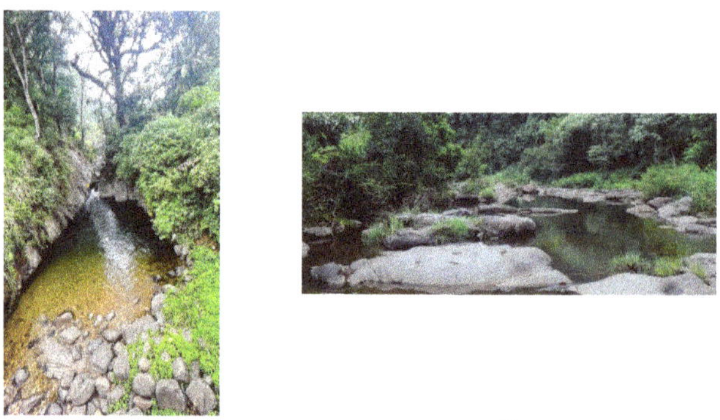

A B

Figure 1. Few natural pools located in the study areas (**A**) Rangala and (**B**): Nillambe.

2.2. Data Collection and Survey Design

The proportionate random sampling technique was employed in selecting a total of 320 locals, who were utilising the natural pools in the two study areas for different purposes. A pre-tested structured questionnaire along with a choice experiment was administered to collect the primary data. The survey instrument focused on three major sections, (1) demographic characteristics; (2) knowledge, awareness, and perception of resource users on conservation and amenity improvement of natural pools; (3) Choice experiment and value elicitation. The perception, awareness and knowledge related questions established a baseline for how much the respondents know about the ecological terminology and its association to the economic and well-being improvement. Furthermore, it also elicited their position on some potential actionable issues relevant to implementation of conservation interventions.

2.3. Analytical Framework of the Choice Experiment

This study employed a DCE to elicit the respondent's preference by presenting sets of choices with varying attributes and the choice set's corresponding price vehicle. WTP is a concept used to measure the value individuals place on certain goods or services, specifically in the context of enhancing recreational facilities. The DCEs allow for estimation and forecasting of individual choice behaviour and provide a way to measure preferences for nonmarket goods. Further, DCEs can generate more precise preference estimates compared to traditional "pick the best" approaches, since it captures decision-rule heterogeneity, allowing for a more accurate representation of respondent behaviour [47].

Choice experiments are survey-based valuation methods used to estimate the marginal values of individual elements in environmental resources. Choice modeling provides decision-makers with richer information on economic values, enhancing the quality and sustainability of natural resources at local, national, and global levels [48,49]. Often, DCE designs consist of a small number of choice sets with a limited number of alternatives to increase response efficiency. Optimal designs, also known as orthogonal designs, are used when prior information about population preferences is not available. The orthogonalisation procedure works in the context of choice card attributes and levels, by introducing column vectors for alternative-specific attributes and forcing their values to be orthogonal with other generic attributes within the same alternative. This maintains orthogonality within individual alternatives, but not necessarily across alternatives [47,50].

Although several non-market valuation techniques have been used to estimate the monetary value of ecosystem services, stated preference approaches are increasingly used as they rely on preferences or values as stated by individuals [29,49]. The major advantage of the stated preference methods is that they possess flexibility to capture both use and non-use values. Choice experiment models allow for the estimation of the relative importance of multiple environmental attributes and their levels [37]. Conditional logit (CL) model can be effectively used to relate the probability of a choice among the alternatives to the characteristics of the attribute levels defining those alternatives, which is consistent with the random utility theory. Further, unlike other regression models, the Conditional logit model avoids sparse data biases, leading to more accurate interpretations [49].

2.4. Theoretical Background

Theoretically, DCEs are based on the idea that respondents gain satisfaction from the features of things they choose rather than the things themselves. People aim to get the most satisfaction by picking the best option from a range of possible choices, which are described by their features, while each feature may possess different levels. Therefore, respondent's choices depend on the combination of these features in the options they are presented with [51].

In a DCE, the satisfaction (or utility) a person (i) gets from a choice (j) is not just about the obvious features (x) of the choice. There are also hidden factors that can affect their satisfaction. These are represented by a random element (ε) in the calculation. This approach follows the random utility theory suggested by Hensher et al. [52]. The theory suggests that this random element is simply added to the utility calculation. Therefore, the utility that person (i) gets from choice (j) is the sum of the utility from the obvious features and this random element [52]. Therefore, individual (i)'s utility (U) from alternative j can be expressed as follows (Equation (1)).

$$U_{ij} = X_{ij} + \varepsilon_{ij} \quad (1)$$

A DCE presents several choice sets (R), each including a status quo (x) and various alternatives (xj). A participant (i) chooses an alternative (j), if its utility (Uij) surpasses that of others (Uij'). The chance that (i) chooses (j) over other alternatives (j') within a set (R) is denoted as probability Pr(j | R), calculated where Uij > Uij' for all j' in R, and j $\neq$ j'. Responses from a survey can be effectively used to find out which option is most preferred by the people. When it is assumed that the random element in the satisfaction calculation is the same across all choices and that the utility people get from the features is linear, a CL model can be used for estimation [53]. Assuming that the error term is independently and identically distributed, and an indirect utility (V) is linearly related with attributes (x), the CL model estimates can be expressed as below (Equation (2)).

$$V_{ij} = ASC + \beta_{ij} \quad (2)$$

In the equation, V is the indirect utility obtained by the $_i$th individual for the $_j$th alternative. β is the marginal utility of the attributes (x). The Alternative Specific Constant (ASC) measures the effect of unobserved factors on the choice of alternatives relative to the status quo.

2.5. Designing of the Choice Experiment

Choice experiments often use cards that list different options with various features for participants to choose from. In the current study, the features to include on these cards were chosen after group discussions and by reviewing literature. Attributes that were used for the DCE were 'Reduction of environmental damage', 'Number of recreational activities', 'Community (who are interested to gain income) income increase from recreational values', 'User labour contribution (hours per visit) for a conservation programme', and 'Willingness to Pay per visit'. Using a design approach that considers all possible combinations, a total of 243 different scenarios were initially generated in SPSS (version 23). Subsequently, a narrow down method was applied to restrict the possible scenarios up to few key combinations, which were used for making choice cards. The final set of options, showcasing five main features and their different levels, are displayed in Table 1.

Table 1. Attributes in the choice card.

Attributes	Levels
Environmental damage Reduction	50%
	20%
	No reduction *
Number of recreational activities	14
	11 *
	Status quo
Community income increase from recreational values	20%
	10%
	No income *

Table 1. *Cont.*

Attributes	Levels
User labour contribution (hours per visit)	1
	0.5
	No contribution *
Fund per adult per visit (LKR)	100
	50
	No fund *

Note: * Status quo option, Number of recreational activities -7 (Walking, Swimming, Playing games, Sightseeing, Singing, Dancing, and Photography), 11 (Walking, Swimming, playing games, Sightseeing, singing, Dancing, Photography, Arts and crafts, Cycling, Meditation, and Yoga), 14 (Walking, Swimming, playing games, Sightseeing, singing, Dancing, Photography, Arts and crafts, Cycling, Meditation, Yoga, Camping, Star-grazing, and Hiking).

The choices included different scenarios that participants could pick from, regarding how to improve recreation in natural pools. Each person could choose from Options A, B, or C, where Option C was to keep things as they are at the pools currently. Options A and B offered different changes or improvements expected in future.

2.6. Data Analysis and Interpretation

All the collected data were double-checked and verified on the same day for completeness and consistency before entering it into Microsoft Excel data sheets (version, 2016). Cross-tabulations and logical checks were done to ensure the accuracy of the data. Any null data were treated as missing data and appropriately removed during the analysis.

2.7. Relative Importance Index

Relative index analysis was selected in this study to rank the criteria according to their relative importance based on participants' replies and prioritise indicators rated on Likert-type scales, as shown in Equation (3).

$$RII = \sum_{i=1}^{5} \frac{W_i X_i}{X_i} \quad (3)$$

where, W_i = the weight given to each factor by respondents, ranging from 1 to 5.

2.8. Estimating the Residents' Willingness-to-Pay

A conditional logit model was fitted to analyse the data using STATA (version 2016) software. The model includes attributes in general linear form as shown in Equation (4).

$$U_i = ASC + \beta_1 In(X_1) + \beta_2 In(X_2) + \beta_3 In(X_3) + \beta_4 In(X_4) + \beta_5 In(X_5) + \epsilon_i \quad (4)$$

U_i = Utility of the $_i$th alternative
ASC = Alternative Specific Constant
$x_1, \ldots, x_5$ = Component attributes of $_i$th alternative
ϵ_i = Error component

The coefficients of the CL model cannot be interpreted directly. Therefore, the following formula (Equation (5)) can be used to calculate the marginal welfare measure for a change in attribute (i), by dividing the coefficient estimate for that attribute by the coefficient estimate for the monetary attribute [42].

$$MWTP = -\left(\frac{\beta_{attribute}}{\beta_{monetary\ attribute}}\right) \quad (5)$$

To estimate the mean MWTP, including the upper bound and lower bound within 95% confidence interval, the Krinsky-Robb (KR) parametric bootstrapping technique was used.

Furthermore, the Log-likelihood and McFadden's pseudo-R-squared were used to assess the goodness of model fit [53].

3. Results

3.1. Socio-Demographic Information of the Respondents

A total of 320 respondents participated in the survey, providing insights into their engagement with and attitudes towards natural pools. The socio-demographic profile of the respondents and their recreational behaviour concerning natural pools is shown in Table 2. The majority of respondents were within the 20–30 year age group (55.3%), indicating a young adult demographic predominance. Those above 60 years were minimally represented (1.67%), suggesting potential barriers or disinterest among the elderly population in engaging in recreational pool activities. Respondents were distributed across various districts, with Kandy (46%), Nuwara Eliya (13.7%), and Colombo (10.3%) being the most represented. This wide geographic coverage ensures diverse insights into the recreational use of natural pools across different regional contexts. A significant majority of respondents (67%) held diplomas as their highest educational qualification, followed by those with secondary education (16.7%), as shown in Table 2. This suggests that the sample had a relatively higher educational attainment, which could correlate with the higher awareness of sustainable practices in recreation. The majority (36%) of respondents were employed in the private sector, followed by farming, reflecting a blend of agricultural and private sector occupational engagement. This could also be due to the fact that farming is the key income source of the locals residing in the study area. The monthly income categories of respondents revealed that the largest segment of respondents earned between Sri Lankan Rupees (LKR) 45,001 to LKR 60,000 (32%), which could influence their discretionary spending on recreational activities.

Table 2. Socio-demographic information of the respondents.

Category	Sub Category	Percentage (%)
Gender	Female	62.7
	Male	37.3
Age (Years)	20–30	55.3
	31–45	25.0
	46–60	18.0
	>60	1.7
District	Kandy	46.0
	Nuwara Eliya	13.7
	Matale	5.7
	Colombo	10.3
	Gampaha	8.7
	Anuradhapura	1.0
	Badulla	4.7
	Galle	2.7
	Matara	0.3
	Kegalle	2.0
	Kurunegala	3.3
	Puttalam	1.7
	Other districts	0.0

Table 2. *Cont.*

Category	Sub Category	Percentage (%)
Education level	Primary education	3.7
	Secondary education	16.7
	Diploma	67.0
	Tertiary education (degree and above)	12.7
Employment status	Farming	32.0
	Private sector job	36.0
	Government sector job	4.67
	Self-employed	11.7
	Unemployed	8.7
	Other	7.0
Monthly income category (LKR)	<15,000	2.3
	15,001 to 30,000	21.0
	30,001 to 45,000	31.3
	45,001 to 60,000	32.00
	≥60,001	14.0
Frequency of visiting natural pool and its surrounding in the past 12 months	Yes. But not now	4.0
	Always	39.7
	Sometimes	29.7
	Rarely	13.7
	No	13.0
Standard of recreational facilities	Very good	7.7
	Good	36.7
	Neither good nor poor	40.3
	Poor	2.3
	Very poor	0
	Do not know	13.0
Willingness to improve sustainable recreational services	Yes	89.0
	No	11.0
Preference on institutional support for improving sustainable recreational services	Community based organisation support	12.0
	Government Support	79.0
	Both	9.0

The natural pool and its surroundings have been consistently frequented by a considerable portion of respondents, with 39.7% visiting 'always' and 29.7% indicating 'sometimes'. This consistent engagement underscores the importance of these natural pools for recreational activities of the community (Table 2). The perception of the standard of recreational services was predominantly deemed 'Neither good nor poor' (40.3%) or 'Good' (36.7%). This indicates the need for improvement in recreational service standards, which aligns with the perception of the substantial majority (89%), who expressed a desire to enhance sustainable recreational services (Table 2). The community's inclination towards external support for improving sustainable recreational services in natural pools was very much in favour of government support (79%), followed by community-based organisation support (12%). This finding suggests a trust in governmental initiatives and a potential underutilisation of community-based resources in recreational development.

The percentage preference of the respondents over different ecosystem services provided by natural pools are shown in Figure 2. Results indicated that the respondents in general highly prioritise ecosystem services provided by natural pools, as over 50% rated 'very important' to all the services. This demonstrates a strong public inclination towards environmental awareness and the necessity for sustainable practices. They tend to believe that maintenance of water quality, availability of recreational activities as well as community benefits to be important factors among the potential ecosystem services.

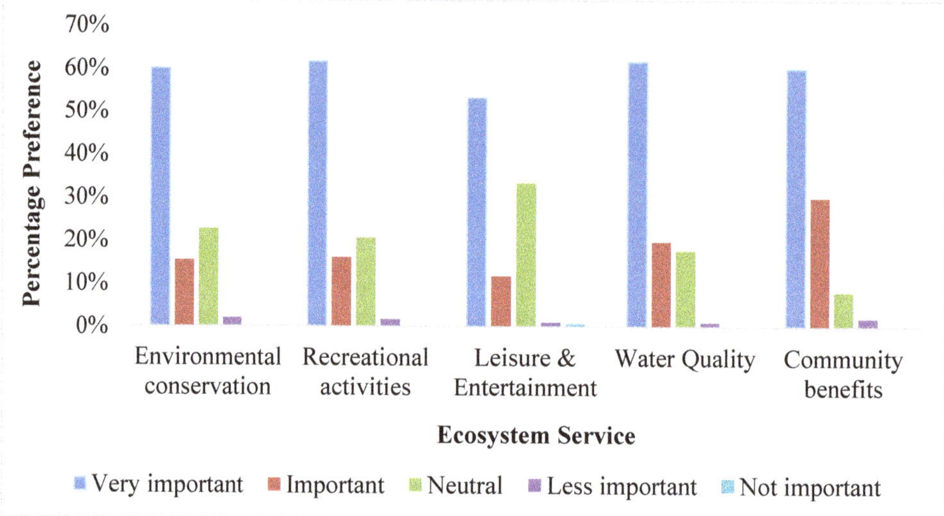

Figure 2. User preferences for ecosystem services of natural pools.

The association of ecosystem services is illustrated by the Principal Component Analysis (PCA) plot, as shown in Figure 3. This ordination biplot is based on the relative importance of services provided by natural pools as perceived by the respondents. The two-dimensional plane of the biplot captures the variance and trade-offs of ecosystem services. PCA1 and PCA2 explained a combined variance of 93.5% of the total variance. The variables, labeled A to L, correspond to different recreational perception-related indicators. The spread of the variables along PCA1 (88.9%), suggested that most variables are strongly associated with this component. Variables closer to the circumference of the circle are well represented in the PCA space. For instance, variable K which is community income generation closely aligns with PCA1, indicating it is a dominant factor in the dataset. Variable A (waste disposal and recycling methods) also extends farther in PCA1, indicating a significant influence. Variables J (security) and L (advertising) extend towards PCA2, which captures a relatively smaller portion of the variance (4.6%), suggesting these factors contribute uniquely to the dataset's variability.

Factors D, C and E lie closer to each other, suggesting a possible correlation among those (Figure 3). Hence providing knowledge and awareness on the importance of natural pool conservation in the forms of education programmes can have significant implications in inculcating positive attitudes and values among users. This shows a clear spatial pattern of tradeoffs between different ecosystem services. Further, all variables were clustered in the positive quadrant of PCA1 indicating a strong association. Therefore, factors such as cultural benefits, spiritual benefits and adverstising seemed to be correlated indicating the potential for developing the natural pools in such a way to attract the visitors seeking such ecosystem services.

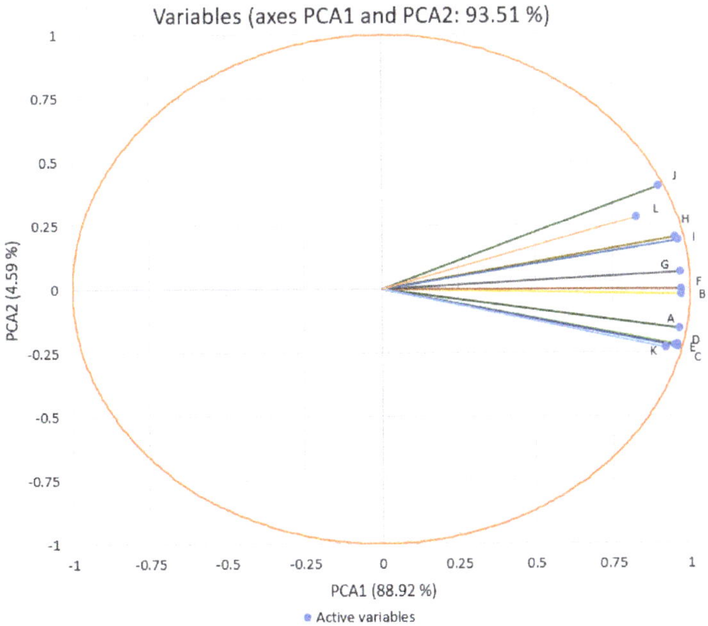

Figure 3. Trade off analysis for ecosystem services. Note: A—Waste disposal and recycling methods; B—Water quality and soil health; C—Education programmes to conserve nature; D—Recreational activities to conserve nature; E—Facilities for recreational activities; F—Physical and mental benefits; G—Social benefits; H—Spiritual benefits; I—Cultural benefits; J—Security; K—Community income generation; L—Advertising.

3.2. Marginal Willingness-to-Pay (MWTP) for Ecosystem Services

Table 3 shows the main effect specifications identified using the CL regression along with standard errors, coefficients, p-values, and the MWTP values for each attribute level. Results show that in terms of environmental damage reduction, a 20% reduction level has a positive coefficient of 0.568, indicating a significant ($p = 0.03$) preference for this level of environmental improvement. Hence, the MWTP of 113.6 suggests that visitors are willing to pay a considerable premium for a 20% reduction in environmental damage. Meanwhile, the 50% reduction level has a larger coefficient (1.488), which reflects a statistically significant stronger preference. The MWTP for 50% reduction is higher at 279.6, which implies that visitors value a 50% reduction of environmental damage to have more environmental benefits. Where the number of recreational activities is of concern, the level of 14 activities shows a positive and significant co-efficient (0.748), which indicates a strong preference and statistical significance for a higher number of activities. The MWTP of 149.62 suggests that visitors might pay substantially more to have more recreational activities in the studied natural pool sites. In terms of number, the level of 11 activities shows a negative non-significant coefficient (−0.536), suggesting a lower number of activities, which might not significantly and necessarily detract from visitors' utility (Table 3).

Table 3. Results of the Conditional Logit Regression.

Attribute	Levels	SE	Co-Efficient	Odds Ratio	MWTP
ASC		0.014	0.018	0.712	
Environment damage reduction	20% reduction	0.456	0.568 *	1.080	113.6
	50% reduction	0.788	1.488 *	1.071	297.6
No of recreational activities	14 activities	0.762	0.748 *	1.312	149.6
	11 activities	0.352	−0.536	0.961	−107.2
Community income increase	10% increase	0.244	−0.826 *	0.813	−165.2
	20% increase	0.312	0.422 *	1.490	84.40
Visitors labor contribution per visit	1 h	0.058	0.028	0.988	5.66
	0.5 h	0.324	0.938	0.992	187.60
Willingness to pay per visit	-	0.058	0.005 *	0.961	

Note: *—Coefficients that are significant at a 95% level of confidence; SE—Standard Error; MWTP—Marginal Willingness to Pay in LKR; log pseudolikelihood—(−556.46803); sample N = 320.

The CL model (fixed effects) assumes homogeneous preferences across respondents as difference in either the strength of the preference or as the direction (i.e., magnitude or sign of the coefficient). ASC in the model represents a composite of respondents' underlying preference for choice alternatives. Respondents consider income improvement of the community to be significantly important. This fact is also confirmed from the results in Figure 3. Both income levels are significant compared to business-as-usual scenario. However, a 10% income increase has a negative significant coefficient (−0.826) suggesting a disutility associated with this level of income increase, with visitors potentially unwilling to pay more (MWTP of −165.2) or possibility willing to accept. Meanwhile, the 20% income increase shows a significant positive coefficient (0.422) denoting a strong positive utility for this level of income increase, with a high MWTP (84.40). This suggests that visitors might pay significantly more for these community benefits for their economic well-being (Table 3). Labour contribution of 1 h had a positive coefficient (0.028) suggesting a higher affinity for this labour contribution, which was non-significant. However, a significant 0.5 h contribution suggested a higher positive impact on the utility for 0.5 h of labour contribution, with a positive MWTP of 187.6. The significant positive coefficient (0.005) indicates that higher payment requirements per adult visit increase the utility for visitors, suggesting a willingness to pay more. An odds ratio of 0.98 for funds per adult per visit suggested that the odds of preferring or choosing a one unit increase in funds contributed per adult per visit are 0.96 times those of the no funds, indicating a lower preference for much higher contributions.

According to the results, community income increment by 20% and number of activities denoted the highest odds ratios. This shows that for example, when income increases, the number of activities improves by one unit compared to the status-quo option, the visitor utility increases and are willing to pay more for the benefit of the local community. For a 20% reduction in environmental damage, the odds ratio was 1.08. This indicates that the odds of this level being preferred are 1.08 times greater than the no reduction level. The 50% reduction reported an odds ratio of 1.07, which was 1.07 times greater than the no reduction level for 50% level of reduction. Preferences slightly favoured environmental damage reduction initiatives, with a marginal increase in the likelihood of choosing a 20% or 50% reduction, over the no reduction scenario (Table 3). Results revealed a total user MWTP of LKR 554.8 per year per respondent for the multiple benefits provided by the pool ecosystem to conserve the ecosystem for its multiple benefits provided.

4. Discussion

This study applied a Discrete Choice Experiment approach to evaluate the recreational value of visitors of natural pools in Sri Lanka. Recreational values are often classified under cultural values [54–56]. Among the multiple ecosystem values provided by the pool ecosystems, cultural ecosystem services are considered as passive use values as these are intangible in nature and can be improved to provide numerous social and economic benefits [54,57]. Results revealed that certain demographic characteristics of users are important factors to assess and understand the recreational value of amenities. The findings of the study are in line with the findings of previous similar studies, which employed popular stated preference techniques such as the Contingent Valuation method [58] and Choice Experiments [55] to explore freshwater ecosystems and their cultural values that provide economic and social benefits to the community.

Horcea-Milcu et al. has shown how cultural uses are strongly dependent on socio-economic characteristics of the users such as education and income, which are comparable to our findings [59]. A previous study conducted by Liu et al. further shows how user attitudes such as bequest motives and environmental consciousness are related to the proximity [60]. The majority of the respondents of this study were from close proximity, which may influence the strong positive coefficients of the choice experiment attributes [55]. According to the findings, respondents preferred a 50% reduction of environmental damage. Therefore, initiatives should target a moderate 50%reduction in environmental damage, as this level significantly enhances the MWTP and underscores the value of respondent's perceptions on environmental conservation. This result complies with the findings of Wallmo and Lew [61], which explains how diminishing marginal utility is linked to water and environmental quality reduction of streams. Hence, a strategic approach focusing on key areas aligning with user preference is essential for natural pool conservation and development initiatives.

Enhancing the visitor experience by maintaining or improving the number of recreational activities is imperative, as this factor notably increases MWTP. In terms of community income derived from recreational activities, a nuanced approach is justified. A 20% increase in community income was highest positively received over a 10% increase, warranting thorough assessments to align community benefits with respondents' expectations. Furthermore, reevaluating the necessity and extent of labour contributions is imperative. Tait et al. has also shown how WTP for improvement in swimming water quality can have a positive relationship with the employment and income generation [62]. Aforementioned studies have further emphasised that users are willing to pay more for alternatives with more job opportunities and improved water quality. This study also explored the funding structure, which could be a combination of direct payment as well as labour. Other forms of contribution for a sustainable management and provision of facilities may yield a more favourable reception [63,64].

The findings of PCA suggest that waste disposal, water quality, conservation education, recreational activities, facilities, and community income generation tend to have a strong influence on user preference for a destination, in this case natural pools. Individual and societal benefits such as physical, mental, social, spiritual, and cultural gains are interrelated and contributed more to the second principal component. Security and advertising denoted a moderate combined influence on both components. It suggests that efforts to improve or invest in these areas may positively affect the users of ecosystem services. Demographics show that the majority of users are from surrounding areas, therefore this may have a strong influence on the preference for community improvement.

The relative importance of recreation related factors suggests that factors related to various aspects of recreational perception are most influential among the younger groups (15–30 years old) of visitors and tend to diminish in importance with age. Community income generation factor, however, maintains relevance across a wider age range, suggesting that it is considered relatively more important. This heterogeneity suggests that planning for sustainable ecosystem management initiatives must cater to various age groups effectively. The number of responses for each importance level suggests that the efforts should focus on bolstering community income generation and environmental conservation initiatives, as these are clearly valued by the community. Enhancing recreational activities and their associated benefits should be undertaken with the aim of elevating their importance, perhaps by demonstrating their economic and social value. Several previous studies have emphasised that such improvements can improve public goods to provide more economic and social benefits to the community [60,61].

Results of the relative importance ranking show that it is imperative to consider conservation of natural pool ecosystem services in a way that improves recreational activities, which can enhance economic and social benefits to the community. Natural pools are ecosystems that provide multiple benefits. This study focuses more on the use values of the system. It is evident that through improvement of facilities and effective conservation methods, pool systems can be improved as sustainable revenue-generating entities creating direct and indirect economic benefits. A comprehensive strategy focusing on waste management, ecological conservation, education, and eco-friendly recreation is essential in this regard. Initiating robust waste disposal and recycling methods is paramount, involving the provision of well-marked waste segregation facilities and the collaboration with local waste management services to ensure responsible waste handling and innovative recycling initiatives. Ensuring water quality and soil health involves regular monitoring of water parameters, and the implementation of soil conservation strategies. Such planning must be done with the involvement of the local community for more sustainable freshwater ecosystem service conservation [64].

It is important to sufficiently enforce government regulations for effective environmental conservation as regulation acts as a strong economic incentive in this regard [60]. Willingness to pay of users for improving recreation and cultural values of freshwater ecosystems such as natural pools are comparatively similar to those by Wallmo and Lew [61]. These studies show how cultural values are usually rated relatively low, compared to other ecosystem services but in a medium range, which is comparable with our findings. These findings emphasise on instituting educational programmes aimed at raising environmental awareness, which encompass interactive learning experiences, hands-on experience in conservation activities, and collaboration with environmental experts to instill values of sustainability among visitors. Integrating recreational activities that promote conservation, such as eco-friendly nature trails and incentivised participation in environmental stewardship initiatives, will further embed an ethos of respect and responsibility towards the natural environment.

The findings of the current study revealed a higher willingness to improve sustainable recreational services of the studied natural pools among the local community. This could be caused by a variety of factors such as the higher education level and monthly income, followed by higher environmental awareness [36,38]. Further, positive attitudes of local communities on the importance of these natural pools for their income, health and wellbeing could also contribute to this tendency [41,42]. However, previous studies have suggested that this WTP for sustainable recreational services can vary significantly among different regions of the country due to several factors such as proximity to the freshwater ecosystem of interest, cultural differences across regions, local environmental conditions and regional income differences [38,39,65–67]. Further, studies are recommended to evaluate the regional differences among the WTP to improve sustainable recreational services and to estimate the maximum limits. This will be of immense importance in making policy decisions regarding the community based conservation of these ecosystems.

Natural pools also hold a significant importance for these types of non-use values such as existence and bequest values [68]. Enhancing water-based activities is beneficial, entailing safe swimming zones, lifeguard services, and the provision of eco-friendly rental equipment for activities. Integrating educational elements through informational signage and organised workshops or guided tours will enrich the visitor experience [69]. Engaging the community in the planning process and actively seeking visitor feedback will not only ensure that facilities are met but shall exceed user expectations, making the natural pools a sustainably managed revenue generating entity [26].

5. Conclusions

The study findings indicate that visitors of the natural pools place a significant value on higher economic improvements, high availability of recreational activities and environmental damage reduction. There is a clear WTP for these enhancements, as evidenced by positive coefficients and MWTP values. For example, the value attached to further improvements tends to be influenced by diminishing returns, as the MWTP for a 50% damage reduction is more than double that of a 20% reduction. When it comes to paying, visitors believe that the community should be made better-off through higher income generation. One of the reasons for this perception could be that they believe improved income generation could boost greater benefits, facilities and amenities for visitors as well.

The findings of this study revealed that users were also willing to pay through labour contribution. Hence, these findings can be effectively used to guide co-management based initiatives for freshwater ecosystem management, which are found to be sustainable in the long run. Users were also willing to accept a payment for certain income generation activities, which could be through direct cash or in-kind measures. Moreover, the significantly higher preference for environmental damage reduction exhibits the user affinity and inclinations towards conservation. This is an indication of the potential for implementing nature-based solutions for ecosystem conservation. If implemented, such programmes should be voluntary and perhaps incentivised with discounts or other benefits. It is essential to consider the negative utility of increased funds per adult per visit. The willingness to pay indicates the maximum price consumers are willing to pay for the ecosystem service, which helps to derive the demand for an environmental good or service. Therefore, such pricing strategies should be carefully evaluated to ensure that they do not become a barrier to entry or visitation. Considering tiered pricing, discounts for advance booking, or membership programmes that offer added value without significantly increasing the single-visit cost are few strategies can be recommended. Consumer surplus can be estimated as a measure to understand the gains and losses of price setting.

Further studies should be conducted to understand quantified trade-offs between conservation, water quality improvement and economic development of natural freshwater ecosystems such as natural pools. Multidisciplinary studies are warranted to understand how monetary valuation of these ecosystems can be integrated into national policy making. Understanding these aspects better could help in drafting policies that align visitor experiences with conservation and community goals. Strategies that can enhance community income are more likely to gain strong public support. Additionally, initiatives should focus on improving environmental conditions and providing education on conservation, as these are also highly valued. In contrast, while still important, spiritual and cultural benefits are seen as less immediate priorities and could be integrated into broader programmes that primarily address the more pressing economic and environmental concerns.

Author Contributions: Conceptualisation, M.U., L.U. and M.M.M.N.; methodology, M.U., L.U. and M.M.M.N.; software, B.A.A. and A.T.; validation, B.A.A. and A.T.; formal analysis, M.U. and M.N.; investigation, M.U. and M.N.; resources, B.A.A.; data curation, M.U. and M.N.; writing—original draft preparation, M.U., M.N. and L.U.; writing—review and editing, M.M.M.N., A.T. and B.A.A.; visualization, B.A.A. and M.M.M.N.; supervision, M.M.M.N. and B.A.A.; project administration, M.M.M.N.; funding acquisition, B.A.A. All authors have read and agreed to the published version of the manuscript.

Funding: This research was funded by Researchers Supporting Project Number (RSP2024R443), King Saud University, Riyadh, Saudi Arabia.

Institutional Review Board Statement: Ethical clearance for the study was obtained from the Ethics Review Committee (ERC) of the Faculty of Agriculture and Plantation Management, Wayamba University of Sri Lanka (ERC/2022/012; Approval Date: 25 November 2022).

Informed Consent Statement: Written informed consent was obtained from all study participants who volunteered for the study.

Data Availability Statement: The raw data supporting the conclusions of this article will be made available by the authors on request.

Acknowledgments: The authors wish to express their profound gratitude to village officers and all the participants for their immense support given. The authors also extend their appreciation to the Researchers Supporting Project number (RSP2024R443), King Saud University, Riyadh, Saudi Arabia.

Conflicts of Interest: The authors declare no conflicts of interest.

Abbreviations

CL: Conditional Logit; CVA: Contingent Valuation Approach; GDP: Gross Domestic Production; DCE: Discrete Choice Experiments; KES: Kenyan Shilling; MWTP: Marginal Willingness-to-Pay; LKR: Sri Lankan Rupees; PCA: Principal Component Analysis; PHP: Philippine Peso; WTP: Willingness to Pay.

References

1. Poloprutská, T.; Nováček, M.; Oppeltová, P. Case Study of Selected Nature Swimming Pools in the South Moravian Region. *Ochr. PríRody Slov. EkolóGia* **2021**, *40*, 312–324. [CrossRef]
2. Hughes, J.; Bond, H.; Knight, C.; Stanley, K. Challenges for Freshwater Ecosystems. In *Water Science, Policy, and Management: A Global Challenge*; John Wiley & Sons Ltd.: Hoboken, NJ, USA, 2019; pp. 75–95.
3. Jocque, M.; Vanschoenwinkel, B.; Brendonck, L.U.C. Freshwater rock pools: A review of habitat characteristics, faunal diversity and conservation value. *Freshw. Biol.* **2010**, *55*, 1587–1602. [CrossRef]
4. De Meester, L.; Declerck, S.; Stoks, R.; Louette, G.; Van De Meutter, F.; De Bie, T.; Michels, E.; Brendonck, L. Ponds and pools as model systems in conservation biology, ecology, and evolutionary biology. *Aquat. Conserv. Mar. Freshw. Ecosyst.* **2005**, *15*, 715–725. [CrossRef]
5. Reid, A.J.; Carlson, A.K.; Hanna, D.E.L.; Olden, J.D.; Ormerod, S.J.; Cooke, S.J. Conservation Challenges to Freshwater Ecosystems. In *Encyclopedia of the World's Biomes*; Elsevier: Amsterdam, The Netherlands, 2020; pp. 270–278.
6. Sánchez-Ríos, C.P.; Trejo-Perea, M.; Sánchez-Ríos, L.D.; Sánchez-Ríos, M.F. Implementation of natural pools: An alternative of improvement for effects in airway by exposure to chlorinated pools. *Neumol. Cir. Torax* **2020**, *79*, 197–203.
7. Venohr, M.; Langhans, S.D.; Peters, O.; Hölker, F.; Arlinghaus, R.; Mitchell, L.; Wolter, C. The underestimated dynamics and impacts of water-based recreational activities on freshwater ecosystems. *Environ. Rev.* **2018**, *26*, 199–213. [CrossRef]
8. Nkwanyana, S. Recreation and leisure in promoting social inclusion: A reflection of documented theory. *Afrrican J. Hosp. Tour. Leis.* **2020**, *9*, 1–9.
9. Litwiller, F.; White, C.; Gallant, K.A.; Gilbert, R.; Hutchinson, S.; Hamilton-Hinch, B.; Lauckner, H. The benefits of recreation for the recovery and social inclusion of individuals with mental illness: An Integrative Review. *Leis. Sci.* **2017**, *39*, 1–19. [CrossRef]
10. Gungor, B.S. Cultural Ecosystem Services and Recreational Use: A Review Study in Belgrad Forest, Istanbul. *J. Multidiscip. Res. Sustain.* **2018**, *1*. [CrossRef]
11. Lloyd-Smith, P. The economic benefits of recreation in Canada. *Can. J. Econ.* **2021**, *54*, 1684–1715. [CrossRef]
12. Wolter, L. *Nature-Based Tourism in Mallorca's Natural Areas: The Benefits of Tourism for Natural Areas*; Springer Science & Business Media: Berlin, Germany, 2013.
13. Acuña, V.; Auró, M.; Campillo, V.; Petrovic, M.; Pueyo, J.; Freixa, A. Natural swimming holes, at the crossroad between conservation and recreation. *Freshw. Biol.* **2024**, *69*, 100–111. [CrossRef]
14. Meyer, N.; Schafft, M.; Wegner, B.; Wolter, C.; Arlinghaus, R.; Venohr, M.; Von Oheimb, G. A day on the shore: Ecological impacts of non-motorised recreational activities in and around inland water bodies. *J. Nat. Conserv.* **2021**, *64*, 126073. [CrossRef]
15. Lynch, A.J.; Cooke, S.J.; Arthington, A.H.; Baigun, C.; Bossenbroek, L.; Dickens, C.; Harrison, I.; Kimirei, I.; Langhans, S.D.; Murchie, K.J.; et al. People need freshwater biodiversity. *WIREs. Water* **2023**, *10*, e1633. [CrossRef]
16. Morino, M. Degradation of Ecosystem Services caused by the Underuse of Commons. *Sociol. Theory Methods* **2014**, *29*, 261–276.
17. Musostov, Z.; Kulakov, K.; Tarkhanova, Z. Tourism and recreation their role in ensuring sustainable development of territories. *E3S Web Conf.* **2023**, *451*, 07007. [CrossRef]
18. Wolman, O.; Edmondson, J.C.; Chan, L. Technology Assessment: The Evaluation of Residential Pool Sanitation Options Using TOPSIS. In *Infrastructure and Technology Management: Innovation, Technology and Knowledge Management*; Springer International Publishing: New York City, NY, USA, 2018; pp. 437–446.
19. Katupotha, J.I.N.A.D.A.S.A.; Gamage, S.A.C.H.I.T.H. Understanding the River Basin Classification of Sri Lanka. *Wildlanka* **2020**, *8*, 175–197.

20. De Moura, I.E.M.O.; Neto, J.M.M.; Da Silva, E.A. Residential swimming pools maintenance under an environmental perspective. *Sci. Total Environ.* **2023**, *903*, 166612. [CrossRef]
21. Fernando, S.; Bandara, J.S.; Smith, C. Regaining Missed Opportunities: The role of tourism in post-war development in Sri Lanka. *Asia Pac. J. Tour. Res.* **2013**, *18*, 685–711. [CrossRef]
22. Jayawardena, C. What innovations would enable tourism in Sri Lanka to Re-Build? *Worldw. Hosp. Tour. Themes* **2022**, *14*, 586–595. [CrossRef]
23. Samaranayake, H.M.S.; Lantra, N.; Jayawardena, C. Forty six years of organised tourism in Sri Lanka (1966–2012). *Worldw. Hosp. Tour. Themes* **2013**, *5*, 423–441.
24. Sumanapala, D.; Wolf, I.D. Think globally, act locally: Current understanding and future directions for nature-based tourism research in Sri Lanka. *J. Hosp. Tour. Manag.* **2020**, *45*, 295–308. [CrossRef]
25. Morrison, K.; Bunch, M.J.; Hallström, L. Public health at the watershed scale. In *Water Policy and Governance in Canada*; Springer International Publishing: New York City, NY, USA, 2017; pp. 337–356.
26. Stough-Hunter, A.; Lekies, K.S.; Donnermeyer, J.F. When environmental action does not activate concern: The case of impaired water quality in two rural watersheds. *Environ. Manag.* **2014**, *54*, 1306–1319. [CrossRef] [PubMed]
27. Shopinski, S.; Tejada, T.; Jenkins, H.; Raad, S.; Quinn, M.; Lachance, L. Paddling Together: Water Trails as Innovative Public Health Strategies. *Health Promot. Pract.* **2023**, *24* (Suppl. S1), 41S–45S. [CrossRef] [PubMed]
28. Anantha, K.H.; Wani, S.P.; Shyam, D.M. Increasing incomes and building climate resilience of communities through watershed development in rainfed areas. In *Community and Climate Resilience in the Semi-Arid Tropics: A Journey of Innovation*; Springer International Publishing: New York, NY, USA, 2020; pp. 203–225.
29. Mellaku, M.T.; Melka, Y.; Ayenew, B.; Taye, T.T.; Tilahun, A. The contribution of local outdoor recreational services to the sustainable management of environmental resources: The case of Tabor Mountain Recreational Park in Hawassa City, Ethiopia. *Sustain. Sci. Pract. Policy* **2022**, *18*, 70–80. [CrossRef]
30. Rathnayake, R.M.W. Economic values for recreational planning at Horton Plains national park, Sri Lanka. *Tour. Geogr.* **2016**, *18*, 213–232. [CrossRef]
31. Alamri, A.S.; Georgiou, S.; Stylianou, S. Discrete choice experiments: An overview on constructing D-Optimal and near-optimal choice sets. *Heliyon* **2023**, *9*, e18256. [CrossRef]
32. Sierra, L.; Marin, W.; Castro, L.G.; Hernández-Manrique, O.L. Economic Valuation of Benefits in Freshwater Ecosystems: Complex Wetlands System Belonging to the San Juan River in the *Magdalena Medio* Region, Colombia. *Sustainability* **2021**, *13*, 5374. [CrossRef]
33. Fu, B.-J.; Su C-o Wei, Y.-P.; Willett, I.R.; Lu, Y.-H.; Liu, G.-H. Double counting in ecosystem services valuation: Causes and countermeasures. *Ecol. Res.* **2011**, *26*, 1–14. [CrossRef]
34. Raudsepp-Hearne, C.; Peterson, G.D.; Bennett, E.M. Ecosystem service bundles for analyzing tradeoffs in diverse landscapes. *Proc. Natl. Acad. Sci. USA* **2010**, *107*, 5242–5247. [CrossRef]
35. Brouwer, R.; Langford, I.H.; Bateman, I.J.; Turner, R.K. A meta-analysis of wetland contingent valuation studies. *Reg. Environ. Chang.* **1999**, *1*, 47–57. [CrossRef]
36. Ureta, J.U.; Ureta, J.C.; Bower, L.M.; Peoples, B.K.; Motallebi, M. The value of improving freshwater ecosystem services: South Carolina residents' willingness to pay for improved water quality. *J. Environ. Manag.* **2024**, *353*, 120260. [CrossRef] [PubMed]
37. Mamboleo, M.; Adem, A. Estimating willingness to pay for the conservation of wetland ecosystems, Lake Victoria as a case study. *Knowl. Manag. Aquat. Ecosyst.* **2022**, *423*, 22. [CrossRef]
38. Bueno, E.A.; Ancog, R.; Obalan, E.; Cero, A.D.; Simon, A.N.; Malvecino-Macalintal, M.R.; Sugui, L. Measuring households' willingness to pay for water quality restoration of a natural urban lake in the Philippines. *Environ. Process.* **2016**, *3*, 875–894. [CrossRef]
39. Haque, M.N.; Saroar, M.; Fattah, M.A.; Morshed, S.R. Environmental benefits of blue ecosystem services and residents' willingness to pay in Khulna city, Bangladesh. *Heliyon* **2022**, *8*, e09535. [CrossRef] [PubMed]
40. Tyngkan, H.; Singh, S.B.; Nongbri, B.; Lyngkhoi, D.R.; Gogoi, J. A Comparative Analysis of Pre and Post Watershed Development Programme: A Case Study of Umngoh Watershed in Ri-Bhoi District of Meghalaya. *Indian J. Econ. Dev.* **2021**, *17*, 584–590.
41. Salampessy, M.L.; Febryano, I.G.; Widhyastini, I.G.A.M. Community perception on the utilization of natural resources in the Cisadane Watershed. *IOP Conf. Series. Earth Environ. Sci.* **2021**, *739*, 012007. [CrossRef]
42. Kasi, E. Marginal Communities in Drought-prone Regions: The role of NGOs in watershed development in South India. *J. Dev. Soc.* **2015**, *31*, 98–124. [CrossRef]
43. Vári, Á.; Podschun, S.A.; Erős, T.; Hein, T.; Pataki, B.; Iojă, I.C.; Adamescu, C.M.; Gerhardt, A.; Gruber, T.; Dedić, A.; et al. Freshwater systems and ecosystem services: Challenges and chances for cross-fertilization of disciplines. *Ambio* **2022**, *51*, 135–151. [CrossRef]
44. Zaman, R.; Ali, S. The Application of Choice Experiment Methodology to the Freshwater Ecosystem Services: A Review. *Int. J. Bus. Econ. Aff.* **2023**, *8*, 200–210.
45. Xuan, B.B.; Sandorf, E.D.; Aanesen, M. Informing management strategies for a reserve: Results from a discrete choice experiment survey. *Ocean Coast. Manag.* **2017**, *145*, 35–43. [CrossRef]
46. Marques, R.; Carvalho, P.T.; Pires, J.; Fontainhas, A. Willingness to pay for the water supply service in Cape Verde—How far can it go? *Water Sci. Technol. Water Supply* **2016**, *16*, 1721–1734. [CrossRef]

47. Connelly, L. Logistic Regression. *Medsurg Nurs.* **2020**, *29*, 353–354.
48. Boyle, K.J.; Holmes, T.P. Choice Experiments and Valuing Forest Attributes. In *Handbook of Forest Resource Economics*; Routledge: London, UK, 2014; pp. 151–164.
49. Greenland, S.; Schwartzbaum, J.A.; Finkle, W.D. Problems due to small samples and sparse data in conditional logistic regression analysis. *Am. J. Epidemiol.* **2000**, *151*, 531–539. [CrossRef] [PubMed]
50. Tang, L.; Luo, X.; Cheng, Y.; Yang, F.; Ran, B. Constructing an optimal orthogonal choice design with alternative-specific attributes for stated choice experiments. *Transp. Res. Rec.* **2014**, *2451*, 50–59. [CrossRef]
51. Lancaster, K.J. A New Approach to Consumer Theory. *J. Political Econ.* **1966**, *74*, 132–157. [CrossRef]
52. Hensher, D.A.; Rose, J.M.; Greene, W.H. *Applied Choice Analysis: A primer*; Cambridge University Press: New York, NY, USA, 2005.
53. McFadden, D.L. Conditional logit analysis of qualitative choice behavior. In *Frontiers in Econometrics*; Zarembka, P., Ed.; Academic Press: New York, NY, USA, 1974.
54. Rooshdi, R.R.R.M.; Majid, M.Z.A.; Sahamir, S.R.; Ismail, N.A.A. Relative importance index of sustainable design and construction activities criteria for green highway. *Chem. Eng. Trans.* **2018**, *63*, 151–156.
55. Doherty, D.; Murphy, M.; Hynes, S.; Buckley, C. Valuing ecosystem services across water bodies: Results from a discrete choice experiment. *Ecosyst. Serv.* **2014**, *7*, 89–97. [CrossRef]
56. Millennium Ecosystem Assessment (MEA). *Ecosystems and Human Well-Being: A Report of the Millennium Ecosystem Assessment*; Island Press: Washington, DC, USA, 2005.
57. Venn, T.J.; Quiggin, J. Accommodating indigenous cultural heritage values in resource assessment: Cape York Peninsula and the Murray–Darling Basin, Australia. *Ecol. Econ.* **2007**, *61*, 334–344. [CrossRef]
58. Perni, Á.; Barreiro-Hurlé, J.; Martínez-Paz, J.M. Contingent valuation estimates for environmental goods: Validity and reliability. *Ecol. Econ.* **2021**, *189*, 107144. [CrossRef]
59. Horcea-Milcu, I.; Jan, H.; Abson, D.; Fischer, J. Cultural Ecosystem Services: A Literature Review and Prospects for Future Research. *Ecol. Soc.* **2013**, *1*, 34.
60. Liu, Y.; Zhang, R.; Zhao, W.; Wang, S.; Fu, B. Comparison between tourists' and inhabitants' willingness to pay for nature in the Tibetan Plateau. *J. Clean. Prod.* **2020**, *255*, 120219. [CrossRef]
61. Wallmo, K.; Lew, D.K. Public Willingness to Pay for Recovering and Downlisting Threatened and Endangered Marine Species. *Conserv. Biol.* **2012**, *26*, 830–839. [CrossRef]
62. Tait, P.; Baskaran, R.; Cullen, R.; Bicknell, K. Nonmarket valuation of water quality: Addressing spatially heterogeneous preferences using GIS and a random parameter logit model. *Ecol. Econ.* **2012**, *75*, 15–21. [CrossRef]
63. Quintas-Soriano, C.; Martín-López, B.; Santos-Martín, F.; Loureiro, M.; Montes, C.; Benayas, J.; García-Llorente, M. Ecosystem services values in Spain: A meta-analysis. *Environ. Sci. Policy* **2016**, *55*, 186–195. [CrossRef]
64. McCartney, M.; Acreman, M.; Bergkamp, G. Freshwater Ecosystem Management and Environmental Security. In *Vision for Water and Nature*; Institute of Hydrology: Wallingford, UK, 2000; pp. 151–203.
65. Lapointe, M.; Cumming, G.S.; Gurney, G.G. Comparing ecosystem service preferences between urban and rural dwellers. *Bioscience* **2019**, *69*, 108–116. [CrossRef]
66. Ren, Y.; Lu, L.; Zhang, H.; Chen, H.; Zhu, D. Residents' willingness to pay for ecosystem services and its influencing factors: A study of the Xin'an River basin. *J. Clean. Prod.* **2020**, *268*, 122301. [CrossRef]
67. Gibson, J.M.; Rigby, D.; Polya, D.A.; Russell, N. Discrete choice experiments in developing countries: Willingness to pay versus willingness to work. *Environ. Resour. Econ.* **2016**, *65*, 697–721. [CrossRef]
68. Oleson, K.L.L.; Barnes, M.; Brander, L.M.; Oliver, T.A.; Van Beek, I.; Zafindrasilivonona, B.; Van Beukering, P. Cultural bequest values for ecosystem service flows among indigenous fishers: A discrete choice experiment validated with mixed methods. *Ecol. Econ.* **2014**, *114*, 104–116. [CrossRef]
69. Song, H.J.; Lee, C.-K.; Park, J.A.; Hwang, Y.H.; Reisinger, Y. The influence of tourist experience on perceived value and satisfaction with temple stays: The experience economy theory. *J. Travel Tour. Mark.* **2014**, *32*, 401–415. [CrossRef]

water

MDPI

Article

La Marina Baja Water Consortium (1950–1978): Hydro-Economic Model of Water Governance behind Tourism Development in *Benidorm* (Spain)

César Sánchez-Pérez *, María-Inmaculada López-Ortiz and Patricia Fernández-Aracil

Institute of Water and Environmental Sciences, University of Alicante, San Vicente del Raspeig, 03690 Alicante, Spain; iortiz@ua.es (M.-I.L.-O.); patricia@ua.es (P.F.-A.)
* Correspondence: csp9@alu.ua.es

Abstract: This paper analyzes the events that originated an integrated water resources management (IWRM) model called *Consorcio de Aguas de la Marina Baja* (CAMB), in the province of Alicante (Spain), in 1978. The impact of tourism and population growth in the second half of the 20th century motivated the need for new management formulas seeking a balance between available resources and a greater need for water resources. The emergence of mass tourism in Benidorm at the end of the 1950s generated a great imbalance between the needs and availability of water resources. Also considering the effect of periods of severe drought, the solution to the deficit was found in the principles of institutional economics and circular water management. Water infrastructure and technology are elements of great importance in this model, allowing the exchange of natural water for reclaimed water, as a result of previous agreements between traditional irrigators and supply users of coastal populations. Its success has guaranteed the coexistence of traditional agriculture and the consolidated tourism activity, making possible the conservation of the cultural landscape. The historical and economic analysis of the model that led to the creation of CAMB can be applied to other regions facing similar challenges.

Keywords: water governance; institutional economy; water exchanges; irrigation; urban water supply; circular economy; *Benidorm*

1. Introduction

This research focuses on the events that led to the gestation of a model of integrated management of water resources, constituting the entity called *La Marina Baja* Water Consortium (*Consorcio de Aguas de La Marina Baja, CAMB*, in Spanish) in 1978, located in the district called *La Marina Baja*, whose head is the city of *Benidorm* (province of Alicante, Spain). The impact of tourism since the second half of the 20th century in this region motivated the need to find new management formulas: the increase in demography, the massive arrival of tourists, urban development with new accommodation, a greater demand for energy resources and the food associated with this growth led the actors involved to seek a balance between available resources and a greater need for water resources. After some frustrated attempts during the first decades of the second half of the 20th century, the need and the experience accumulated over the years to deal with water scarcity, recurrent periods of drought and increasing demand resulted—almost intuitively—in a management model that responded to the water supply problems of this region in southeastern Spain according to the principles of good water governance [1].

The main economic activities in *La Marina Baja* until the 1950s were fishing and agriculture and, from a demographic point of view, the district had hardly experienced any changes since 1840. Nevertheless, from the second half of the 1950s, the Spanish economy experienced a process of international reintegration and internal liberalization that resulted in a period of unprecedented economic growth. These facts propitiated the appearance of mass tourism in *Benidorm*. As a consequence, urban development and demographic growth took place, which in just a few decades generated a great imbalance between the needs for and availability of water resources. This scarcity, together with different periods of severe drought, such as those that occurred in 1968–1969 and 1978–1984, motivated the implementation of this water governance model based on the principles of institutional economics [2] and circular water management [3]. Water infrastructure and technology were of great importance, allowing a system of exchanges of natural water for reclaimed water between traditional irrigators and users in the primary phase. These social agreements and the formalization of *La Marina Baja* Water Consortium allowed the configuring, after a historical process, of a model of integrated water resources management (IWRM) [1] that bet on what, decades later, was called technological neutrality: the use of all available technologies to achieve the objectives. This success has allowed two economic activities to coexist in the district in a way that is compatible with the conservation of the cultural landscape: traditional agriculture and the currently consolidated tourism industry.

The hypothesis put forward in this research study is based on demonstrating how dry or semi-arid territories, traditionally dedicated to agriculture and with water scarcity and periods of severe drought, experiencing a rise in new economic activities that require a high demand for resources can find a balance between demand and supply, thanks to governance and IWRM, for the benefit of all stakeholders. Thus, the main aim of this work is to complete the analysis of the case study in *La Marina Baja* district with a historical perspective to find interrelationships between tourism-driven economic development and the economic background, focusing on the period prior to its implementation and founding years (1950–1978), as well as institutional decisions determining the constitution of this IWRM model.

2. Methodology

The methodology of this research combined qualitative analysis of literature and archive documents of the *Benidorm* City Council, such as meeting minutes or correspondence, together with interviews with stakeholders and a historiographer, whose names have been included in the acknowledgements section. Moreover, based on a close analysis of the statistical sources and the academic literature, the case study will provide a valuable insight about the gestation of the consortium. Methods are based on institutional analysis underpinnings which link method to synthesis and theory building, through a process of rigorous screening in which institutions and society have played an important role in producing local socioeconomic outcomes or structural changes.

Public and private statistical databases have been gathered to fulfill the analysis. On the one hand, the private database obtained from *Fundación Banco Bilbao Vizcaya Argentaria* is specified in section number 4. On the other hand, the public database is compiled by the *National Statistics Institute of Spain*. Both institutions made intensive efforts to formulate methodological notes in their respective documents or datasheets, reflecting the potential limitations or biases in the economic data published. Nonetheless, by assuming they contain the most accurate information available, these documents and datasets make it possible for the macroeconomic evolution behind management changes to illustrate how effective good water governance is in terms of institutional economy.

3. Study Area, Historical Droughts and Geographical Context

The main climatological characteristic of the southeastern peninsular region is aridity, which results in the existence of an intense water deficit in the region, considering the meager and irregular rainfall, the high potential evapotranspiration and the persistence of continuous periods of drought [4]. In the district of *La Marina Baja*, two historical moments related to droughts marked its evolution: the first occurred during the seventeenth century and is interrelated with the implementation of a piece of infrastructure known by the name of *Séquia Mare*; the second was the articulation of an institution, *La Marina Baja* Water Consortium, in 1978.

Little is known about the importance of water in *La Marina Baja* district and *Benidorm* before the second half of the twentieth century. During much of the sixteenth century, *Benidorm* had only 6 or 7 inhabitants to take care of the Castle of *Benidorm*, as the site had been depopulated as a result of the Berber attacks in 1503. It was in 1666 when Beatriz de Fajardo, who had inherited the lordships of *Polop* and *Benidorm* in the Kingdom of Valencia, completed the piece of infrastructure commonly called *Séquia Mare*, which crossed much of the district. The first investment she made was the *Séquia Mare* [5], in order to increase the population of the affected land and collect more manorial rents in *Benidorm*, *La Nucía* and *Alfaz del Pi*, settlements repopulated since then. This water infrastructure was the main vector that allowed the urban and demographic development of the district [6].

Periods of drought proved to be a powerful incentive for the improvement of the management of the scarcity of water resources, as in 1968–1969 and 1978–1984 in the district of *La Marina Baja*. In this vein, a second key moment is linked to the definitive establishment of *La Marina Baja* Water Consortium in 1978, when the city that "invented" modern tourism was about to close its doors because of the lack of water. The problem, described as an "ordeal" by Esquembre [7], mobilized Rafael Ferrer, the mayor of *Benidorm*, and even the central government. An interministerial commission proposed, in the first days of June, "closing *Benidorm*" to the entry of tourists, diverting them to other coastal enclaves of Spain, in order to avoid "a dreaded and more than likely epidemic, in addition to a host of health risks due to lack of hygiene" [7]. That drought induced the water depletion of the reservoirs and dried up or salinized the wells, giving rise to a critical scenario. Finding solutions different from a mere restriction, in the summer of 1978, tankers distributed water among neighbors, but the most remarkable thing was the speed with which all the administrations worked to achieve it: the government had to seize some boats that were transporting peanut oil to Morocco and they proceeded to clean them to bring water to *Benidorm* through a 3 km emergency pipeline to the reservoir [8].

Analyzing the drought period of the late 1960s in *La Marina Baja*, the *Guadalest* dam did not even reach half of its total capacity annually in the years 1965, 1966, 1967 and 1968. The need to increase urban water resources without compromising the needs of agricultural lands led users to consider the creation of a community of communities [9]. Prior to the 1968 drought and after several meetings in the civil government and the provincial council with the aim of setting up an organization that could provide a solution to the problems, in March 1968 the decision was formalized to establish a consortium for the water supply and sanitation of the municipalities of *Alfaz del Pi*, *Altea*, *Benidorm*, *Benisa*, *Benitachell*, *Calpe*, *Gata de Gorgos*, *Jávea* and *Teulada* [8]. The meeting was held under the chairmanship of the Minister of Public Works and was attended by the Civil Governor, the Director General of Hydraulic Works, the President of the Provincial Council, the government delegate in the Water Basin Authority (*Confederación Hidrográfica del Júcar*) and the mayors of the affected municipalities. During previous years the need to provide the region with an organization to manage water resources, with an integrated approach, had already been spoken of, as reflected in the minutes of the *Benidorm* City Council, and on 18 November 1967, the *Benidorm* City Council in full agreed to join the consortium for the supply of drinking water. The consortium agreement was signed on 12 March 1968 [10], even including the possibility to include more neighboring populations. However, on 4 July 1969, in the *Benidorm* City Council, the determination was made to cover with the consortium only the towns of *Altea*, *Benidorm* and *Villajoyosa*, as the most important of the coast, in addition to *Alfaz Pi*, *La Nucía*, *Polop*, *Callosa d'En Sarriá* and *Finestrat*, in order to satisfy the demands for irrigation of the agricultural area of *La Marina Baja* district and make the legal compensation viable, as the irrigation community of the *Canal Bajo del Algar* has the right to a flow of 1000 L/s of available water [11]. On 6 August 1969, the full city council agreed to seek all possible resources and began the drilling for the collection of drinking water, hiring a businessman who owned a machine for the development of these works [12].

Years later, the drought from 1978 to 1984 marked the definitive turning point and was the trigger for the implementation of a new good governance body in *La Marina Baja*, in a sort of instinctive process, in which the institution provided itself with management rules and regulations. This was necessary as increasing the amount of water or developing new infrastructure, which is not always enough to improve the balance of available resources with water requirements. The crisis, due to a lack of water, led to a consolidation of the management model of exchange, agreed and consensual, of natural water for supply, under the ownership of irrigators, for reclaimed water suitable for irrigation. Both the need to be supplied by tankers and to suffer restrictions threatened to create a third-world image far removed from the modernity of the tourist destination par excellence of the province and could generate a reputational crisis that would result in a loss of competitiveness of the tourism sector in international markets. The authorities involved strove to promote a solution that would solve and prevent the situation from repeating itself in the future. It was a question of guaranteeing the urban supply of the tourist centers of *La Marina Baja* and to remove uncertainties regarding water safety, being also advantageous for the irrigators involved in the agreements described above. Gaviria et al. [13] emphasized this novel and innovative character of *Benidorm*, which implied potentialities that should be exploited from an ecological perspective, which would place *Benidorm* "at the forefront of Spanish planning and execution with ecological criteria".

From a hydrographic perspective, *La Marina Baja* district is located between the minor basins of the *Algar-Guadalest* and *Amadorio-Sella* rivers, a context with a marked shortage of water that presents frequent cyclical periods of drought, generating peaks of crisis [4,14], which made it more challenging to address concerns between 1950 and 1978, a period in which *Benidorm* became "one of the most spectacular examples of tourism development imaginable: the flagship of tourism in the Valencian Community and the most efficient mass tourism factory on the Spanish coast" [15]. It should be noted that from 1840 onwards and until the fifties of the twentieth century, there was no demographic growth in *La Marina Baja* district. It was between 1950 and 1991 when this area experienced an extraordinary demographic increase, with a 557% population increase, from 22,845 inhabitants (2726 in *Benidorm*) to more than 127,000 (75,322 in Benidorm) [8], directly linked to urban and tourism development.

4. The Case Study within the Economic Background

According to the statistical database obtained from Alcaide Inchausti [16], an analysis of the macroeconomic variables explaining interrelationships derived from the hydro-economic model proposed in this research was carried out, from the national to the local scale. The Spanish economy underwent transformations during the second half of the last century, which is the period in which it experienced sustained growth without precedent in its history. From 1960 to 1975, certain phenomena played a very important role in the province of *Alicante*: the tendency for the Spanish population to locate preferentially in the insular areas and the Mediterranean periphery, the progress of industrialization and the appearance and expansion of tourism as the first national industry. Gross domestic product (GDP) at constant market prices grew by 146.34%, while the resident population increased by 16.41%, which meant that GDP per capita grew by 111.61% in fifteen years, equivalent to a cumulative annual rate of 5.12%. The change in the economic policy of the Franco regime after the application of the Stabilization Plan of 1959 contributed to all this, which meant a process of liberalization and progressive opening towards the exterior and allowed Spain to benefit from the favorable situation that the European economy was experiencing after the Second World War. The expansion of tourism took place, compensating the balance of payments in those years, and was favored by investment in infrastructure, especially highways.

The labor market experienced a profound change (Figure 1). The number of jobs in the primary sector fell by 37.7%, while industry, construction and services registered a joint growth of 41% (53.5% in construction, 45.1% in services and 30.5% in industry). The convergence index with respect to the first 15 countries that today form the European

Union (EUR-15), which in 1960 stood at 59.2%, rose to 79.82% in 1975, making Spain a semi-developed country [16].

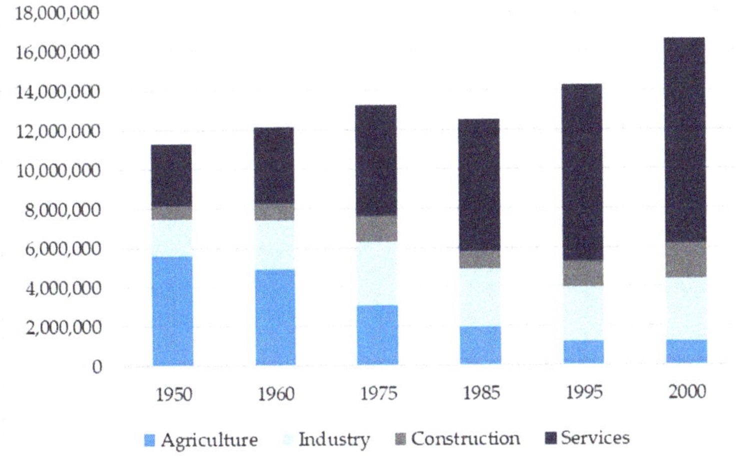

Figure 1. Evolution of total employment and employment by sector of activity in Spain (in full-time equivalent units), 1950–2000. Source: own elaboration from [16].

From 1975 onwards, the political transition together with the energy crisis led to a very significant delay in the process of European convergence, the index of which for the EUR-15 fell to 71.60 in 1985, the same position of 1962. However, the 1985–1995 decade represented a considerable advance for the Spanish economy, with growth higher than that recorded by the European Union as a whole, bringing the convergence index to 80.2% of the EUR-15 [16], as a new expansion took place once democratic institutions were consolidated and the country joined the European Union. During this decade, there was an intense increase in the Spanish resident population as a result of immigration, which led to a notable growth in the employed population while the opening of the Spanish economy to the outside world advanced considerably. At this time, *Benidorm* was the maximum icon of mass tourism, making it necessary to increase resources for urban supply. The last five years of the 20th century, from 1995 to 2000, was one of the most brilliant periods for the Spanish economy, reaching 85.8% in the 2000 convergence index, driven by the requirements established for access to the euro as a single currency within the European Union [16].

The changes that took place in the Spanish economy between 1950 and 2000 were reflected in the country's productive structure (Figure 1). Employment in the primary sector went from 49.7% in 1950 to 23.2% in 1975 and 7.3% in 2000, which was offset by increases in the remaining sectors: industrial, construction and, mainly, services, according to the process of tertiarization of the Spanish economy. In terms of GVA (Figure 2), the agricultural sector has reduced its share of the total from 15.3% in 1950 to 4.8% in 2000. The rural exodus was the fact that most influenced economic evolution in the twentieth century, allowing the improvement of total factor productivity, partly achieved through increased industrialization, as well as the expansion of tourism and of all services. According to this trend, the Valencian Region was the third in terms of GDP growth at constant prices between 1930 and 2000 in Spain, only surpassed by the Madrid Region and the Canary Islands.

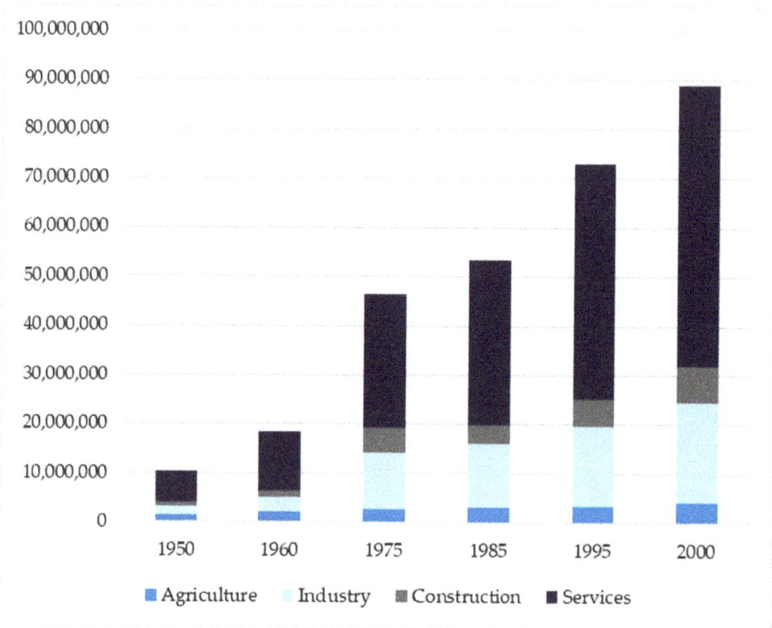

Figure 2. Evolution of gross value added (GVA) by sector of activity in Spain (in millions of constant 1995 pesetas), 1950–2000. Source: own elaboration from [16].

Singularly, the province of *Alicante* experienced notable demographic growth from the mid-1950s until 2000, which was greater in intensity than that experienced by the country as a whole; especially in the period 1960–1975, when the annual growth rate of the province was 2.48% compared to 1.02% in Spain (Figure 3). Even in the years of the crisis of the mid-seventies of the twentieth century, *Alicante*'s demographic dynamics were positive (1.7% compared to 0.83% in Spain). The behavior of employment was also much more positive in the province during the entire period, and the growth rate of the number of jobs in the period 1975–1985 was 0.99% in the province compared to negative figures (−0.59%) in Spain. This means that the economy of *Alicante* withstood the onslaught of the oil crisis better and that, although its rate of job creation slowed, it did not reverse the positive trend that it had been experiencing, which is a sign of the greater capacity for adaptation and flexibility of the provincial economic fabric (Figure 4).

The importance of tourism in this geographical area should also be taken into account in this "less negative" trajectory. Although the growing trend in the number of passengers at *Alicante* airport was interrupted from 1979 onwards (Figure 5), from the mid-1980s onwards, the figures recovered strongly.

Specifically, the district of *La Marina Baja* (Table 1 and Figure 6) was converted from being a district that expelled population until the mid-twentieth century—which was related to the limited opportunities for welfare offered by its traditional economy based on primary sector activities—to a group of municipalities (with the city of *Benidorm* as the main destination) that gradually became attractive to immigration in the heat of the development of a mass tourism model.

During the period between 1950 and 2000, the economy of *Alicante* evidenced a strong structural change, going from having an eminently agricultural base, both in terms of employment (43.4% of the total in 1950) and in terms of GVA (16.3% in 1950), to an economy with a diversified economic structure, centered on the tertiary sector (Figure 7).

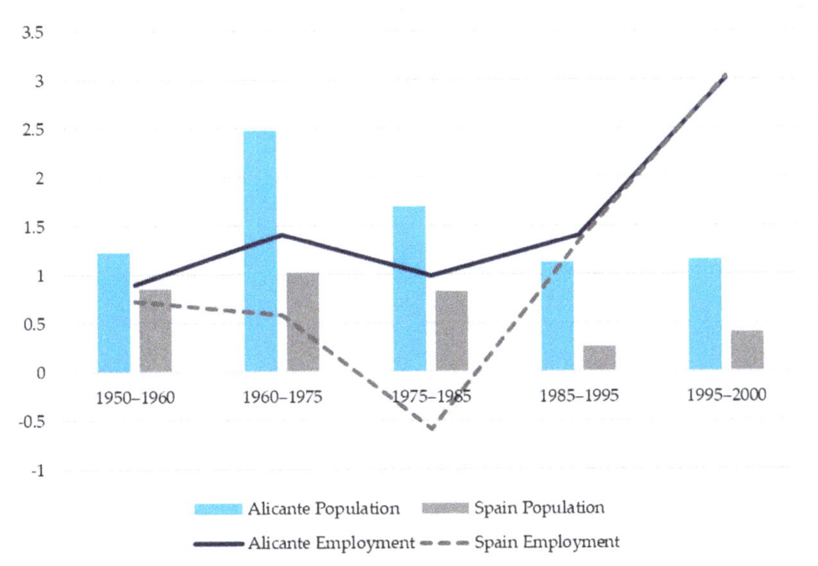

Figure 3. Average cumulative rate of change in population and employment in Spain and *Alicante* (in percent), 1950–2000. Source: own elaboration from [16].

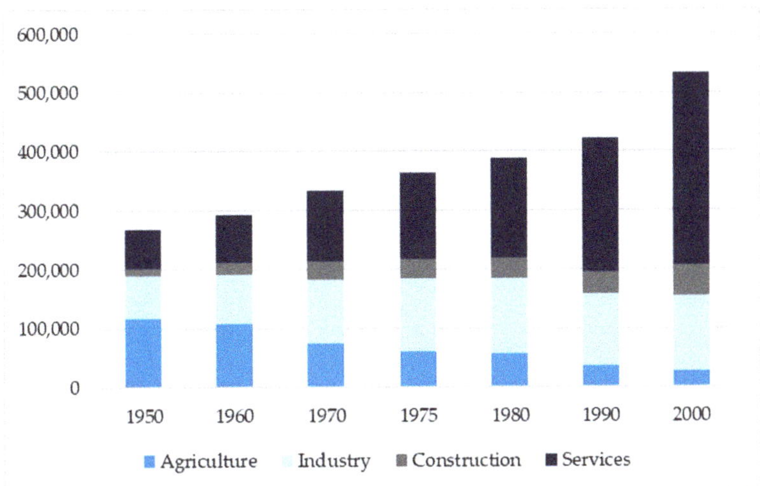

Figure 4. Evolution of employment by sector of activity in the province of *Alicante* (in full-time equivalent units), 1950–2000. Source: own elaboration from [16].

Table 1. Evolution of the population of Spain, province of *Alicante* and district of *La Marina Baja*, 1900–1991. Source: own elaboration from [17].

Year	Spain	*Alicante* Province	*La Marina Baja*
1900	18,618,086	470,149	38,595
1910	19,995,686	497,616	37,770
1920	21,389,686	512,186	35,483
1930	23,677,794	545,838	34,685

Table 1. *Cont.*

Year	Spain	*Alicante* Province	*La Marina Baja*
1940	26,015,907	607,562	34,726
1950	27,976,755	634,065	33,296
1960	30,528,539	711,942	33,834
1970	34,040,989	920,105	44,548
1981	37,683,362	1,148,597	55,276
1991	38,872,268	1,334,545	64,274

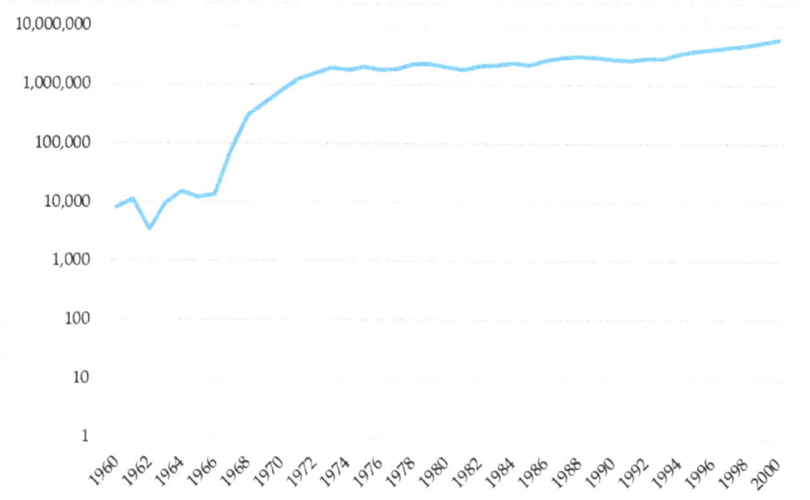

Figure 5. Evolution of the number of passengers at *Alicante* airport (in logarithmic scale), 1960–2000. Source: own elaboration from [17].

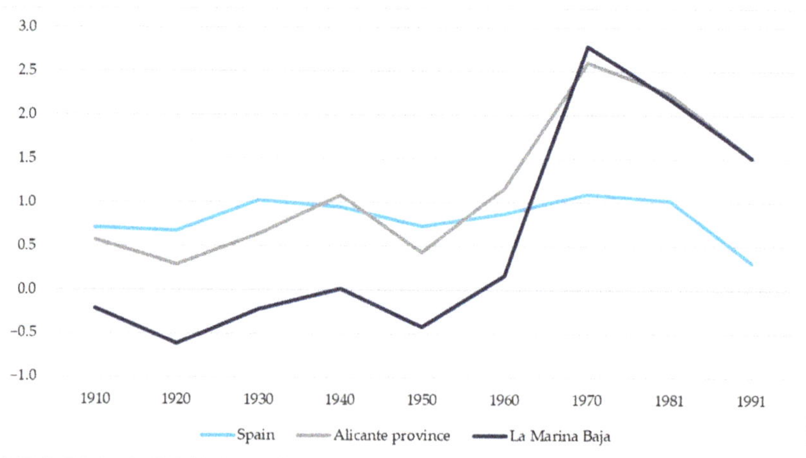

Figure 6. Average cumulative variation rate of the population of Spain, the province of *Alicante* and the region of *La Marina Baja*, 1910–1991. Source: own elaboration from [17].

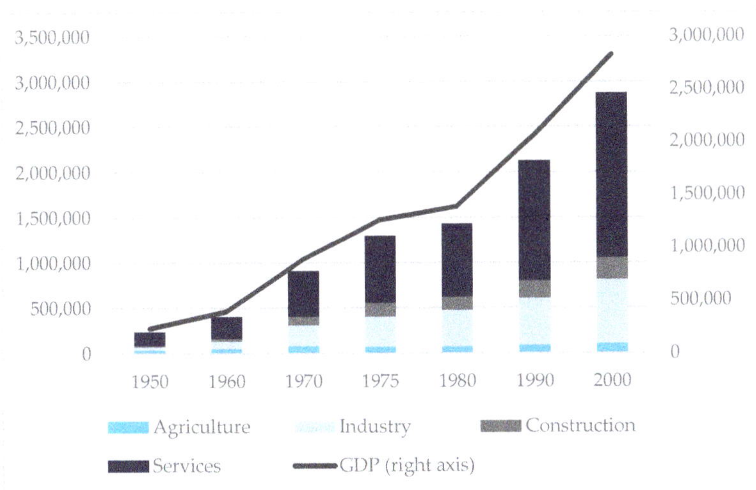

Figure 7. Evolution of gross domestic product (GDP) and gross value added (GVA) by sector of activity in the province of *Alicante* (in millions of constant 1995 pesetas), 1950–2000. Source: own elaboration from [16].

Thus, the primary sector went from representing more than 43% of employment and more than 16% of GVA in 1950 to reducing its share of employment to less than half in 1975 and to 5% of employment and 3.7% of provincial GVA in 2000. This decline in agricultural and fishing activities has been offset by the prominence of other productive sectors, particularly services, with the percentage of industrial employment remaining stable. Construction has more than doubled the percentage of jobs generated in the province (from 4.4% in 1950 to 9.6% in 1975), also increasing the percentage of GVA from 5.4% in 1950 to 11.5%. But the sector that has increased its share of provincial employment the most has been services; while in 1950 it accounted for a quarter of total employment (25.3%), in 1975 it was already 40% and in 2000 it exceeded 61%. The average annual growth rate of provincial GDP between 1950 and 1975 was 7% and between 1975 and 2000 it was 3.2%, both of which are not insignificant figures.

The Spain of the 1950s presented a backward economic model, predominantly agrarian [18] and from the mid-1950s, the situation became unsustainable due to the internal and external imbalances of the Spanish economy: inflation crisis, lack of foreign reserves to finance the required inputs for the industrialization process and serious problems in the balance of payments. After the 1959 Stabilization Plan, in just one year, the current account balance improved substantially, the state's accounts were cleaned up and inflation was controlled [19]. Spain was entering the path of growth, industrialization and internationalization of its economy, finally overcoming the long and deep crisis caused by the civil war and above all by the disastrous policies adopted by Franco's authorities during the post-war period [20]. One of the driving forces behind Spain's economic development and liberalization to the outside world during the 1960s and 1970s was the sustained boom in tourism, remarkably from abroad. Tourism not only allowed the Spanish economy to advance, but also became an accelerator of social modernization [21].

This period of growing liberalization was directly reflected in the province of *Alicante*, which became one of the main sun and beach tourist destinations in the country, and proof of this was the notable growth in the number of passengers at *Alicante* airport: from 8230 in 1960 to 1,253,555 in 1971, mainly after the opening of the new airport in 1967. It can be seen that the number of passengers at *Alicante* airport has experienced an exponential evolution up to the present day, with some exceptions, such as between 1978 and 1981, when the number of passengers fell from 2,033,008 in 1978 to 1,818,974 passengers in 1981, which was possibly influenced by the reputational crisis of *Benidorm*—the water supply crisis of 1978 resulted in serious economic losses for *Benidorm* and damaged its image as a holiday destination [22]— in addition to the effects of the second oil crisis.

Coastal territories were facing the hatching of mass tourism from Europe, which opened a new model of north–south relations [23]. In addition to its environmental and social value on the territory, water proved to have a high economic value, as the management of water resources was decisive for the economic and demographic development of *Benidorm* and the region: "water management, as an economic good, is an important means to achieve an efficient and equitable use and to promote the conservation and protection of water resources" [24]. At present, almost all the coastal municipalities of *La Marina Baja* district and the coast of *Alicante* have tourism as their main economic activity.

Complementary institutional decisions in *Benidorm*, such as the approval of the first General Urban Development Plan in 1956 and previously the approval of the New Alignment Project for the Levante Beach, were decisive for its subsequent urban, touristic and demographic growth, as exposed in *Así será Benidorm*, published in 1955, by the visionary mayor of the city, Pedro Zaragoza. During the early years of the 1950s, the city was already experiencing an increase in vacationers [25]. But this first urban development generated serious imbalances between the available resources, not always related to precipitation levels but correlated to a greater extent with increased demand [23], driven by the higher per capita consumption resulting from the new consumption standards associated with urbanization. In the case of *Benidorm*, unitary consumption went from 80 L/s in 1969 to 600 L/s in 1974 and the evolution of the potable water charged shows a significant growth associated with the urban development (Table 2).

Table 2. Evolution of drinking water billing charged in *Benidorm* in current prices, 1964–1975. Source: own elaboration from [13].

Year	Water Billing (Current Pesetas)	Increase Index
1964	2,212,000	1
1965	4,137,000	1.9
1966	5,056,000	2.3
1967	7,254,000	3.3
1968	8,485,000	3.8
1969	11,944,000	5.4
1970	15,501,000	7.0
1971	15,206,000	6.9
1972	20,624,615	9.3
1973	31,837,000	14.4
1974	34,726,325	15.7
1975	40,424,615	18.3

5. The Circular Hydro-Economic Model of Water Exchanges in *La Marina Baja*: Win–Win Solutions

We find a first reference to setting up a consortium to manage water resources in *La Marina Baja* in 1967 [25], promoted by the *Benidorm* City Council to supply the city of *Benidorm* on a regular basis during the summer months, when water demand increases with tourism. But, during the first years of the seventies of the last century, attempts were frustrated by political vicissitudes at the end of the Franco regime. The suitability of forming a consortium of municipalities, which would be beneficiaries of a model of integrated water management in a district with few natural water sources to meet the requirements of strong demographic growth, is based on the fact that the supply of drinking water is qualified in Spanish legislation as a public service of local competence, contained in Article 25 of the Local Government Bases Act, where inter-municipal water consortiums for the supply of water to towns are contemplated, even in the precedent law from 1955 [26].

The choice of the legal formula for creating a consortium is based on cooperation between public agents, as one of the most important aspects that characterize consortia is their flexibility by allowing other types of institutions, beyond the public administrations themselves, to participate in them [27]. In this sense, "the characteristic element of the consortium consists in the fact that its constitution has as a basic presupposition an identical objective situation for all those who participate in it and from which, precisely, derives that common need that it tries to satisfy jointly through its creation" [28].

It was in October 1977 when the consortium was formally constituted, under the legal form of a local associative entity [4,8] with the following objectives: the study of the water supply and sanitation needs of *La Marina Baja*; the elaboration, in collaboration with the Water Basin Authority (*Confederación Hidrográfica del Júcar*), of the plans for water use and sanitation; the listing of studies, preliminary projects and projects to satisfy the water needs of the district; the application for concessions or authorizations for water supply and wastewater treatment; the execution of works and installations for water treatment, evacuation, purification, discharge and use of wastewater; and the coordination of the consortium's own activities, as well as those of the town councils, with the Ministry responsible for water matters.

Among its most relevant activities are the collection and regulation of surface and groundwater, the integrated management of surface and groundwater resources for different uses, the reuse of wastewater and the exchange of natural groundwater for reclaimed wastewater through agreements, a pillar on which the success of the consortium's own water management is based. The rights to agricultural water use concessions were reoriented to guarantee all users the supply of the resources necessary for irrigation and for supplying the municipalities in the consortium. Long before reclaimed water gained prominence in the heat of circular economy in the field of water management, *La Marina Baja* had already made evident the need to give more than one use to the available water resources, responding to scarcity and making the resource an element of environmental, social and economic opportunity. It has been necessary to wait until the second decade of the 21st century for the European Union to institutionally incorporate circularity in the field of water [29].

In most places in the world that combine scarcity and periods of severe drought with increasing demand there are water governance issues and critical challenges that are still unresolved, as reflected in a European communication [30]. In this context, the consortium's management model becomes relevant: effective in solving scarcity problems, in guaranteeing users by eliminating uncertainties in relation to economic activities and promoting environmentally sustainable behavior in line with circular economy. Social trends and legislative action establish that the transition to a circular economy is an opportunity to transform our economy and make it more sustainable, contribute to climate objectives and the conservation of global resources, create jobs at the local level and generate competitive advantages for Europe [3]. The management model in *La Marina Baja* has made it possible to protect typical ecosystems of the cultural landscape of a traditionally agricultural region, as well as the benefits for the preservation of biodiversity.

If we delve into the history and origins of *La Marina Baja* Water Consortium, and the reasons that drove the search for solutions, we find a commitment to dialogue, agreements and decisions, typical of institutional economy, given that "institutions allow to resolve the tensions posed by human cooperation" [2]. Under the leadership of the *Benidorm* City Council, decisions were taken by organizations such as the Provincial Council of *Alicante*, the Government of Spain, the Water Basin Authority and the other affected municipalities, as well as the traditional irrigators of the area, who had held concessions for irrigation use since long before 1970. As was demonstrated years later with the success of CAMB, "without appropriate institutions, policies will not work; without appropriate policies, institutions will not work" [20]. Having the same needs morally obliges all the participants of the consortium to have a common interest that ends up having a notable repercussion for social interest and this results in the liability to proportionally sustain the burdens by all the actors participating in the consortium, all of them being co-participants in the decisions taken [28]. Consequently, this is an integrated, solidarity-based, participatory, and financially co-responsible management model, financed according to the return generated.

The consortium was constituted on the principles accepted in IWRM, such as management unity, the recognition of individual stakeholders and the capacity for interrelation between them. The management body gives a social dimension to water management, providing transparency in decision making, committing financing from all those who participate and incorporating cost compensation and a fair redistribution of the water resources managed. Also, it guarantees the satisfaction of demand in terms of quantity and quality of water as an economic value, in the terms established by the principles of the Dublin Declaration [31]. This Declaration states that "water has an economic value in all its competing uses and should be recognized as an economic good", highlighting the urgent need to give responsible participation to all users, planners and decision-makers.

The linkages of problems associated with water to other facets of society require a holistic approach, as Biswas [32] points out when referring to IWRM, where the participation of the actors involved (local, provincial, and national administrations, civil society and the private sector) is promoted, responding to each one of the problems and needs that could arise in the territory. Good governance was not only adopted by the institutions, but all the actors also had a relevant role, from the users themselves or the public authorities, to the technicians who carried out the actions. Among the roles of the technicians, the figure of José Ramón García Antón should be highlighted: García Antón was chief engineer of the *Benidorm* City Council at the end of the seventies and was later appointed counselor of the regional government, assuming management of, among other departments, environment and water in the government of the Valencian Region. García Antón, was aware of the problems that afflicted the district and *Benidorm* and was a visionary who placed water at the center of his policies for the province of *Alicante* and, in particular, for the success of a tourism icon like *Benidorm*. He pointed out the need to anticipate crisis scenarios, such as droughts, to act on the reuse of wastewater and to complement the dwindling local resources with the contribution of foreign resources: the axes that form the backbone of the successful response to the area's problems.

Most of the groundwater in the area had concessions for agricultural use, and the holders of these concessions, all of which were granted before 1970, were irrigation communities in the district. Since the second half of the fifties, water swap agreements have been a constant in the articulation of the water management model in *La Marina Baja*. The agreements allow the exchange of rights that the irrigators had on their concessions on natural waters in order to ensure water for urban water supply, although these agreements have not always been fruitful. In fact, the incidence of the 1969 drought caused a discrepancy between the parties which, although it meant the theoretical rupture of the agreements, did not prevent the *Canal Bajo del Algar* from continuing to be "the aqueduct that the *Benidorm* City Council needed to receive water from the *Guadalest* Reservoir" [21].

These first agreements between irrigators and municipalities contemplated the transfer of the use of natural waters to supply the coastal municipalities in exchange for financial compensation and/or as investments, and were recorded in [10]. They included the collaboration contract for the execution of works, signed by the town council and the *Canal Bajo del Algar* irrigators community, dated 3 January 1967, for the construction of the necessary connection infrastructure. The agreement was defended by the councilor responsible for the drinking water service on the grounds of the need to guarantee the supply during the summer season, given the insufficient reserves in the *Guadalest* reservoir, which made it necessary to contract hours of water from private wells. The result of the exchange enabled that "the supply of the population has been totally regular", as recorded in [10]. Collaboration between irrigators and municipalities that needed water to meet the growing demand for water supply was a constant and existed prior to the creation of the consortium. In 1970, a meeting was held in *Alicante* between representatives of the Provincial Council, the Water Basin Authority and the municipalities affected by the drought of 1969 to establish water flows and the financial contributions of municipalities (*Altea, Alfaz del Pi, Benidorm, Finestrat, Villajoyosa, Polop, La Nucía* and *Callosa d'En Sarriá*) [13].

In the case of *La Marina Baja* Water Consortium, which is technically and geographically described in [4,33], the voluntary cession by irrigators of natural water in exchange for reclaimed water is a sort of "informal" or asystematic water market [4,27], that has been operating on the basis of collaboration agreements that have allowed exchanges in a peaceful and efficient manner for decades [34,35]. These swap agreements with irrigators for supply in exchange for reclaimed water were described as "picturesque" and "useful" by Van Looy [36] and encompass the historic agreement between *Beniardá* and *Benidorm*, which initially had no compensation, but was later made in exchange for financing *Beniardá*'s festivities, maintained throughout more than 40 years.

Institutional decisions marked the future of water management, already before the constitution of the consortium, during the sixties and seventies of the twentieth century, when the Ministry of Public Works recognized that the district was affected by a water deficit and, consequently, in order to alleviate it in 1973, granted in favor of the Water Basin Authority (*Confederación Hidrográfica del Júcar*) the reservation of 1500 m^3/day of surplus water from the Algar river for the supplies of *Altea, Alfaz del Pi, Benidorm, Finestrat, Polop, La Nucía, Vilajoyosa* and *Callosa d'En Sarriá* [8]. To this concession, 1000 m^3/day were added once the consortium was formed. Since then, the consortium has the reserve of two water uses, one of 7 hm^3/year and the other of 11 hm^3/year, registered in the water registry of the Water Basin Authority, by the resolution of 6 June 2011. These reserves of use respected the rights of irrigators, titles prior to 1970, although the use was subordinated to the release of natural surface water, assigned to irrigation, which is replaced by reclaimed water. In addition to these uses of surplus surface water, there is the contribution of the Beniardá, Sella and Benimantell groundwater wells (Figure 8).

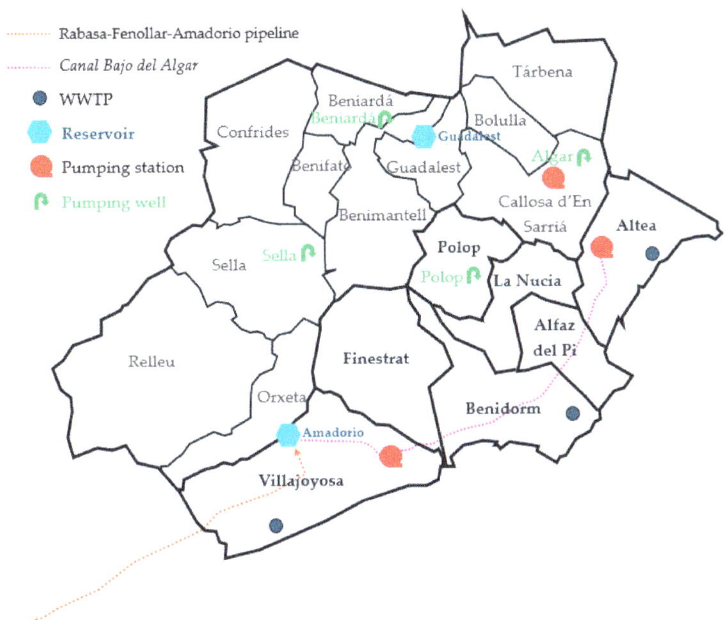

Figure 8. Schematic description of the main infrastructure elements of *La Marina Baja* Water Consortium in the geographical context of *La Marina Baja* district, which are interconnected thanks to pipelines and supply tanks (municipalities integrated in *La Marina Baja* Water Consortium are written in blue). Source: own elaboration based on [4].

The use of all available technologies allowed the reuse of wastewater, increasing the resource supply. A key piece of infrastructure for carrying out the consortium's objectives was the *Benidorm* wastewater treatment plant (WWTP) which began in 1982, even before reused waters were regulated at a national scale, which occurred in 2007. The plant implemented a tertiary water treatment and ultrafiltration system in 2007, complemented by reverse osmosis, generating high-quality regenerated water for agriculture—a pioneer solution for a WWTP, without which the salinity intolerance of most crops would have prevented treated water to be used. Its strategic location in Sierra Helada, at an altitude of more than 140 m, meant that there were fewer odors derived from the treatment process and that, by gravity, the reclaimed water could be sent to the irrigation communities that were to receive the resources. This WWTP, with a capacity of 25,000 m^3/day, treats the sludge with a complex process of anaerobic digestion, which allows its subsequent agricultural use and the generation of biogas together with cogeneration to supply electricity to the plant itself. The *Villajoyosa* and *Altea* WWTPs complement the supply of water for irrigation (Figure 8).

Historically, the water supply guarantee of *La Marina Baja* Water Consortium is based on three fundamental water systems: the *Algar-Guadalest* and *Amadorio-Sella* rivers, and the pioneer reuse of treated wastewater. Nevertheless, over the last few years, external desalination resources have come to complement the system. The search for new exogenous supplies has been undertaken since 1998—when a water crisis similar to that in 1978 occurred—by developing the *Rabasa–Fenollar–Amadorio* pipeline which enabled the partial use of the infrastructure of the Tajo–Segura aqueduct to bring water from the Alarcón reservoir (located in the province of Cuenca, but in the Júcar River Basin Authority) to the Amadorio reservoir. The further contribution of new external resources received a boost in 2009, when the Ministry of the Environment and Rural and Marine Affairs approved the project for the construction of the *Mutxamel* desalination plant (located out of the area of study, southward of the district), which has been used since 2015 in periods of extreme scarcity, taking advantage of the *Rabasa–Fenollar–Amadorio* pipeline. These management practices together with the current outcomes in technical terms are described in detail in the work of Berenguer Ponsoda [37]. Previously, the expectations placed on the Júcar–Vinalopó water transfer (a potential exogenous new resource for the district) were left behind, as a political decision on changing the water intake point implied a very poor quality of the transferred water, which would have required a prior potabilization process with a resulting unfeasible cost for urban consumption [38].

At present, the population served by the consortium is 159,000 inhabitants on a continuous basis, which in the summer season can increase to between 234,000 and 600,000 inhabitants [4]. Therefore, the axis on which the success of *La Marina Baja* Water Consortium will be based on in the future will continue to be the agreement that allows the exchange of natural water for reclaimed wastewater, i.e., the use of quality groundwater for supply, in exchange for the use of reclaimed water for irrigation in the district, together with the granting of compensation, such as storage and operation infrastructure, as well as financial compensation to the transferors of quality resources. The conceptual model is shown in Figure 9:

Consciously or fortuitously, during the years prior to the creation of the consortium, an integrated water management system was forged in response to the equation of water scarcity versus increased demand. This gave rise to patterns of behavior that, to a large extent, anticipate a model of institutional economics, which fits the definition of Oliver Williamson and Elinor Ostrom. In this regard, it should be noted that Ostrom [39] challenged the idea that individuals act in their own self-interest to the point of destroying a shared resource. With numerous field studies, she demonstrated that local communities, when faced with shared problems, develop governance models for sustainable resource management and that institutions provide a better response to the challenges they face with inclusive policies. For his part, Oliver Williamson [40] argues that the key insight is that the value of conflict resolution depends on two main factors: first, there is no point in being able to resolve conflicts that never arise. Accordingly, there was a need to respond to the strong demand for water resources arising from the boom in tourism in *Benidorm*, and especially in times of drought as indicated during the years 1968–1969 and 1978–1984. Secondly, as Williamson [40] points out, there is no reason to be able to resolve conflicts if the disagreement has no cost. In this case, the cost would have been catastrophic for the interests of *Benidorm*, and for the district as a whole, since *Benidorm* acted as a growth pole for the rest of the coastal municipalities.

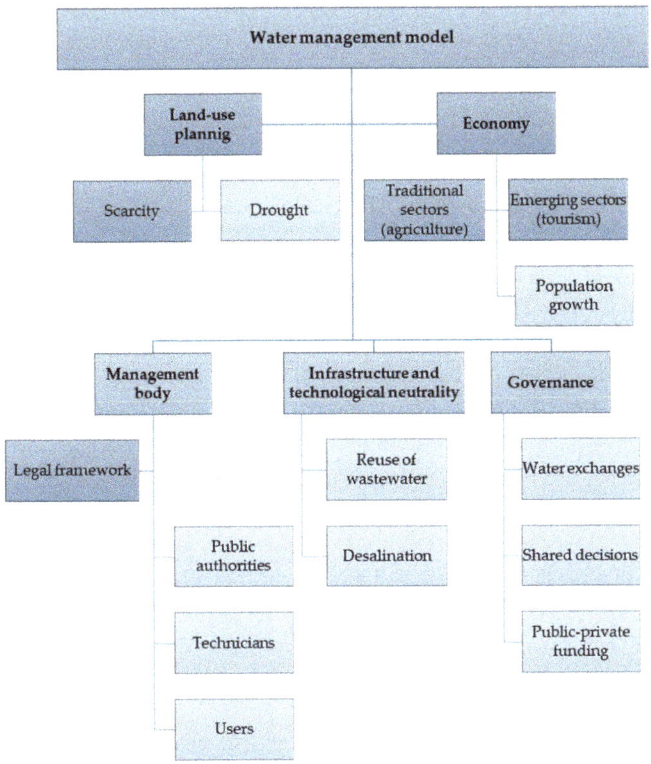

Figure 9. Conceptual map of the hydro-economic model implemented in *La Marina Baja* Water Consortium. Source: own elaboration.

Water was considered a common good that could be exchanged between those who had the administrative concession to use it and those who potentially wanted to acquire that right in a sort of water market, with a broad historical tradition in the area [41]. All stakeholders have gained from the shared management agreements within the framework of the hydro-economic model described above, which conferred water an economic, social and environmental value for the benefit of *La Marina Baja* as a whole, generating contexts of opportunity. After the historical process described from the 1950s, an IWRM system was set up in a territory with water scarcity, which suffered periods of severe drought and which was experiencing urban and demographic growth derived from mass tourism, preserving the cultural landscape and generating an ecosystem of joint wealth, achieving symbiosis between apparently opposing areas—coast versus interior, tourism versus agriculture, urban versus rural—where all the parties involved satisfied their demands. This underlined the continued commitment to the preservation of agriculture, environmental sustainability, conservation of biodiversity and the maintenance of a unique cultural landscape.

During the 1950s and 1960s, IWRM become attractive for developing nations for their modernization, with river basin authorities established in many countries of the Global South, but by the 1970s, concerns over the 'engineering' paradigm started to emerge, due to its technocratic nature and environmental impacts [42,43]. Nevertheless, one of the main advantages of IWRM models is the ability to accommodate local culture, norms or traditions, as a development process towards adaptive solutions to water-related problems, thereby preserving natural resources and ecosystems along with a wide level of participation, users' representation and voluntary local organization with guaranteed water resources [43,44]. Some success stories can be found in the Lower Jordan Rift Valley (Near East) or in the USA, with holistic approaches including the use of different sources of water (such as natural groundwater or surface, reclaimed, desalinated and water for artificial recharge of aquifers); understanding the interactions between water, environment and society; and being extremely sensitive to national, political, cultural and socioeconomic conditions [44,45].

Moreover, the case study could be compared with other significant examples in the world that have implemented an IWRM model, as explained by Dardati [46] for Israel or Australia. Israel is a country with water scarcity, whose management is carried out centrally through the *Water Authority* based on permanent incorporation of advanced technology and infrastructure. The case of Australia exemplifies a decentralized administration where, under Australia's 1901 Constitution, states have the power to allocate water resources [47]; nevertheless, there are discussions about the degree and nature of privatization in relation to water, considering the concept of public ownership rather than querying the initial vesting of the resource in the state [48]. In the 1990s, Australia began reforms to address environmental impacts, in which the figure of an independent administration appears to coordinate the management of the water resources [49]. One of the most important changes was the relocation of water resources to the most agriculturally productive places, analogous to *Benidorm* with its tourism boom. As in the *La Marina Baja* model, public institutions, users and legislation are empowered to be a management instrument, according to the principles of institutional economics, as adequate governance can respond to the problems of dry or semi-arid territories through a holistic IWRM approach, making it possible to face the most important challenges of societies, such as environmental, social and economic sustainability.

6. Conclusions

This paper demonstrates that the historical process that took place in *La Marina Baja* district, in the province of *Alicante* (Spain), resulted in a successful model of water governance, which reached its greatest success with the formal constitution of *La Marina Baja* Water Consortium in 1977. Two historical moments should be emphasized with regard to water as the main resource factor in the economic progress, environmental development and social cohesion of this district, and, particularly, of its main city *Benidorm*. Firstly, the events of the early seventeenth century, when Beatriz de Fajardo ordered the construction of the canal popularly known as *Séquia Mare*, which allowed the repopulation of the coastal municipalities of the district. Secondly, the 1978 drought and the need to bring water by tankers to *Benidorm* marked a turning point in the city known as an icon of international tourism in Spain. Tourism had an unprecedented influence on the awakening of the Spanish economy; it opened Spain to the world and allowed, with carry-over effects, the takeoff of the Spanish economy in other areas such as services, construction and related industries.

In these vibrant economic scenarios faced by the area of study—in which periods of severe drought were combined with structural shortages—the governance model that led to the creation of CAMB, based on integrated water resources management, was the basis for achieving a balance between demand and available resources. Likewise, there was a clear influence of the principles of institutional economics in the case studied, on account of the mobilization and channeling of resources by different administrations working together, launching equitable management rules and integrating the participation of all stakeholders in decision making. The central axis of this successful model of governance is the exchange of natural water for reclaimed water. Natural water is transferred by irrigators to consumers in the primary phase of coastal municipalities, while reclaimed water is transferred to irrigators through advanced purification infrastructure and technologies, making possible the coexistence of economic activities as different as agriculture and tourism.

Finally, it is concluded that this governance model can be applied to other locations with arid territories and similar characteristics from an economic, geographic and climatic point of view, as some studies have shown that the evolution of legal and institutional frameworks of urban water services in Spain could positively impact on water management in developing countries [50]. Largely, water resource planning has been separated from land-use planning [51] and opportunities for explicitly linking planning policies to water availability in Europe were unexamined until the planning framework issued by Directive 2000/60/EC of the European Parliament and of the Council of 23 October 2000, establishing a framework for community action in the field of water policy [52]. *La Marina Baja* was well ahead of its time by establishing a direct relationship between water and territory since the 1960s, an experience which significantly contributes to a management model that could be applied elsewhere. There are countries with scarce water resources and periods of severe drought which have traditionally based their economy on activities such as agriculture and are now experiencing the arrival and expansion of developing economic activities. This could be the case in other Mediterranean locations such as Egypt, Tunisia or Morocco, where many urban water management problems may be a consequence of the absence of an effective integrated approach where water management and land use have not been jointly planned [43,53,54]; such imported strategies, summarized in Figure 9, would be able to address increasing scarcity, gaps in access, legislative changes, lack of infrastructure or new technologies and population growth. However, the consequences of climate change may force us to redefine IWRM models, on which further research is required.

Author Contributions: Introduction, historic sources, investigation, analysis of relevant dynamics and writing—original draft preparation, C.S.-P.; data analysis, validation and supervision, M.-I.L.-O.; formal analysis, validation and supervision, P.F.-A. All authors have read and agreed to the published version of the manuscript.

Funding: This research was funded by the Cátedra del Agua of the University of Alicante and the Diputación Provincial de Alicante (https://catedradelaguaua.org/, accessed on 18 May 2024), grant number CATEDRADELAGUAUA2024.

Data Availability Statement: All researchers involved approve the availability of the data.

Acknowledgments: This work was supported by the University Institute of Water and Environmental Sciences of the University of Alicante. Data and files provided by the Benidorm City Council have been essential. The authors also acknowledge Paco Amillo, Rafael Ferrer, Editor, and anonymous reviewers, whose assistance and comments contributed significantly to improve this work.

Conflicts of Interest: The authors declare no conflicts of interest. The funders had no role in the design of this study; in the collection, analyses or interpretation of data; in the writing of the manuscript; or in the decision to publish the results.

References

1. Lautze, J.; de Silva, S.; Giordano, M.; Sanford, L. Putting the cart before the horse: Water governance and IWRM. *Nat. Resour. Forum* **2011**, *35*, 1–8. [CrossRef]
2. Mercado León, L.A. La nueva economía institucional. Orígenes, bases teóricas y desafíos. *Aglala* **2022**, *12*, 304–317. Available online: https://revistas.uninunez.edu.co/index.php/aglala/article/view/1848 (accessed on 24 April 2024). (In Spanish).
3. Melgarejo Moreno, J.; Lopez Ortiz, M.-I.; Molina Giménez, A. *La Economía Circular y el Sector del Agua en España. Análisis Jurídico-económico*; Tirant lo Blanch: Valencia, Spain, 2023. (In Spanish)
4. Melgarejo Moreno, J.; Fernández Mejuto, M. *El Agua en la Provincia de Alicante*; Diputación Provincial de Alicante: Alicante, Spain, 2020. (In Spanish)

5. Amillo, F.; La Séquia Mare y la Llegada del Agua a Benidorm. Interview in Cadena Ser Benidorm. Available online: https://cadenaser.com/comunitat-valenciana/2023/03/30/la-sequia-mare-y-la-llegada-del-agua-a-benidorm-radio-benidorm/ (accessed on 9 April 2024).
6. Fabián, B. *Report on La Marina Baixa in 1791*; Associació d'Estudis de la Marina Baixa: Alicante, Spain, 2015. (In Spanish)
7. Esquembre, J.; El día que Benidorm Estuvo a Punto de Desplomarse. Diario Información. 2019. Available online: https://www.juntacentral.es/sites/default/files/prensa/2019-07/05-07-19_infor2.pdf (accessed on 18 April 2024). (In Spanish).
8. Gil Olcina, A.; Rico Amorós, A.M. *Consorcio de Aguas de la Marina Baja. Gestión Convenida, Integral y Sostenible del Agua*; Instituto Universitario de Geografía, University of Alicante: Alicante, Spain, 2015. (In Spanish)
9. Gil Olcina, A.; Rico Amorós, A.M. *Canal Bajo del Algar*; Instituto Universitario de Geografía, University of Alicante: Alicante, Spain, 2018. (In Spanish)
10. Benidorm City Council. *Minutes of the Plenary Session of the City Council of 26 September 1968*; Benidorm City Council: Benidorm, Spain, 1968. (In Spanish)
11. Benidorm City Council. *Minutes of the Plenary Session of the City Council of 4 July 1969*; Benidorm City Council: Benidorm, Spain, 1969. (In Spanish)
12. Benidorm City Council. *Minutes of the Plenary Session of the City Council of 6 August 1969*; Benidorm City Council: Benidorm, Spain, 1969. (In Spanish)
13. Gaviria, M.; Iriba, J.M.; Sabbath, F.; Sanz Ramón, J.R. *Benidorm: Ciudad Nueva*; Editorial Nacional: Madrid, Spain, 1977; Volume I and II. (In Spanish)
14. Gil Olcina, A.; Rico Amorós, A.M. *Acueducto Júcar-Vinalopó*; Instituto Universitario de Geografía, University of Alicante: Alicante, Spain, 2023. (In Spanish)
15. Mazón Martínez, T. *Benidorm Un Destino Turístico de Altura*; Cátedra Pedro Zaragoza Orts, Instituto Universitario de Estudios Turísticos, Universty of Alicante: Alicante, Spain, 2010. (In Spanish)
16. Alcaide Inchausti, J. *Evolución Económica de las Regiones y Provincias Españolas en el Siglo XX*; Fundación BBVA: Bilbao, Spain, 2003. (In Spanish)
17. National Statistics Institute of Spain (Instituto Nacional de Estadística, INE). Anuario Estadístico de España. Available online: https://www.ine.es/inebaseweb/treeNavigation.do?tn=180661 (accessed on 23 April 2024).
18. National Statistics Institute of Spain (Instituto Nacional de Estadística, INE). Fondo Documental. 1951. Available online: https://www.ine.es/inebaseweb/25687.do (accessed on 22 April 2024).
19. Barciela, C.; López, M.I.; Melgarejo, J.; Miranda, J.A. *La España de Franco (1939–1975) Economía*; Síntesis: Madrid, Spain, 2005. (In Spanish)
20. Barciela, C. *Autarquía y Mercado Negro. El Fracaso Económico del Primer Franquismo, 1939–1959*; Crítica: Barcelona, Spain, 2003. (In Spanish)
21. Sánchez Sánchez, E.M. El auge del turismo europeo en la España de los años sesenta. *Arbor* **2001**, *170*, 201–224. (In Spanish) [CrossRef]
22. Martínez Ibarra, E. Climate, water and tourism: Causes and effects of droughts associated with urban development and tourism in Benidorm (Spain). *Int. J. Biometeorol.* **2015**, *59*, 487–501. [CrossRef] [PubMed]
23. Vera Rebollo, J.-F. El turismo alicantino: Trayectoria y claves para su análisis. *Canelobre* **2016**, *66*, 9–12. Available online: https://www.cervantesvirtual.com/nd/ark:/59851/bmc0941188 (accessed on 8 May 2024). (In Spanish).
24. Torregrosa, T. *La Gestión del Agua en la Marina Baja (Alicante)*; Corts Valencianes: Valencia, Spain, 2009; Available online: https://www.cortsvalencianes.es/sites/default/files/migrated/publication_book/doc/temas19.pdf (accessed on 11 April 2024). (In Spanish)
25. Moreno Lara, X. *Comunidad de Regantes del Canal Bajo del Algar: Agua para un Desarrollo Sostenible en el Litoral de La Marina Baja*; Javier Boronat: Valencia, Spain, 2012. (In Spanish)
26. LGBA. *Local Government Bases Act (Ley 7/1985, de 2 de Abril, Reguladora de las Bases del Régimen Local)*; Spanish Gobernment: Madrid, Spain; Available online: https://www.boe.es/eli/es/l/1985/04/02/7/con (accessed on 17 April 2024). (In Spanish)
27. Molina Giménez, A. Permutas de agua natural y agua regenerada: Un modelo de aprovechamiento integral en entornos de escasez. In *Mercado de Derechos al Uso Privativo de las Aguas en España. Su Papel en la Gestión de Cuencas Deficitarias*; Navarro Caballero, T., Ed.; Aranzadi: Pamplona, Spain, 2018; pp. 213–249. (In Spanish)
28. Pérez Pérez, E. *La Figura del Consorcio Aplicada a la Gestión de las Aguas Subterráneas*; Confederación Hidrográfica del Segura: Murcia, Spain, 1983. (In Spanish)
29. European Parliament. *Draft Report on Resource Efficiency: Moving towards a Circular Economy European Parliament Committee on the Environment, Public Health and Food Safety*; European Parliament: Brussels, Belgium, 2015. Available online: http://www.europarl.europa.eu/meetdocs/2014_2019/documents/envi/pr/1055/1055309/1055%20309en.pdf (accessed on 19 April 2024).
30. European Commission. Closing the Loop—An EU Action Plan for the Circular Economy. *COM 2015, 614*. Available online: https://eur-lex.europa.eu/legal-content/EN/TXT/?uri=CELEX:52015DC0614 (accessed on 18 April 2024).
31. World Meteorological Organization. *Conferencia Internacional de Dublín sobre Agua y Medio Ambiente CIAMA*; World Meteorological Organization: Geneva, Switzerland, 1992.
32. Biswas, A.K. Integrated Water Resources Management: A Reassessment: A Water Forum Contribution. *Water Int.* **2004**, *29*, 248–256. [CrossRef]

33. Ricart, S.; Rico-Amorós, A.M. To Be, to Do, to Share: The Triple-Loop ofWater Governance to Improve UrbanWater Resilience—Testing the Benidorm' Experience, Spain. *Land* **2022**, *11*, 121. [CrossRef]
34. Torregrosa, T.; Sevilla, M. La integración del medio físico en la gestión integrada de recursos hídricos de la Marina Baja (Alicante). *Investig. Geogr.* **2009**, *48*, 39–76. (In Spanish) [CrossRef]
35. Sanchis-Ibor, C.; García-Mollá, M.; Torregrosa, T.; Ortega-Reig, M.; Sevilla-Jiménez, M. Water transfers between agricultural and urban users in the region of Valencia (Spain). A case of weak governance? *Water Secur.* **2019**, *7*, 100030. (In Spanish) [CrossRef]
36. Van Looy, N. Agua a Cambio de Fiestas, el Histórico Acuerdo Entre Beniarda y Benidorm. Todo Alicante. 2023. Available online: https://www.todoalicante.es/alicante-provincia/agua-cambio-fiestas-historico-acuerdo-beniarda-benidorm-20230802091121-nt_amp.html (accessed on 17 April 2024). (In Spanish).
37. Berenguer Ponsoda, J. El Consorcio de Aguas de La Marina Baja: Un ejemplo de economía circular en la garantía del abastecimiento urbano ante el reto continuo de las sequías. In *Seguridad Hídrica*; Melgarejo, J., López Ortiz, M.-I., Fernández-Aracil, P., Eds.; University of Alicante: Alicante, Spain, 2023; pp. 409–436. (In Spanish)
38. Richart Díaz, V.J. Energía fotovoltaica y conducción Júcar-Vinalopó. In *Agua, Energía y Medioambiente*; Melgarejo, J., López Ortiz, M.-I., Fernández-Aracil, P., Eds.; University of Alicante: Alicante, Spain, 2022; pp. 1241–1261. (In Spanish)
39. Ostrom, E. *Governing the Commons. The Evolution of Institutions for Collective Action*; Cambridge University Press: Cambridge, UK, 1990.
40. Williamson, O.E. The Economics of Governance. *Am. Econ. Rev.* **2005**, *95*, 1–18. [CrossRef]
41. Melgarejo, J.; López Ortiz, M.-I. Los mercados del agua como instrumento para la gestión de la escasez en cuencas deficitarias en España. In *Mercado de Derechos al Uso Privativo de las Aguas en España. Su Papel en la Gestión de Cuencas Deficitarias*; Navarro Caballero, T., Ed.; Aranzadi: Pamplona, Spain, 2018; pp. 183–211. (In Spanish)
42. Fritsch, O.; Benson, D. Mutual Learning and Policy Transfer in Integrated Water Resources Management: A Research Agenda. *Water* **2020**, *12*, 72. [CrossRef]
43. Martínez Santos, P.; Aldaya, M.M.; Llamas, M.R.; Thuy, L.A.D.R. *Integrated Water Resources Management in the 21st Century: Revisiting the Paradigm*; CRC Press: London, UK, 2014.
44. Watson, N.; Shrubsole, D.; Mitchell, B. Governance Arrangements for Integrated Water Resources Management in Ontario, Canada, and Oregon, USA: Evolution and Lessons. *Water* **2019**, *11*, 663. [CrossRef]
45. Wolff, H.P.; Wolf, L.; Subah, A.; Guttman, J.; Tamimi, A.; Jarrar, A.; Salman, A.; Karablieh, E. Methodological challenges in evaluating performance, impact and ranking of IWRM strategies in the Jordan Valley. *Water Sci. Technol.* **2012**, *66*, 1407–1415. [CrossRef] [PubMed]
46. Dardati, E. La gestión hídrica en Australia e Israel: Dos modelos, un solo fin. *Puntos Ref.* **2021**, *587*, 1–22. (In Spanish)
47. Wheeler, S.A.; Owens, K.; Zuo, A. Is there public desire for a federal takeover of water resource management in Australia? *Water Res.* **2024**, *248*, 120861. [CrossRef] [PubMed]
48. Godden, L. Property in urban water: Private rights and public governance. In *Troubled Waters: Confronting the Water Crisis in Australia's Cities*; Troy, P., Ed.; ANU E Press, The Australian National University: Canberra, Australia, 2008; pp. 157–185.
49. Smith, D.I. *Water in Australia: Resources and Management*; Oxford University Press: Melbourne, Australia, 1998.
50. Navarro Ortega, A.; Burlani Neves, R. Legal Aspects of Urban Water and Sanitation Regulatory Services: An Analysis of How the Spanish Experience Positively Would Contribute to the Brazilian New Regulation. *Water* **2021**, *13*, 1023. [CrossRef]
51. Shandas, V.; Lehman, R.; Larson, K.L.; Bunn, J.; Chang, H. Stressors and Strategies for Managing Urban Water Scarcity: Perspectives from the Field. *Water* **2015**, *7*, 6775–6787. [CrossRef]
52. European Parliament, European Union. *Directive 2000/60/EC of the European Parliament and of the Council Establishing a Framework for the Community Action in the Field of Water Policy 2000*; European Parliament: Brussels, Belgium, 2000; Available online: https://eur-lex.europa.eu/legal-content/EN/ALL/?uri=celex:32000L0060 (accessed on 4 December 2023).
53. Carter, N.; Kreutzwiser, R.D.; de Loë, R.C. Closing the circle: Linking land use planning and water management at the local level. *Land Use Policy* **2005**, *22*, 115–127. [CrossRef]
54. Martín García, I. *La Gestión Integrada de los Recursos Hídricos en Andalucía y el Norte de Marruecos*; Fundación Centro de las Nuevas Tecnologías del Agua, CENTA: Seville, Spain, 2015. (In Spanish)

water

MDPI

Article

Multi-Dimensional Collaborative Optimization Model for Agricultural Water Rights Based on Water Price Reform under Changing Environment

Linlin Song [1], Hongshu Wang [1,*] and Liang Ding [2]

[1] College of Economics and Management, Northeast Forestry University, No. 26 Hexing Road, Xiangfang District, Harbin 150040, China; songlinlin_nefu@163.com

[2] College of Science, Northeast Forestry University, No. 26 Hexing Road, Xiangfang District, Harbin 150040, China; dl@nefu.edu.cn

* Correspondence: wanghongshu_nefu@163.com

Abstract: Agricultural water rights trading has become an effective means to solve the shortage of agricultural water. However, in the context of uncertainty, the key elements of the water rights trading system and their interactions remain unclear. Therefore, this study constructs a multi-dimensional collaborative optimization model for agricultural water rights based on water price reform under a changing environment. The model quantitatively characterizes the synergistic effects of resource, economic, social, environmental, and ecological objectives on initial water rights allocation and trading. At the same time, the model uses a system dynamics model and intuitionistic fuzzy number to reflect the impact of a changing environment and uncertainty of the management system on water rights allocation and trading. The results show that through water rights trading, the overall coordinated development of farms has been improved, and the economic benefits and water resources utilization efficiency have been improved.

Keywords: management of agricultural water rights; system dynamics; multi-dimensional evaluation system; multiple uncertainty

1. Introduction

This study proposed a multi-dimensional collaborative optimization model for agricultural water rights based on water price reform under a changing environment (MCO-AWR-WPRCE) to weigh the contradictions among multiple objectives of economic benefits, energy consumption, and water use efficiency of agricultural water rights trading. MCO-AWR-WPRCE can effectively manage water rights in irrigated areas to reduce agri-cultural water use and enhance agricultural benefit value while ensuring agricultural production, providing valuable insights and guidance for current and future water resources management.

Population growth, intensive economic activities, and environmental changes have led to a rapid increase in water demand [1]. Agriculture is the industry that consumes the most freshwater, accounting for about 70% of the total global freshwater consumption [2]. In China, more than half of the cultivated land depends on irrigation to ensure cultivation [3]. As agricultural water use continues to increase, better management of water resources is an effective means to address agricultural water stress [4]. Water rights trading is an important way to optimize water resource allocation by using market mechanisms [5]. Water rights trading can promote the optimal allocation of water resources, maintain the relative balance of agricultural ecosystems, and realize the sustainable use of water resources [6]. Therefore, the management of agricultural water rights is one of the important means to realize the sustainable utilization of agricultural water resources.

Reasonable initial allocation of agricultural water rights is a prerequisite for implementing water rights trading and improving water use efficiency [7]. An effective water rights regime not only lays the foundation for water demand management, but also helps provide a degree of flexibility for water users and other stakeholders to hand over readily available water in the market [8]. However, the initial allocation of agricultural water rights often contains subjectivity and uncertainty, and it is particularly important to objectively determine the initial allocation method of agricultural water rights [9]. The existing initial allocation methods of agricultural water rights mostly use the weighting method, which has distinct regional characteristics and subjective will [10]. The objective construction of the initial water rights evaluation system is an effective way to solve the subjective empowerment problem [11]. Initial water rights allocation is often influenced by multiple dimensions such as resources (water footprint), economy (economic benefits), society (Gini coefficient), environment (greenhouse gas emissions), and ecology (ecological footprint) [12]. Most of the current studies ignore the influence of multi-dimensional factors on the initial water rights allocation scheme, or only consider the response of a few dimensions, which obviously cannot provide effective guidance for water rights allocation in a comprehensive way. The establishment of the initial water rights allocation evaluation index weight system, assigning index weights to the initial water rights allocation, and evaluating the initial water rights in each region can quantitatively characterize the influence of multi-dimensional closely linked indicators on the initial water rights allocation, which has important practical significance for obtaining a reasonable water rights allocation scheme.

Initial agricultural water rights allocation and water rights trading are two important parts of agricultural water rights management, and the water rights trading process is the core of agricultural water rights management [13]. The improvement of water use efficiency can improve the effectiveness and feasibility of water rights trading, thus promoting the sustainable use of water resources. In the process of initial water rights allocation and water rights trading, water intake, water transfer, and other processes will inevitably lead to energy consumption. However, few studies have considered the impact of water use efficiency and energy consumption on the sustainable management of water rights during water rights trading.

Water right transaction is actually the redistribution of water resources. The redistribution of water resources can improve economic benefits, but some people are conservative because they exaggerate their economic benefits, because the increase in economic benefits will do harm to other aspects (such as environment and resource consumption). According to Liptrot and Hussein, redistribution may reduce farmers' income and increase food prices. In addition, the affected farmers themselves may not benefit from the growth of the water-receiving sector. Therefore, the transaction price and reasonable formulation of water rights are particularly important. The trading price of water rights can solve the contradiction between the static nature of initial water rights allocation and the dynamics of social and economic development [14], and play a key role in the smooth realization of water rights trading. A too low trading price not only damages the interests of the transferor of water rights, but also is detrimental to the conservation and protection of water resources. An excessively high trading price may increase the water cost of the water rights transferor and make the transaction difficult to realize [5]. Therefore, determining the trading price of water rights is not only conducive to creating an effective water rights market, but also is beneficial for solving the contradiction of spatial and temporal distribution of water resources and promoting the optimal allocation of water resources.

The management of agricultural water rights is affected by the initial water rights allocation scheme considering multiple dimensions, energy consumption, and water price setting in the process of water rights trading, and it is inevitably affected by multiple factors such as a changing environment and management system, resulting in uncertainty. Therefore, it is very important to reduce the impact of uncertainty on water rights allocation [15]. In terms of the multi-dimensional initial water rights allocation scheme, the driving factors of each dimensional goal change with time and are related to other dimensional goal-driving factors [15]. In the initial water rights allocation process, considering the dynamic and correlation of the driving factors of each dimension goal is helpful to the accurate adjustment of initial water rights and the effective balance of multi-dimensional goals. The system dynamics (SD) method can solve complex system structure, handle multi-dimensional variables, multiple feedback, and time-varying problems, and is an effective method to solve the above problems [16]. However, there are few studies on coupling the SD method with the multi-dimensional optimization model of initial water rights allocation. This coupling can optimize and predict the multi-dimensional influencing factors sustainably from the perspective of system theory, and more accurately reflect the impact of future environmental changes on multiple dimensions such as resources, economy, society, environment, and ecology. The management system will cause the deviation or insufficiency of data statistics, increase the uncertainty of data, and then affect the water rights trading model, thus affecting the output water rights allocation scheme. The comprehensive consideration of the changing environment and the uncertainty of the management system are of practical significance for the objective and true management of agricultural water rights.

The MCO-AWR-WPRCE model quantifies the synergistic effects of resources, economy, society, environment, and ecology on the initial water rights allocation, and considers the impacts of multiple uncertainties of a changing environment and management system on the model, so as to obtain a reasonable agricultural water rights allocation scheme. The MCO-AWR-WPRCE model is a theoretical model of water rights trading considering initial water rights allocation and water price reform. By managing water rights trading schemes, agricultural water consumption is reduced, thus achieving the purpose of water saving, ensuring the agricultural production demand in water-deficient areas.

2. Materials and Methods

This section is divided into five main modules, including (1) data module; (2) evaluation module: SD is used to construct evaluation models for the five dimensions of resources, economy, society, environment, and ecology, in which water footprint index is adopted for resources dimension, economic benefit index is adopted for economic dimension, Gini coefficient index is adopted for social dimension, greenhouse gas emission index is adopted for environmental dimension, and ecological dimension index is adopted for ecological dimension. (3) Optimization module: an agricultural water rights trading model is constructed. MCO-AWR-WPRCE sets the water rights trading mechanism. When the water rights of a certain farm are not enough to meet the irrigation needs of the current year, the farm needs to buy additional water rights from other farms. The aim of this mechanism is to encourage agriculture in the region to implement water-saving measures to improve the efficiency of regional water resources. On the other hand, the surplus water rights can be sold at a reasonable price, converting the surplus water rights into additional economic benefits. The research builds a water rights trading network, which stipulates that water rights trading should be conducted from other regions nearest to the water shortage area, thus realizing the development of trading strategies under distance constraints. If there are no surplus water rights in the nearby region, MCO-AWR-WPRCE's trading strategy will shift to the next region slightly farther away. Through the evaluation module, the initial allocation weight of water rights is output, the trading price of water rights is output through the total water price model, and the initial allocation volume and trading price of water rights are brought into the optimization model. The whole process is carried out under uncertain conditions. (4) Uncertainty module: SD is used to predict the parameters of each dimension of the evaluation system, intuitive fuzzy number is used to quantify the uncertainty of parameters in management, and fuzzy information is more strongly expressed to more accurately express the subjective attitude of decision makers. (5) Model output module: the specific technology roadmap is shown in Figure 1:

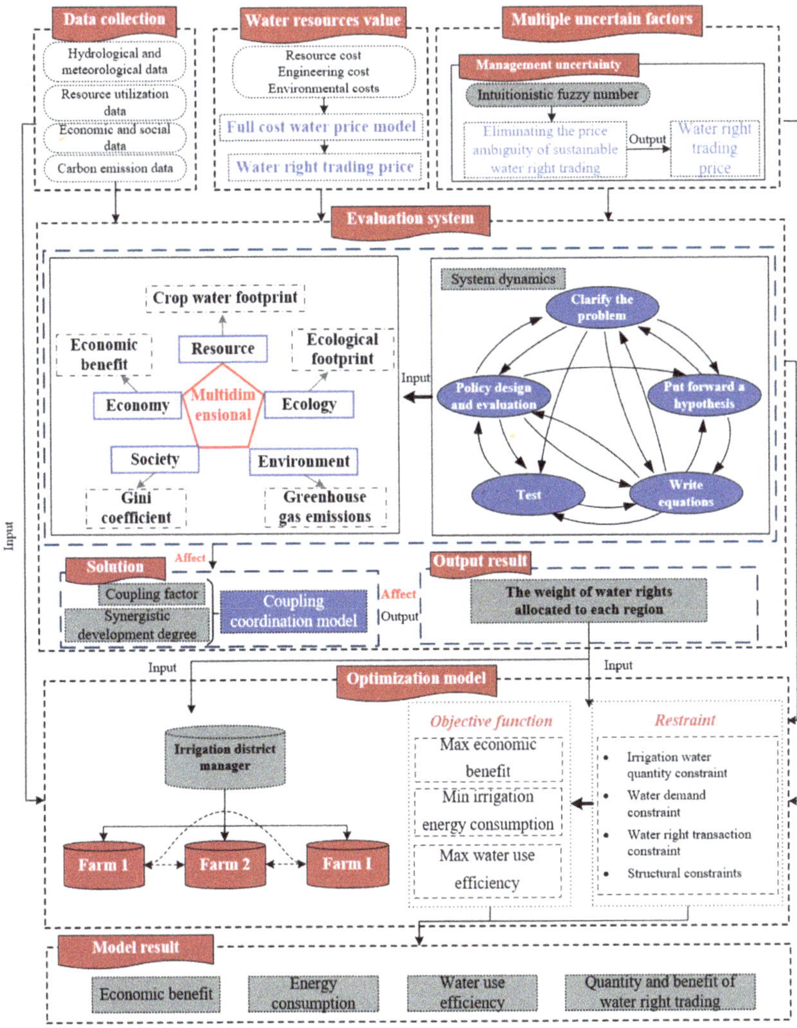

Figure 1. Research technology roadmap.

2.1. Optimization Mode

2.1.1. Economic Benefit Target Based on Water Rights Trading

In order to better cope with the problem of water scarcity, research is conducted to mitigate the impact of water scarcity by allowing different regions to trade water rights in a decentralized manner [17]. The development of water rights trading can be actively promoted through reasonable initial water rights allocation and water price formulation, which can better manage agricultural water resources and optimize resources utilization efficiency, thus improving the sustainable development of agriculture [18]. Therefore, the water rights trading model is selected as one of the objective functions, and the water rights trading model considering the initial water rights allocation and water price setting is as follows [13]:

$$\max EB^* = \left(\sum_{i=1}^{I} (P_i^* Y_i^* - C_i^*) A_i - WPF_i \cdot WR_i^* A_i - WPB_i \sum_{i=1}^{I} WRB_i A_i + WPS_i WRS_i A_i \right) \quad (1)$$

where $*$ means that the parameter is processed by intuitionistic fuzzy number; i is the farm index, $i = 1 \ldots I$; EB^* is total economic benefit, Yuan; P_i^* is the crop unit price in farm i, Yuan/kg; Y_i^* is the crop yield in farm i, kg/ha; A_i is the crop area in farm i, ha; WPF_i is the current agricultural water price in farm i, Yuan/m^3; WR_i^* is the initial allocation of water rights in farm i, m^3/ha; WPB_i is the water purchase price in the water rights trading in farm i, Yuan/m^3; WRB_i is the amount of water rights purchased by farm i from other farm, m^3; WPS_i is the price at which water is sold in the water rights trading in farm i, Yuan/m^3; WRS_i is the amount of water rights that farm i sells to other farm, m^3.

The trading price of water rights, taking into account the transportation cost of water rights, is calculated by the following formula [19]:

$$WPB_i = WPS_i + PE_i \cdot \sum_{i=1}^{I} 1000 \times \left(\sum_{i=1}^{I} \frac{WRB_i hf_{ii} \cdot g}{3.6 \times 10^6} \right) \quad (2)$$

$$hf_{ii} = ph \times TR_{ii} \quad (3)$$

$$ph = 10.294 \times n^2 \times Q^2 \div d^{5.333} \quad (4)$$

where PE_i is the electricity price in farm i, Yuan/kWh; hf_{ii} is the head loss along the distance between farm i and other farms, m; g is the acceleration of gravity, N/kg; ph is head loss per unit pipe length, m/m; TR_{ii} is the distance between farm i and other farm i, km; n is the roughness rate of the channel in the transportation process, without dimension; Q is channel traffic, m^3/s; d is the inner diameter of the channel, m.

When determining the water rights trading, the research takes into account three aspects: resources cost, engineering cost, and environmental cost of water resources [5]. By comprehensively considering resources cost, engineering cost, and environmental cost, the determination of water price in water rights trading can be evaluated and decided more comprehensively. The full-cost water price model can be expressed as follows [20]:

$$WPS_i = WPS_i^R + WPS_i^E + WPS_i^S \quad (5)$$

where WPS_i^R is the cost of water rights resources in farm i, including the cost of water resources management and protection, Yuan/m^3; WPS_i^E is the engineering cost of water rights in farm i, including depreciation cost of fixed assets, maintenance cost of water conservancy facilities, and project operation and management cost, Yuan/m^3; WPS_i^S is the environmental cost of water rights in farm i, including financial costs, water pollution treatment costs, and water environment compensation costs, Yuan/m^3.

Resources cost refers to the quantification of the economic relationship between water resources managers and consumers, reflecting the scarcity value of water resources. The acquisition and treatment of water resources require a certain cost, including the development, collection, transportation, and treatment of water resources. The formula is as follows [20]:

$$WPS_i^E = \frac{Z_i + M_i + S_i}{IQ_i^{mean}} \quad (6)$$

where Z_i is the depreciation cost of fixed assets in farm i, Yuan; M_i is the maintenance cost of large equipment in farm i, Yuan; S_i is the project operation and management cost in farm i, including employee compensation, project maintenance cost, office cost, land use cost, financial cost, and management cost, Yuan.

Engineering cost refers to the quantification of the relationship between production cost and property right, which covers the cost of each link in the process of water resources supply, including the cost consideration of collection, treatment, distribution, and other links. The allocation, transportation, and treatment of water resources need to carry out related engineering construction and operation, which will generate engineering costs. The formula is as follows [20]:

$$WPS_i^S = F_i \cdot WPS_i^R \quad (7)$$

where F_i is the water resources scarcity degree coefficient in farm i, without dimension.

Environmental cost refers to the quantification of the compensation degree of water supply agencies to the water environment. The development and utilization of water resources may have an impact on the surrounding ecological environment, so we must pay attention to the impact of water resources on the environment, and take corresponding measures to compensate and protect it. The formula is as follows [20]:

$$F_i = \frac{Q_{nation}}{WR_i} \tag{8}$$

where Q_{nation} is the national average water consumption for agricultural irrigation, m^3/ha.

The distribution of initial water rights takes into account the coordinated development degree of each region. Refer to Section 2.4 for the calculation of the coordinated development degree. The formula for calculating initial water rights is as follows:

$$WR_i^* = D_i^* \cdot IQ_i \tag{9}$$

where IQ_i is the amount of water rights allocated to farm i, m^3/ha.

2.1.2. Energy Consumption Targets Considering Water Rights Trading Distance

The process of agricultural irrigation and water rights trading involves energy consumption, and the energy consumption of agricultural irrigation mainly comes from pumping, transportation, irrigation, and other links [21]. This study quantifies the energy consumption in the pumping and conveying process, but does not consider the energy consumption in the irrigation process because of the artesian irrigation method in the study area. However, water rights trading may cause certain energy consumption in other links related to water resources. For example, water rights trading leads to the transfer of water resources, which may require additional pumping equipment (such as pumps) to provide water, thus increasing energy consumption. Therefore, one of the objective functions of the model is to consider the minimum electric energy consumption in the process of irrigation water use and water rights trading, and the calculation formula is as follows [19]:

$$\min P = \sum_{i=1}^{I}\sum_{i=1}^{I} \frac{m_i g h f_{ii}}{3.6 \times 10^6} \tag{10}$$

$$m_i = 1000 \times \left(WR_i + \sum_{i=1}^{I} WRB_{ii} - WRS_i \right) \times A_i \tag{11}$$

where P is the energy consumption value of water transmission, kWh; m_i is the quantity of water delivery in farm i, kg.

2.1.3. Water Use Efficiency

Water use efficiency can reflect the relationship between soil and water resources utilization and crop yield in agricultural production. It is an important indicator to measure the effect of crops on water resources utilization and a key parameter to evaluate agricultural water management [22]. Improving water use efficiency can not only save water resources, but also reduce energy consumption, reduce environmental pollution, and improve agricultural production efficiency. Therefore, as one of the objective functions of the model, the larger the value of water use efficiency, the better the model. The calculation formula is as follows [22]:

$$\min WUE = \frac{\sum_{i=1}^{I} Y_i^* A_i}{\sum_{i=1}^{I}\left(\left(WR_i + \sum_{i=1}^{I} WRB_{ii} - WRS_i\right) A_i\right)} \tag{12}$$

2.2. Model Constraints

The optimal design of MCO-AWR-WPRCE includes the variable of demand solution (i.e., the decision variable), and the limiting condition of the decision variable is the constraint condition, which can ensure that the model is solved within the feasible boundary. The constraints studied in this chapter include irrigation water quantity, water demand, water rights trading, structure, etc.

(1) Irrigation water constraint

The constraint of irrigation water refers to the restriction and control of the water used in agricultural irrigation to ensure reasonable utilization of water resources and protect the ecological environment. The sum of the initial allocation of water rights for all users should not be greater than the total allocation of water in the irrigation area, thus ensuring water resources security. Constraints can be expressed as follows [5]:

$$\sum_{i=1}^{I} \frac{WR_i A_i}{\eta_{water}} \leq Q^{sur} \tag{13}$$

where η_{water} is the water resources availability coefficient, without dimension; Q^{sur} is the available quantity of surface water, m^3.

(2) Water demand constraint

Water demand constraint refers to the restriction and control of the water required by the growth and development of crops in each region to ensure the normal growth of crops. The amount of water that can be allocated in each farm needs to meet the water demand of crops to ensure the safe production of food. Constraints can be expressed as follows [5]:

$$W_i^{\min} \leq \left(WR_i + \sum_{i=1}^{I} WRB_{ii} - WRS_i \right) \leq W_i^{\max} \tag{14}$$

where $W_i^{\min}$ is the minimum water demand of crops in farm i, m^3/ha; $W_i^{\max}$ is the maximum water demand for crops in farm i, m^3/ha.

(3) Water rights trading constraints

The amount of water rights purchased by each farm from other farms cannot be greater than the amount of water rights sold by other farms, and the amount of water rights sold by each farm cannot be greater than the amount of water rights initially allocated. Constraints can be expressed as follows [5]:

$$0 \leq \sum_{i=1}^{I} WRB_{ii} \leq WRS_i \tag{15}$$

$$0 \leq WRS_i \leq WR_i \tag{16}$$

The model and decision variables should meet the actual situation, that is, the allocation of water rights should not be negative. Constraints can be expressed as follows [5]:

$$WRB_{ii} \geq 0 \quad \forall i \tag{17}$$

$$WRS_i \geq 0 \quad \forall i \tag{18}$$

2.3. Model Solution

MCO-AWR-WPRCE is constructed to weigh the three objective functions of economic benefit, energy consumption, and water use efficiency. To couple multiple objectives together, it is necessary to introduce membership function framework [23]. In this paper, a fuzzy algorithm is used to introduce satisfaction variables λ to transform the multi-objective problem into an equivalent fuzzy linear programming problem with a single objective. The transformed model is as follows [23]:

$$\max = \lambda \tag{19}$$

For the objective function that is larger and better, the following membership degree formula is used for quantitative characterization. Maximizing the objective function includes economic benefits and water use efficiency [23]:

$$F(x) - F_{\min}(x) \geq \lambda[F_{\max}(x) - F_{\min}(x)] \tag{20}$$

For the membership function that is smaller and better, the following formula is used for quantitative characterization. The minimization objective function includes the energy consumption objective function [23]:

$$F_{\max}(x) - F(x) \geq \lambda[F_{\max}(x) - F_{\min}(x)] \tag{21}$$

$$\begin{cases} G(x) \leq h \\ x \geq 0 \\ 0 \leq \lambda \leq 1 \end{cases} \tag{22}$$

where λ is the satisfaction of the membership function, the larger the λ is, the greater the satisfaction of the coordination of each goal and the better the optimization; $F_{\min}(x)$ and $F_{\max}(x)$ are the lowest and highest acceptable levels of the objective function, respectively; $G(x) \leq h$ includes irrigation water constraints, water demand constraints, water rights trading constraints, and structural constraints, which are consistent with the constraints expressed in Section 2.2 above. The model process is shown in Figure 2.

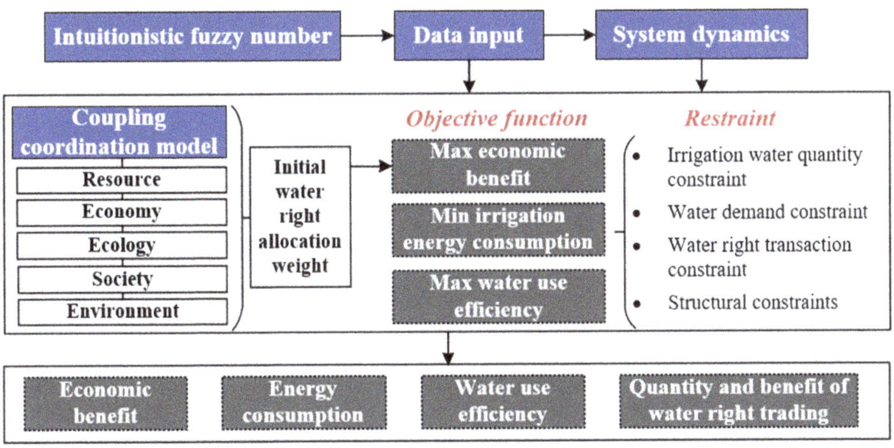

Figure 2. Model concept map.

2.4. Evaluation Index System for Sustainable Use of Agricultural Water Rights Trading

The evaluation system of agricultural water-saving potential is divided into five subsystems including resources, economy, society, environment, and ecology. This hierarchical structure is helpful to better evaluate the dynamic change characteristics and evolution law of regional agricultural water-saving potential, which will help guide agricultural water use decision making and water-use planning, and promote the sustainable use of regional water resources. The explanations of parameter variables in each dimension are shown in Table 1.

Table 1. Definition of rating system parameters.

Variable Symbol	Variable Interpretation
i	Farm index
sur	Upper corner mark of surface water
gro	Upper corner mark of groundwater
$*$	Parameters are fuzzified
RES	Resource dimension related parameters
ECO	Economic dimension related parameters
SOC	Social dimension related parameters
ENV	Environmental dimension related parameters
$ECOL$	Ecological dimension related parameters
D_i^*	Coordinated development degree in farm i, without dimension
C_i	Coupling development index in farm i, without dimension
T_i	Comprehensive development index in farm i, without dimension
F_i^{RES}	Resources development indicators in farm i, m^3/kg
F_i^{ECO}	Economic development indicators in farm i, Yuan
F_i^{SOC}	Social development indicators in farm i, without dimension
F_i^{ENV}	Environmental development indicators in farm i, without dimension
F_i^{ECOL}	Ecological dimension development index in farm i, without dimension
a^{RES}	Resources dimension weight, without dimension
a^{ECO}	Economic dimension weight, without dimension
a^{SOC}	Social dimension weight, without dimension
a^{ENV}	Environmental dimension weight, without dimension
a^{ECOL}	Ecological dimension weight, without dimension
WFP_i	Water footprint in the resources dimension in farm i, m^3/kg
WFP_i^{blue}	Blue water footprint in farm i, m^3/kg
WFP_i^{green}	Green water footprint in farm i, m^3/kg
WFP_i^{grey}	Gray water footprint in farm i, m^3/kg
WC_i^{blue}	Blue water usage in farm i, m^3
WC_i^{green}	Green water usage in farm i, m^3
$Yield$	Total production in farm i, kg
A_i	Crop planting area in farm i, ha
$ET_{c,i}$	Actual evapotranspiration of crops in farm i, mm
PR_i	Precipitation in farm i, mm
Y_i	Yield per unit area in farm i, kg/ha
WC_i^{grey}	Grey water usage in farm i, m^3
θ	Nitrogen leaching coefficient, %
FER_i	Crop fertilizer usage in farm i, kg/ha
c_{nat}	Nitrate concentration under normal circumstances, mg/L
c_{max}	Maximum nitrate concentration, mg/L
ET_o	Reference evapotranspiration of crops, mm
K_s	Water stress coefficient of crops, without dimension
K_{cb}	Basic crop coefficient of crops, without dimension
K_e	Soil evaporation coefficient of crops, without dimension
ECO_i	The economic benefits in farm i in economic dimension, Yuan
P_i	Crop selling price in farm i, Yuan/kg
C_i	Crop planting costs in farm i, Yuan/ha, including seeds, fertilizers, pesticides, machinery, labor, etc.
CGF_i	Crop planting costs in farm i, Yuan/ha
CWF_i	Crop water cost in farm i, Yuan/ha
δ_i^{fe}	Crop fertilizer cost in farm i, Yuan/ha
δ_i^{pe}	Crop pesticide cost in farm i, Yuan/ha
δ_i^{ma}	Cost of crop machinery diesel in farm i, Yuan/ha
δ_i^{fil}	Cost of agricultural film for crops in farm i, Yuan/ha
δ_i^{se}	Crop seed cost in farm i, Yuan/ha
δ_i^{lab}	Labor cost of crops in farm i, Yuan/ha
WPR_i^{sur}	Surface water prices in farm i, Yuan/m^3
IQ_i^{sur}	Surface water irrigation quota in farm i, m^3/ha

Table 1. *Cont.*

Variable Symbol	Variable Interpretation
WPR_i^{gro}	Groundwater prices in farm i, Yuan/m^3
IQ_i^{gro}	Groundwater irrigation quota in farm i, m^3/ha
$Gini_i$	Gini coefficient in the social dimension in farm i
PO_i	Population in farm i, persons
CFP_i	Carbon footprint in the environmental dimension in farm i, kg CO_2-eq/ha
$CE_i^{CO_2}$	CO_2 emissions in farm i, kg CO_2-eq/ha
$CE_i^{N_2O}$	N_2O emissions in farm i, kg N_2O-eq/ha
$CE_i^{CH_4}$	CH_4 emissions in farm i, kg CH_4-eq/ha
SCS	CO_2 soil carbon sequestration in farm i, kg CO_2-eq/ha
PES_i	Pesticide dosage in farm i, kg/ha
DIE_i	Agricultural diesel consumption in farm i, kg/ha
ELE_i	Irrigation electricity consumption in farm i, kWh/ha
ε^{fer}	Carbon emission coefficient of fertilizers, kg CO_2-eq/kg
ε^{pes}	Carbon emission coefficient of pesticides, kg CO_2-eq/kg
ε^{die}	Carbon emission coefficient of agricultural diesel, kg CO_2-eq/kg
ε^{ele}	Carbon emission coefficient of irrigation electricity, kg CO_2-eq/kg
ς^{CH_4}	CH_4 emission coefficient of rice field, kg/ha
γ^{vol}	Nitrogen volatilization coefficient, %
ς^{fer}	N_2O emission coefficient in fertilizers, kg N_2O-eq/kg
ς^{vol}	N_2O emission coefficient of nitrogen volatilization in fertilizers, kg N_2O-eq/kg
ς^{leach}	N_2O emission coefficient of nitrogen leaching, kg N_2O-eq/kg
ς^{SCS}	Soil carbon sequestration rate, kg/ha
cef_i^{crop}	Ecological footprint of farmland in farm i, ha
cef_i^{ene}	Ecological footprint of fossil energy in farm i, ha
cef_i^{water}	Ecological footprint of freshwater resources in farm i, ha
$EECI_i$	Ecological coordination index in the ecological dimension, without dimension
CEF_i	Crop ecological footprint in farm i, ha
$CECC_i$	Ecological carrying capacity of crops in farm i, ha
γ^{crop}	Equivalent factor of farmland, without dimension
Y_{rice}	National rice yield per unit area, kg/ha
γ^{ene}	Equivalent factors of fossil fuels, without dimension
δ^{FER}	Conversion coefficient of fertilizer, without dimension
δ^{PES}	Conversion coefficient of pesticides, without dimension
δ^{FIL}	Conversion coefficient of agricultural film, without dimension
δ^{DIE}	Conversion coefficient of diesel, without dimension
δ^{ELE}	Conversion coefficient of electricity consumption, without dimension
γ^{water}	Equivalent factor of freshwater resources, without dimension
CV_c	Average calorific value of crops, J/T
FO	Global freshwater resources output capacity, J/M^3
FD	Global freshwater depth, m
η	Freshwater resources conversion coefficient
j	The energy index, with a total energy of J
PA_{ij}	Per capita ecological productivity area of energy j in farm i, ha
γ_{ij}	Equivalence factor of energy j in farm i, without dimension
y_{ij}	Yield factor of energy j in farm i, without dimension
β	Biodiversity coefficient, %

The agricultural water rights management model covers two key parts, namely initial water rights allocation and water rights trading, between which there is a relationship of mutual influence and restriction [13]. The initial water rights allocation directly affects the amount and frequency of water rights trading that can be conducted. Conversely, an increase in the volume of water rights trading may lead to a decrease in the initial water rights allocation. In order to determine the final allocation of initial water rights, the multi-dimensional agricultural water-saving potential evaluation system constructed in this study is used to conduct a comprehensive assessment of each region. The evaluation system comprehensively considers many factors and can reasonably allocate initial water rights and ensure the reasonable allocation of resources to meet the agricultural needs of each region.

The degree of correlation of an evaluation system can be measured by the degree of coupling, which is the tightness of multiple connections in the whole [24]. Therefore, the construction of the coordinated development degree model can reflect the level of sustainable coordinated development in various agricultural regions, evaluate the coordination degree of interaction and coupling among various dimensions, and reasonably evaluate the sustainable development level of water rights distribution in various regions [25]. It is composed of coupling degree model and comprehensive development index, and the formula is as follows [25]:

$$D_i = \sqrt{C_i \cdot T_i} \tag{23}$$

The calculated D_i are the data from 2015 to 2020. The intuitionistic fuzzy number is used to reflect the fuzziness, and the accuracy function is used to quantify the definite number and solve it (Section 2.6). Finally, D_i^* is obtained.

The concept of coupling is originally derived from capacity coupling in physics to describe how tightly different parts interact [26]. The coupling degree of this study realizes the dynamic correlation of coordinated development through the interaction and influence of the development indices of five dimensions, namely resources, society, economy, environment, and ecology, and can reflect the degree of interdependence and mutual restriction among the systems. The formula is as follows [26]:

$$C_i = \frac{F_i^{RES} \times F_i^{ECO} \times F_i^{SOC} \times F_i^{ENV} \times F_i^{ECOL}}{\left(\frac{F_i^{RES}+F_i^{ECO}+F_i^{SOC}+F_i^{ENV}+F_i^{ECOL}}{5}\right)^5} \tag{24}$$

Coordination degree refers to the degree of benign coupling in the coupling interaction relationship, which can reflect the quality of coordination [26]. It can be obtained by the weights corresponding to the five dimensions of development index of resources, economy, society, environment, and ecology. The formula is as follows [26]:

$$T = a^{RES} \times F_i^{RES} + a^{ECO} \times F_i^{ECO} + a^{SOC} \times F_i^{SOC} + a^{ENV} \times F_i^{ENV} + a^{ECOL} \times F_i^{ECOL} \tag{25}$$

2.4.1. Resource Dimension Index

Water footprint is an effective index to measure total water resources consumption [27]. Therefore, crop water footprint is included in the evaluation of agricultural water-saving potential rating index system. The crop water footprint family generally includes blue water footprint, green water footprint, and grey water footprint. In the resource dimension, multivariate water footprint is used to quantify the comprehensive consumption of water resources. The formula is as follows [28]:

$$F_i^{RES} = WFP_i = WFP_i^{blue} + WFP_i^{green} + WFP_i^{grey} \tag{26}$$

where WFP_i^{blue} is the blue water footprint of crops, that is, the amount of blue water absorbed from the soil during the growth of crops. Blue water refers to water resources in the surface and soil, usually supplied by deep water sources such as groundwater and rivers [28]. The larger the blue water footprint, the higher the utilization of blue water resources by crops, and the formula is as follows [28]:

$$WFP_i^{blue} = \frac{WC_i^{blue}}{Yield} = \frac{A_i \cdot \max\{0, ET_{c,i} - PR_i\}}{A_i \cdot Y_i} \tag{27}$$

WFP_i^{green} is crop green water footprint, which refers to the water resources stored by natural precipitation in soil and absorbed by crops [28]. The larger the green water footprint index, the higher the green water resources occupied by crops. The formula is as follows [28]:

$$WFP_i^{green} = \frac{WC_i^{green}}{Yield} = \frac{A_i \cdot \min\{ET_{c\_i}, PR_i\}}{A_i \cdot Y_i} \tag{28}$$

WFP_i^{grey} is the crop grey water footprint, that is, the amount of water required to absorb pollutant load according to water quality standards [28]. The formula is as follows:

$$WFP_i^{grey} = \frac{WC_i^{grey}}{Yield} = \frac{A_i \cdot \theta \cdot FER_i / (c_{\max} - c_{\text{nat}})}{A_i \cdot Y_i} \tag{29}$$

2.4.2. Economic Dimension Index

Agricultural economic benefit is the difference between agricultural production labor results and labor consumption, and is a metric to measure the economic distribution of agricultural water rights [29]. Here, labor achievements are mainly quantified by the economic income generated by the sale of crops, while labor consumption is mainly quantified by the economic cost of crops in the planting process. The cost composition involves water, seeds, fertilizers, pesticides, machinery, labor, and electricity consumption, etc. The formula is as follows [29]:

$$F_i^{ECO} = ECO_i = (P_i Y_i - C_i) A_i \tag{30}$$

$$C_i = CGF_i + CWF_i \tag{31}$$

$$CGF_i = A_i(\delta_i^{fe} + \delta_i^{pe} + \delta_i^{ma} + \delta_i^{fil} + \delta_i^{se} + \delta_i^{lab}) \tag{32}$$

$$CWF_i = WPR_i^{sur} \cdot IQ_i^{sur} \cdot A_i + WPR_i^{gro} \cdot IQ_i^{gro} \cdot A_i \tag{33}$$

2.4.3. Social Dimension Index

As a function reflecting objective equity, Gini coefficient can effectively measure the difference degree of agricultural water resources allocation between regions [30]. Therefore, the Gini coefficient is chosen as one of the indicators of social dimension. The Gini coefficient values are between 0 and 1, and the smaller the Gini coefficient values, the fairer the distribution is. The formula is as follows:

$$F^{SOC} = Gini_i = \frac{1}{2I\ A_i/PO_i} \sum_{l=1}^{I} \sum_{k=1}^{I} \left| \frac{A_l}{PO_l} - \frac{A_k}{PO_k} \right| \tag{34}$$

2.4.4. Environmental Dimension Index

Taking greenhouse gas emissions as an environmental dimension indicator, the aim is to minimize greenhouse gases produced in the process of agricultural production [31]. Therefore, in this study, greenhouse gas emissions are selected as the environmental dimension index for accounting, and the calculation formula is as follows [31]:

$$F_i^{ENV} = CFP_i = \frac{CE_i^{CO_2} + 298CE_i^{N_2O} + 25CE_i^{CH_4} - SCS_i}{A_i \cdot Y_i} \tag{35}$$

where CO_2 emissions mainly come from agricultural inputs, including fertilization, pesticide application, agricultural diesel, etc. The calculation formula is as follows [31]:

$$CE_i^{CO_2} = A_i\left(\varepsilon^{fer} \cdot FER_i + \varepsilon^{pes} \cdot PES_i + \varepsilon^{die} \cdot DIE_i + \varepsilon^{ele} \cdot ELE_i\right) \tag{36}$$

CH_4 emissions are mainly from rice fields, and the calculation formula is as follows:

$$CE_i^{CH_4} = A_i \cdot \varsigma^{CH_4} \tag{37}$$

N_2O emissions are mainly from soil emissions and emissions from fertilizer application, and the calculation formula is as follows:

$$CE_i^{N_2O} = A_i \cdot FER_i \cdot \left(\varsigma^{fer} + \gamma^{vol} \cdot \varsigma^{vol} + \theta \cdot \varsigma^{leach} \right) \tag{38}$$

Carbon fixation can be estimated using empirical coefficients, calculated by the following formula:

$$SCS = A_i \cdot \varsigma^{SCS} \tag{39}$$

2.4.5. Ecological Dimension Index

Agricultural water-saving potential is closely related to ecological benefits, and excessive water saving will lead to regional ecological degradation crisis [32]. The ecological coordination index mainly reflects the coordination degree between regional ecological environment and social and economic development. The closer the ecological coordination index is to 1.414, the better the coordination is. On the contrary, the closer the ecological coordination index value is to 1, the lower the coordination. The ecological index consists of two parts: one is ecological footprint; the other part is ecological carrying capacity [32].

$$F_i^{ECOL} = EECI_i = \frac{CEF_i + CECC}{\sqrt{CEF_i^2 + CECC^2}} \tag{40}$$

The research mainly focuses on the quantification of ecological footprint in the agricultural field. The formula for calculating ecological footprint is as follows [32]:

$$CEF_i = cef_i^{crop} + cef_i^{ene} + cef_i^{water} \tag{41}$$

$$cef_i^{crop} = \gamma^{crop} \frac{A_i \cdot Y_i}{Y_{rice}} \tag{42}$$

$$cef_i^{ene} = \gamma^{ene} \cdot \frac{\left(FER_i \cdot \delta^{FER} + PES_i \cdot \delta^{PES} + FIL_i \cdot \delta^{FIL} + DIE_i \cdot \delta^{DIE} + ELE_i \cdot \delta^{ELE} \right)}{\varepsilon} \cdot cef^{crop} \tag{43}$$

$$cef_i^{water} = \gamma_{water} \frac{A_i \cdot Y_i \cdot CV}{\eta \cdot FO \cdot FD} \tag{44}$$

The formula for ecological carrying capacity is as follows:

$$CECC = (1 - \beta) \times PO \times \sum_{i=1}^{I} \sum_{j=1}^{J} (PA_{ij} \times \gamma_{ij} \times y_{ij}) \tag{45}$$

2.5. System Dynamics (SD)

Future climate change will affect the calculation results of water-saving potential. SD model is used to simulate the driving parameters of agricultural water-saving evaluation system in various dimensions of resources, economy, society, environment, and ecology. The core idea of SD is to study the dynamic connection between various elements within the whole system [33]. Compared to other methods, SD has the outstanding advantage that it can accurately represent the behavior and performance of a system without prior inspection and testing of the system [34]. In the evaluation of agricultural water-saving potential system, the application of SD has shown great potential. By constructing the SD model, the detailed simulation and comprehensive simulation analysis of each key driving factor in the multi-dimensional evaluation system of agricultural water-saving potential can be realized, and then the dynamic evolution process of the system can be fully grasped. Through the operation and adjustment of the model, various potential impacts of agricultural water-saving potential under different future environmental change conditions can be predicted.

SD Simulation Modeling Procedure

To build an SD model, follow these steps to ensure its integrity [34].

1. Identify problem and system boundaries:
   (1) Choose the problem: Clearly define the problem to be solved, including the background and cause of the problem.
   (2) Key variables: Identify the key variables involved, considering the interrelationships between these variables and related concepts.
   (3) Time frame: Clarify the time dimension of the problem, including history, present, and future time periods.
   (4) Reference model: Analyze historical data and behavior of key variables to understand past trends and expected future behavior of the system.
2. Propose dynamic hypothesis:
   (1) Examine existing theories and research to understand how to explain the dynamic behavior of problems.
   (2) Propose the dynamic change hypothesis based on the internal feedback structure of the system.
   (3) Draw diagrams based on initial assumptions, key variables, reference models, and other available data, including system boundary diagrams, subsystem diagrams, causal loop diagrams, stock flow diagrams, policy structure diagrams, etc.
3. Write an equation:
   (1) Master decision rules.
   (2) Specify parameters, behavior relationships, and initial conditions.
   (3) Check if the target is consistent with the boundary.
4. Conduct test:
   (1) Comparison with reference models: Assess whether the model adequately reproduces past behavior patterns.
   (2) Robustness analysis under extreme conditions: In extreme cases, verify if the model's behavior results are consistent with reality.
   (3) Sensitivity analysis: Study how sensitive the model is to parameters, initial conditions, boundaries, and model assumptions.

2.6. Intuitionistic Fuzzy Number

Parameter input is required during MCO-AWR-WPRCE construction. Uncertainty and imprecision of input parameters are unavoidable. The constructed MCO-AWR-WPRCE involves many factors such as natural conditions, socio-economic conditions, and human activities, which leads to multi-factor uncertainties in the research process. In the determination of parameters, due to changes in the environment and policies, some parameters lack clear data boundaries, and data information will be omitted if expressed with definite numbers, such as coordinated development degree, crop yield, planting cost, initial water rights allocation, and other parameters change in different times. Intuitionistic fuzzy numbers have more flexible modeling capabilities, stronger interpretability, stronger reasoning ability, and comprehensive integration of uncertainty and fuzzy effects on data [35]. Therefore, intuitionistic fuzzy numbers are used to deal with the uncertainty of the input data of MCO-AWR-WPRCE. However, the intuitionistic fuzzy number method is introduced to transform the time series data into a fuzzy data set, and the mathematical method of precision function can effectively transform the fuzzy data set into the final value.

In 1965, Zadeh proposed fuzzy set theory [36], and then Atannassov proposed the concept of intuitive fuzzy sets [37]. The proposed intuitionistic fuzzy set admits that data have contradictory attributes, which makes the description of data attributes more comprehensive and the performance ability more prominent. In fuzzy decision theory, intuitionistic fuzzy numbers are used to describe the attributes of decision units. In order to consider the fuzzy multi-attribute decision problem, it is necessary to rank the advantages and disadvantages of the intuitionistic fuzzy numbers, and compare the sizes through the precision function, whose basic formula is referred to in [38].

2.7. Sensitivity Analysis and Harmonicity Model

To investigate the impact of various factors on the model's objectives, we conducted sensitivity analysis for each parameter. A sensitivity threshold of $|\text{sensitivity}| \geq 0.1$ was employed, where values exceeding this threshold indicate significant influence on the system and close correlation, while values below it suggest minor influence and relative insensitivity. Furthermore, sensitivity analysis reveals both positive and negative sensitivities. A positive value signifies that the variable and parameter change in the same direction, meaning an increase or decrease in the parameter results in a corresponding increase or decrease in the variable. Conversely, a negative value indicates an inverse relationship between the variable and parameter.

$$S = (\Delta x)/(\Delta y) \tag{46}$$

where S is a sensitive result; (Δx) is the change value of independent variable (parameter) and (Δy) is the change value of dependent variable (multi-objective result).

This study used a two-line average indicator to gain insight into the trade-off between system economic, environmental, and social effects by crop pattern adjustment, and harmony degree was used to express their comprehensive effect on system sustainability, as follows:

$$EES = \frac{1}{2}(Econ \cdot Ene + Ene \cdot Res + Res \cdot Econ)\sin 120^{\circ} \tag{47}$$

The EES metric integrates three main indices of economic ($Econ$)—energy (Ene)—resources (Res).

3. Applications

3.1. Study Area

To verify the feasibility of building MCO-AWR-WPRCE, a real-world case study is used. The case study involves the XKH irrigation area, located in Mishan and Hulin, Heilongjiang province, with geographical coordinates of 132°45′–133°17′ east longitude and 45°01′–45°41′ north latitude. The irrigation area is adjacent to Songacha River and Wusuli River, north to BWL farm Tongsan Highway and Dalian Baohe River, west to Xiaohei River. There are five farms in the region: BWL farm, BWQ farm, BWB farm, QF farm, and XKH farm. The total area is 2.36×10^4 ha, with 2.11×10^4 ha of arable land (0.63×10^4 ha of paddy field and 1.48×10^4 ha of dry field) currently available. The five farms under study are state-owned farms, which have management areas, operation stations, and forest farms. Now it has developed into an all-round development of agriculture, forestry, animal husbandry, sideline, and fishery; the national important commodity grain base, which is integrated with science, education, culture, health, and sports, has gradually developed into a specialized farm with rice cultivation as the leading industry. The irrigated area has a continental monsoon climate in the middle and temperate zone, with a large variation in the range of cold and hot air and frequent invasion by cold air. The average annual precipitation is 565 mm, the reference evapotranspiration is 1240 mm, the precipitation distribution is extremely uneven, and the average annual temperature is 2.8 °C, as shown in Figure 3. Five farms have perfect irrigation channels and water diversion and drainage facilities, but the extensive management of water resources leads to the waste of water resources, so XKH irrigation area is selected for water resources management. The above information was obtained through field investigation.

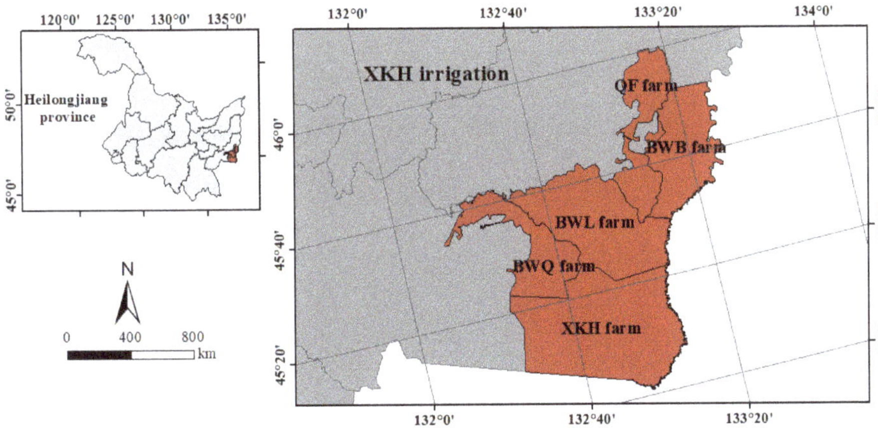

Figure 3. Overview of the XKH irrigation.

3.2. Model Parameters and Data

MCO-AWR-WPRCE data mainly include the following categories: socio-economic-related parameters, energy-related data, and hydrometeorological-related data. Data sources include China Geospatial Data Cloud, China Earth System Science Data Sharing Network, China Meteorological Science Data Sharing Service network, feasibility study report of XKH irrigation area, planning report, and field investigation.

3.2.1. MCO-AWR-WPRCE-Related Data

The MCO-AWR-WPRCE input includes data on economic targets, energy consumption, and water use efficiency, as shown in Tables 2 and 3. The planting cost of each farm in the XKH irrigation area is 7716.89 Yuan/ha, the transportation price is 0.48 Yuan/m^3, and the current water price is 0.003 Yuan/m^3. The maximum and minimum constraints for irrigation water are 4500 m^3/ha and 2500 m^3/ha, respectively. The coordination degree is obtained by solving the model established in Section 2.3, and the initial allocation of water rights in various regions can be determined by the coordination development degree. The above data are all from the field investigation and feasibility study report of the XKH irrigation area.

Table 2. Economy-related parameters.

Name Unit	Crop Price Yuan/kg	Engineering Water Prices Yuan/m^3	Environmental Cost Yuan/m^3	Selling Water Price Yuan/m^3
BWL farm	4.36	0.077	0.013	0.093
BWQ farm	4.57	0.039	0.016	0.057
BWB farm	5.37	0.043	0.012	0.059
QF farm	4.49	0.035	0.012	0.050
XKH farm	3.71	0.048	0.012	0.062

Table 3. Society-related parameters.

Name Unit	Area ha	Water Rights Allocation m^3/ha	Yield kg/ha	Coordinated Development Degree Di	Initial Water Rights m^3/ha
BWL farm	57,453	3001	9585	0.80	2411.90
BWQ farm	28,927	2580	9196	1.52	3924.06
BWB farm	32,627	3247	8713	0.44	1443.82
QF farm	26,600	3451	8751	0.99	3431.69
XKH farm	35,813	3451	8817	1.24	4266.96

3.2.2. Rating Model-Related Data

The weight values of a^{RES}, a^{ECO}, a^{SOC}, a^{ENV}, and a^{ECOL} in each dimension of the model are 0.2. The SD model is used to simulate the driving parameters of the agricultural water-saving evaluation system in the dimensions of resources, economy, society, environment, and ecology. The above data are all from the field investigation and feasibility study report of the XKH irrigation area. Social dimension parameters are simulated by data from 2011 to 2019, and other dimension data are simulated by data from 2015 to 2019, as shown in Tables 4–7.

Table 4. SD model simulation parameters—society dimension.

	Time	2011	2012	2013	2014	2015	2016	2017	2018	2019	Unit
	Actual evapotranspiration	632	615	633	636	699	647	718	745	790	mm
BWL farm	Precipitation	573	603	573	464	584	865	642	653	985	mm
	Fertilizing amount	227	275	250	227	206	139	138	146	168	kg/ha
	Actual evapotranspiration	632	615	633	636	699	647	718	745	790	mm
BWQ farm	Precipitation	573	603	573	464	584	865	642	653	985	mm
	Fertilizing amount	228	276	251	228	207	182	234	253	135	kg/ha
	Actual evapotranspiration	632	615	633	636	699	647	718	745	790	mm
BWB farm	Precipitation	573	603	573	464	584	865	642	653	985	mm
	Fertilizing amount	166	200	182	166	151	164	202	151	134	kg/ha
	Actual evapotranspiration	632	615	633	636	699	647	718	745	790	mm
QF farm	Precipitation	573	603	573	464	584	865	642	653	985	mm
	Fertilizing amount	187	226	206	187	170	121	116	121	136	kg/ha
	Actual evapotranspiration	632	615	633	636	699	647	718	745	790	mm
XKH farm	Precipitation	573	603	573	464	584	865	642	653	985	mm
	Fertilizing amount	141	171	155	141	128	492	492	257	372	kg/ha

Table 5. SD model simulation parameters—economic dimension.

	BWL Farm		BWQ Farm		BWB Farm		QF Farm		XKH Farm	
	Yield (kg/ha)	Crop Price (Yuan/kg)	Yield (kg/ha)	Crop Price (Yuan/kg)	Yield (kg/ha)	Crop Price (Yuan/kg)	Yield (kg/ha)	Crop Price (Yuan/kg)	Yield (kg/ha)	Crop Price (Yuan/kg)
2015	9375	3.55	9195	3.72	8895	4.36	8700	3.59	9060	2.77
2016	9200	4.93	9179	5.15	8881	6.04	8850	4.97	8700	3.84
2017	9304	2.54	9742	2.73	9022	3.3	9150	2.6	9405	3.38
2018	12366	3.45	9138	3.68	7966	4.26	8669	3.87	7580	3.13
2019	8934	6.44	9136	6.73	8632	7.89	8668	6.5	9191	5.02
2020	8957	5.62	8868	5.88	8708	6.89	8640	5.68	8775	4.39

Table 6. SD model simulation parameters—environmental dimension.

	BWL Farm		BWQ Farm		BWB Farm		QF Farm		XKH Farm	
	Pesticide Dosage (kg/ha)	Diesel Oil Consumption (kg/ha)	Pesticide Dosage (kg/ha)	Diesel Oil Consumption (kg/ha)	Pesticide Dosage (kg/ha)	Diesel Oil Consumption (kg/ha)	Pesticide Dosage (kg/ha)	Diesel Oil Consumption (kg/ha)	Pesticide Dosage (kg/ha)	Diesel Oil Consumption (kg/ha)
2015	4.08	0.12	2.36	0.12	8.69	0.1	4.68	0.08	1.74	0.09
2016	3.87	0.16	2.34	0.13	8.44	0.1	5.85	0.07	1.73	0.09
2017	3.75	0.16	2.28	0.13	8.44	0.1	5	0.07	1.73	0.09
2018	3.83	0.15	2.22	0.12	8.44	0.1	5.78	0.06	1.73	0.09
2019	4.54	0.14	7.15	0.12	9.91	0.11	5.99	0.07	3.41	0.09
2020	4.35	0.14	7.07	0.1	9.32	0.11	5.94	0.08	3.43	0.09

After establishing the system dynamics model, it is crucial to assess its validity. This entails testing the model's accuracy by comparing historical data with simulation results to determine their consistency and gauging the reliability of the model. Subsequent to the system dynamics model test, evaluating the model is essential to ensure the precision of its parameter calculations [39,40]. The root mean square error (RMSE) method is employed for this evaluation.

Table 7. SD model simulation parameters—social dimension.

	BWL Farm	BWQ Farm	BWB Farm	QF Farm	XKH Farm
			Total Population (Person)		
2015	20,497	17,113	12,707	13,483	9702
2016	20,931	17,280	13,585	13,584	12,814
2017	20,765	17,210	14,332	13,670	12,736
2018	21,881	17,092	14,930	13,708	12,736
2019	22,722	17,337	15,362	13,643	9017

4. Results

4.1. SD Prediction Result

The evaluation system of agricultural water-saving potential is a comprehensive multi-dimensional system, including five sub-systems of resources, economy, society, environment, and ecology. In order to better evaluate the water-saving potential of each region, the evaluation system consists of 69 variables, which interact with each other and jointly affect the calculation of agricultural water-saving potential, as shown in Figure 4. Among them, the effective irrigated area, total population, grain output value, carbon emission, and ecological footprint are state variables. Population increase, population decrease, carbon emission increase, carbon emission reduction, biological footprint increase, and farmland area change are rate variables. Fertilizer consumption and grain yield are auxiliary variables. The fertilizer conversion coefficient and land balance factor are constants. It can be clearly seen from the figure that there are intricate internal connections among various dimensions. For example, the total population can be quantified not only by the value of the Gini coefficient, but also by the calculation of the ecological footprint.

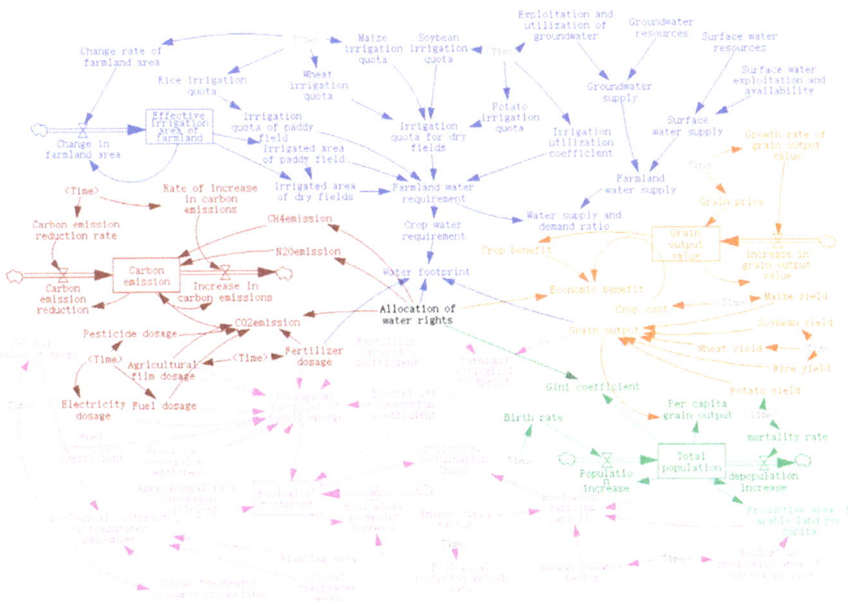

Figure 4. Multi-dimensional evaluation of SD flow charts. Note: Blue represents the environmental dimension, red represents the resource dimension, pink represents the economic dimension, green represents the social dimension, and yellow represents the ecological dimension, Gray is the starting point of each dimension and has no practical significance.

In this study, the SD model is used to model and predict each parameter variable in the multi-dimensional agricultural water-saving potential evaluation system. In the resource dimension, the SD model chooses 2011 as the starting time of model operation, and 2011–2019 as the time of the model operation and actual test. In the dimensions of economy, environment, and society, the SD model chooses 2015 as the starting time of the model operation, and 2015–2020 is used to test the correctness of the model, as shown in Figure 5. Since the parameters of the ecological dimension do not have long historical series values, the current annual data are used to calculate in the model.

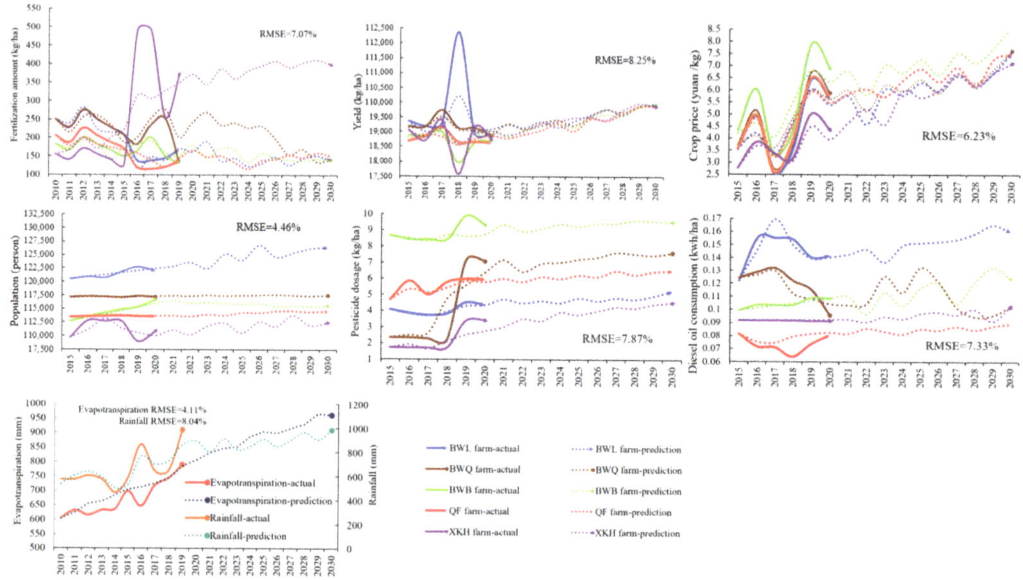

Figure 5. Water allocation map after model optimization. Note: Crop growth period 1–5 refers to the dividing stage, jointing stage, heading stage, milk-ripening stage, and yellow-ripening stage of rice.

The error of the simulation results is controlled within 10%, which verifies the reliability of the model. In the resource dimension, key indicators such as actual evapotranspiration, precipitation, and fertilizer application are selected for simulation prediction. Compared with the historical values, it can be seen that the actual evapotranspiration, precipitation, and fertilizer application showed a gradual upward trend, among which the change trend of actual evapotranspiration is relatively gentle, and the change trend relatively between the historical minimum actual evapotranspiration and the predicted maximum actual evapotranspiration is 56.81%. The variation frequency between the historical minimum precipitation and the predicted maximum precipitation is 70.25%. In the economic dimension, the output and crop price are selected to simulate the forecast, and the output and crop price show a gradually rising trend. Yields vary from 6.67% to 14.94%, with different farms varying in frequency. The change trend of the crop price shows a wave growth, with a range of 83.68% to 152.39%. In the social dimension, the index of the population number is selected for the simulation prediction. The variation range of the population number of each farm is between 11.29% and 46.36%, indicating that the change frequency of the population flow is also different in different farms due to their different development. This difference is closely related to the economic development of each farm. Farms with higher economic benefits have greater demand for personnel and greater adhesion to talents. Conversely, farms with lower economic benefits have lower adhesion to talents. In the environmental dimension, pesticide consumption and diesel oil consumption are simulated. The variation range of pesticide consumption is 9.29% to

239.42%, and that of diesel oil is 10.16% to 34.74%. The amount of pesticide and diesel oil shows a gradually increasing trend, and there are obvious differences among different farms. The change trend of pesticide consumption first increases and then decreases, and finally tends to a stable growth trend.

4.2. Resource, Economic, Environmental, Social, and Ecological Dimensions Evaluation System Results Analysis

Coordinated development degree D is a standard for evaluating the level of coordinated development among five dimensions of resources, economy, society, environment, and ecology. The obtained coordinated development degree of the evaluation system is analyzed according to the criteria in Table 8.

Table 8. Degree of coordinated development D.

Coordinated Development Level	0.9–1.00	0.8–0.9	0.7–0.8	0.6–0.7	0.5–0.6	0.4–0.5	0–0.4
Coordination level	High-quality coordination	Good coordination	Intermediate coordination	Primary coordination	Barely coordination	Borderline disorder	Imbalance

According to the constructed evaluation system, the coordinated development degree of each dimension index in different periods can be calculated, as shown in Figure 6. By analyzing the data results from 2015 to 2020, the average coordinated development degree of each farm and the average growth proportion of each year can be obtained. During this period, the average coordinated development degrees of the five farms are 0.25, 0.47, 0.15, 0.31, and 0.39, respectively. It can be seen that the development status of different farms is quite different. Among them, the BWQ farm has maintained a high level of coordinated development degree, and the BWB farm, although the annual average is the lowest, continues to rise, and its growth rate ranks first among the five farms. Among them, the coordinated development degree of the XKH farm is relatively high and in a positive growth state, with a growth rate of 5.98%. In contrast, the coordinated development degrees of the BWB or BWL farms are relatively low, but their growth rates are high, and they are in a state of positive development. Overall, all five farms are in a state of uncoordination or near uncoordination. To this end, farm managers need to always adhere to the scientific development concept, attach importance to and give play to the unique advantages of each farm in different leading industries and resources fields, and optimize the layout on this basis to achieve the coordinated improvement of economic, social, and environmental benefits. In the process of promoting sustainable agricultural development, factors such as population change and ecological environmental protection should also be taken into account to formulate more scientific and rational development plans and policies.

4.3. Analysis of Water Rights Trading Scheme

MCO-AWR-WPRCE considers the influence of the trading distance of water rights on the allocation of water rights, and realizes the efficient allocation of water resources. By minimizing trading distance constraints, the model achieves efficient water rights allocation and energy consumption savings. MCO-AWR-WPRCE not only helps save energy consumption, but also helps improve the economic benefits of agricultural water rights. As shown in Figure 6, through model optimization, it is found that the use of water rights in the BWL and the BWB farm is in a relatively tight state, and water rights need to be purchased from other farms to meet their agricultural development needs. The amount of water rights purchased by the BWL farm is 5.06×10^6 m^3, and the amount of water rights purchased by the BWB farm is 2.48×10^7 m^3 and 9.98×10^6 m^3, respectively, from the QF farm and the XKH farm, in Figure 7. However, the BWL farm, the QF farm and the XKH farm do not carry out water rights trading because the initial water rights provided by them are greater than the water rights demanded under the boundary conditions of the model.

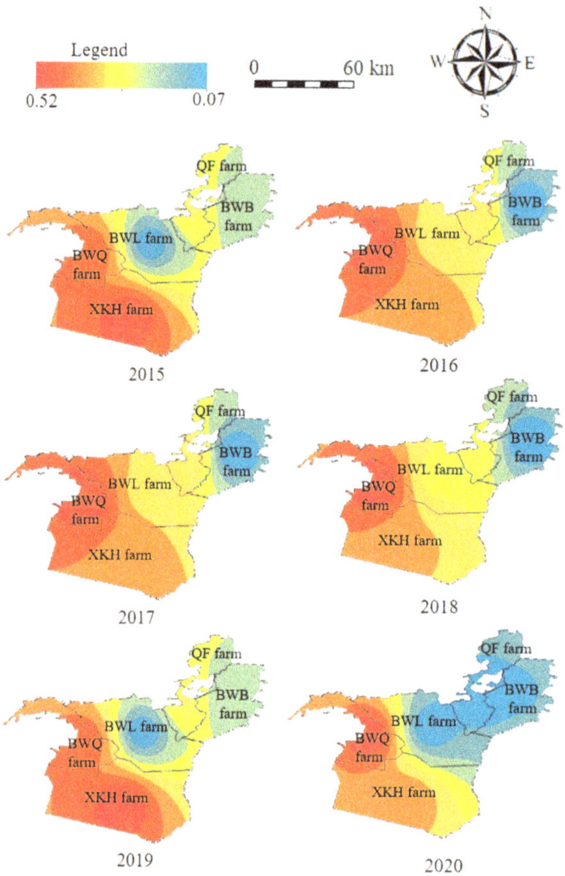

Figure 6. Calculation results of coordinated development degree of each farm from 2015 to 2020.

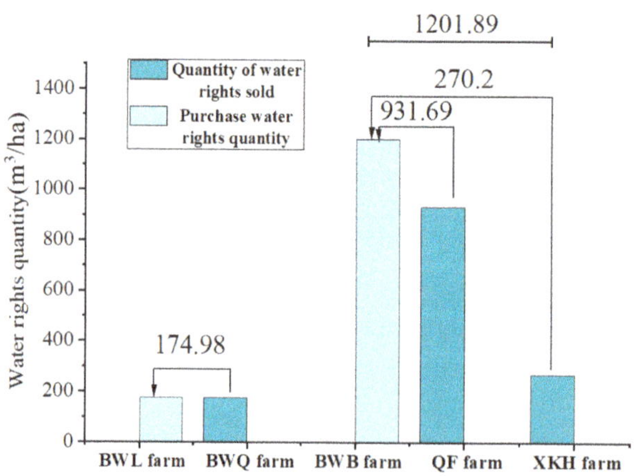

Figure 7. Water rights allocation schemes for individual farms.

4.4. Objective Function Result Analysis

Based on the water rights trading scheme, this study studied the optimal tradeoff model between multiple objectives such as economic benefit, energy consumption, and water use efficiency, and explored the impact of water rights trading on water resources management and agricultural production. In this chapter, the direct fuzzy number processing method is used to solve each target, and a series of data about each farm is obtained, as shown in Figure 8. Through comparative analysis, it is found that the total economic benefit of the BWL farm is the highest, which is 1.95×10^9 Yuan, while that of the QF farm is the lowest, which is 8.42×10^8 Yuan; the economic benefit per unit area of the BWQ farm is the highest, which is 3.82×10^4 Yuan/ha, and the lowest is the Ba Wuba farm, at only 2.50×10^4 Yuan/ha. The reasons for these differences are mainly the differences in the planting area and the degree of coordinated development of each farm. The BWQ farm has the highest total energy consumption and the lowest energy consumption per unit area, while the BWB farm has the lowest total energy consumption and the highest energy consumption per unit area. This is mainly because energy consumption considers the initial allocation of water rights and the energy allocation of water rights trading. The highest water use efficiency is 1.95 kg/m^3 in the BWL farm, and the lowest is in the BWB farm, at only 1.84 kg/m^3. The differences in each indicator confirm the differences in the management of water rights between farms. On this basis, this study further discusses the impact of water rights trading on water resources management and agricultural production in irrigated areas. Through comparison, it is found that the total economic benefit of each farm increased by 2.25% and the water interest efficiency increased by 7.43% compared with the actual situation. This indicates that water rights trading can reduce agricultural water use and increase agricultural benefit value on the premise of ensuring agricultural production. Therefore, the introduction of a water rights trading model in the management of water rights in irrigated areas can provide valuable insights for current and future water resources management. Water rights trading can reduce agricultural water use and increase agricultural benefit value on the premise of ensuring agricultural production. This is of great significance to the practice of water right management in irrigated areas.

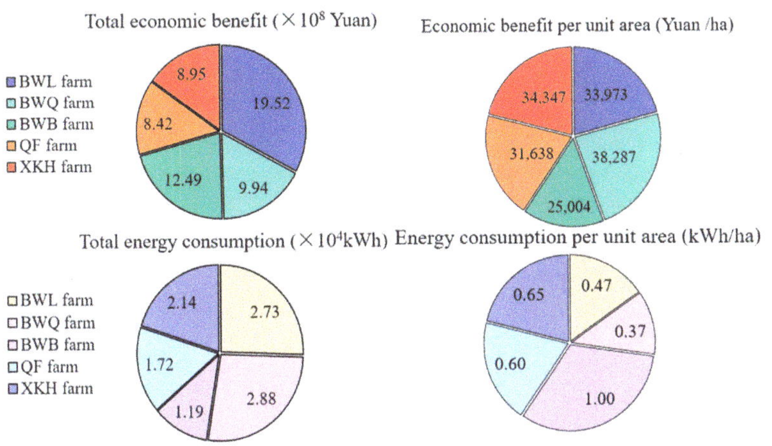

Figure 8. Individual farm energy target results.

4.5. Analysis of Coordinated Development Degree under Future Change

The research predicts the future coordinated development degree of agriculture from 2021 to 2030, as shown in Figure 9. The average coordinated development degree of the five farms from 2021 to 2025 is between 0.13 and 0.47. And the average annual growth rate is between −18.46% and 3.93%. The comparison shows that the coordinated development degree of the BWL farm continues to decline, while the coordinated development degree of the BWQ farm shows a trend of first stability and then decline. Although the overall development of the BWQ farm is still the most balanced among the five farms, its downward trend needs to be vigilant. However, the BWB farm, the QF farm, and the XKH farm all show a trend of first increase and then decrease. Among them, the coordinated development degree of the BWB farm is the lowest, while the coordinated development degree of the XKH farm is the highest. On the whole, there are still great contradictions and problems in the balance between resources, economy, society, environment, and ecology in the five farms. Overall, significant contradictions and challenges persist in achieving a balanced equilibrium among resources, economy, society, environment, and ecology within the five major farms. This underscores the imperative for farm managers to actively promote coordinated development across multiple dimensions while concurrently reinforcing organic coordination among various facets, all while ensuring sustained harmony within their respective systems. Such efforts are essential to engendering a synergistic and interactive momentum, facilitating the sustainable and coordinated advancement of agriculture across multiple dimensions. In light of this, farm managers must steadfastly adhere to the principles of scientific development. They should prioritize and leverage the unique strengths of each farm within diverse leading industries and resource domains. Building upon this foundation, they can optimize operational layouts and continually refine industrial structures. Through these measures, the coordinated enhancement of economic, social, and environmental outcomes can be realized.

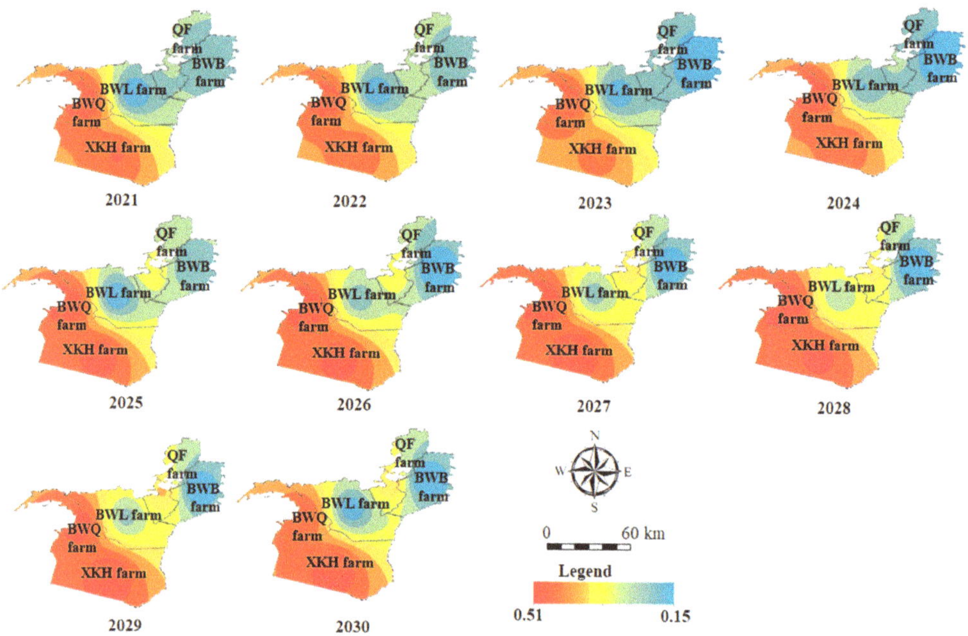

Figure 9. Calculation results of the coordinated development degree of each farm in 2021–2030.

4.6. Analysis of Water Rights Trading under Changing Environment

The changing environment in the future will have a significant impact on MCO-AWR-WPRCE. The SD model is used to simulate and forecast the evaluation indicators, and the coordinated development degree of each farm in 2021–2030 is obtained. The results are brought into MCO-AWR-WPRCE, and the results of water rights trading under future change scenarios are obtained, as shown in Figure 10. In 2021–2030, the BWL farm has been in a state of water shortage, and the situation continues to grow. The priority of purchasing water rights is as follows: the BWQ farm, then the XKH farm. In 2021, the initial water rights of the farm can meet the farm demand, but in 2022–2030, the initial water rights allocation gradually fails to meet the farm's water demand, and it begins to purchase water rights from other farms. The priority levels of water rights purchased by the BWB farm are as follows: the QF farm, then the XKH farm. In the period of 2021–2030, the initial water rights allocation of the BWQ farm, the QF farm, and the XKH farm can always meet the needs of their own agricultural development, and the surplus water rights can be sold to obtain additional economic benefits.

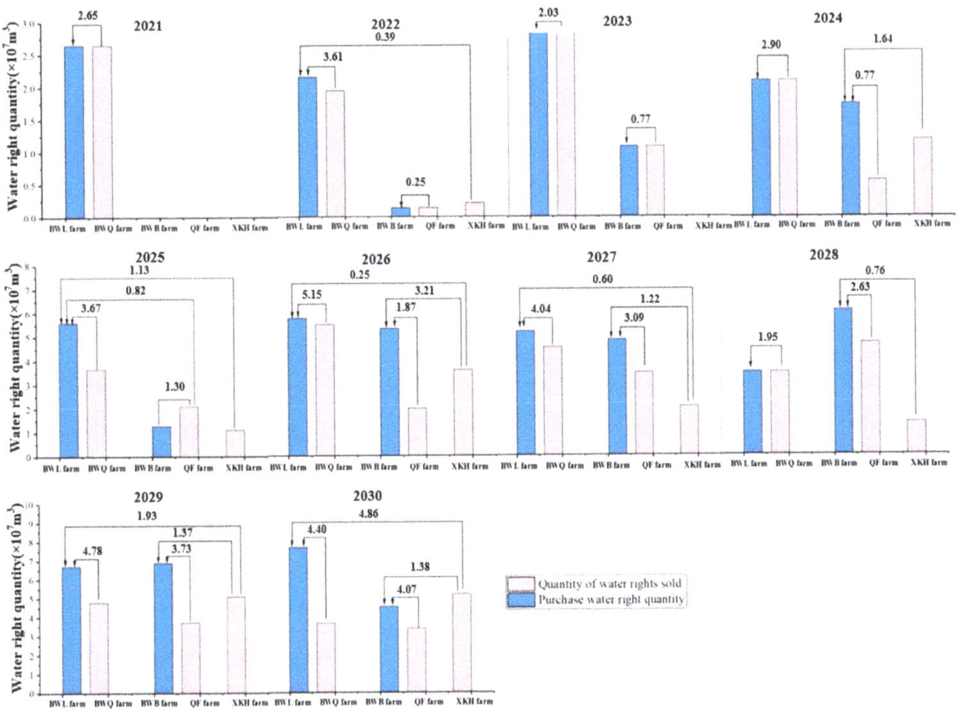

Figure 10. Results of water rights trading by farms in 2021–2030.

5. Discussion

At present, some studies try to take the local water shortage level as the basis to improve the water price model, and they are only limited to calculating the regional average water availability. These models are restricted by the current regional supervision water price paradigm [41,42]. In addition, in the current water price paradigm, all stations in a specific administrative unit will share the same charging standard. This price system violates the fair principle of sustainable development of water resources. Therefore, the whole water price model is adopted in the pricing process of water resources, and the trading distance of water rights in various regions is considered. It is reasonable to bring these factors into the pricing process, which can express the principle of fairness and rationality.

Among the parameters, the initial water right allocation weight exhibits the highest positive sensitivity to the optimization model (sensitivity = 4.31), indicating a substantial impact. Conversely, the water right transaction distance demonstrates the most prominent negative sensitivity to the optimization model (sensitivity = −1.63), in Table 9. While parameters of other coefficient types show correlations, their influence is comparatively weaker. To assess the overall sustainability of the model, considering the comprehensive development level of the economy, resource utilization efficiency, and energy consumption, we employed the harmony model. The harmony model calculated an initial harmony degree of 0.32, reflecting the balance between economy, resource utilization efficiency, and energy consumption. Following optimization, the harmony degree of the model increased to 0.41, indicating enhanced overall sustainability and improved comprehensive benefits. These findings underscore the positive impact of model optimization on sustainability metrics, signifying an advancement in the balanced development of economy, resource utilization efficiency, and energy consumption.

Table 9. Sensitivity result.

Variable	Sensitivity Result
Initial water right weight	4.31
Cost	−0.001
Price	−0.01
Water right transaction distance	−1.63
Yield	3.94
Planting area	2.85
Water availability coefficient	2.54

A key assumption of the model is that the transfer of water resources is affected by distance, and the energy consumption of water resources cannot be ignored in the process of transfer. In existing research, it is assumed that a virtual water bank will sell the surplus water resources from various areas to the water bank, and water-deficient areas will buy water rights from the water bank to achieve water savings. However, the water bank is merely a conceptual entity, providing only a theoretical basis for the process of water rights transactions. Additionally, there is no consideration of energy and resource consumption in the process of buying and selling water rights through the water bank, which does not align with reality. In this study, the channel is considered as the network for water rights trading, and the consumption of energy and resources in the process of water rights trading is taken into account, providing a robust theoretical foundation for the actual implementation of water rights trading schemes. Moreover, the theoretical model is analyzed using the actual irrigation area XHK, yielding positive results in terms of improved water resource utilization and economic benefits.

In this paper, the MCO-AWR-WPRCE model is proposed, and the model is studied on the scale of the irrigation area. Although this work is meaningful to all aspects of environmental management, some limitations need to be solved in the future. Secondly, the proposed MCO-AWR-WPRCE model has a strong connection with the current water price system, which is based on the overall rationality of the current water price system. The current water price system in the study area may have limitations. For example, the current system only considers the water price cost of agricultural water, which may be at a low level for the water price setting of industry and the service industry. In future studies, the researchers can adjust the model for specific regions and analyze the possibility of more water sources and treatment for the various processes of water intake, transport, use, and drainage.

6. Conclusions

In this study, an optimization model framework of agricultural water rights management based on a multi-dimensional evaluation system is constructed. The biggest highlight of this paper is to build a sound system of assessment and optimization of sustainable management of agricultural water rights under the environment of multiple uncertainties of the hydrological environment and management system and to weigh the economic benefits, energy consumption, and water use efficiency of agricultural water rights trading. The synergistic effects of multiple dimensions such as resources, economy, society, environment, and ecology on the initial allocation of water rights are quantified. The model is applied to the XKH irrigation area in Heilongjiang province, northeast China. The main conclusions are as follows:

(1) The use of water rights in the farms of BWL and BWB is in a relatively tight state, and water rights need to be purchased from other farms to meet their agricultural development needs. The transfer of water rights will tend to areas with higher comprehensive benefits and higher sustainable development level.
(2) The total economic benefit of each farm increased by 2.25% compared with the actual situation, and the water interest efficiency increased by 7.43%. The improved benefits indicate that MCO-AWR-WPRCE can improve agricultural water efficiency and increase economic benefits.
(3) In the case of future changes, the BWL farm has always been in a state of water shortage, and purchases water rights from the BWQ farm and the XKH farm. The initial water rights allocated by the BWB farm in 2021 can meet its own requirements, and then it needs to purchase water rights from the QF farm and the XKH farm to meet its own development needs.

Author Contributions: Conceptualization, L.S. and H.W.; methodology, L.S.; software, L.S.; validation, H.W.; formal analysis, L.D.; investigation, H.W.; resources, L.S.; data curation, L.S.; writing—original draft preparation, L.S.; writing—review and editing, H.W.; visualization, L.S.; supervision, H.W.; project administration, H.W.; funding acquisition, L.D. All authors have read and agreed to the published version of the manuscript.

Funding: This research was funded by Heilongjiang Province Postdoctoral Research Launch Fund, grant number LHB-Q16008.

Data Availability Statement: The original contributions presented in this study are included in the article; further inquiries can be directed to the corresponding author.

Conflicts of Interest: The authors declare no conflicts of interest.

References

1. Zhang, Q.; Shen, J.S.; Sun, F.H. Spatiotemporal differentiation of coupling coordination degree between economic development and water environment and its influencing factors using GWR in China's province. *Ecol. Model.* **2021**, *462*, 109794. [CrossRef]
2. Li, J.; Fei, L.; Li, S.; Shi, Z.; Liu, L. The influence of optimized allocation of agricultural water and soil resources on irrigation and drainage in the Jingdian Irrigation District, China. *Irrig. Sci.* **2020**, *38*, 37–47. [CrossRef]
3. Zhang, C.; Dong, J.; Ge, Q. Mapping 20 years of irrigated croplands in China using MODIS and statistics and existing irrigation products. *Sci. Data* **2022**, *9*, 407. [CrossRef] [PubMed]
4. Srivastav, A.L.; Dhyani, R.; Ranjan, M.; Madhav, S.; Sillanpää, M. Climate-resilient strategies for sustainable management of water resources and agriculture. *Environ. Sci. Pollut. Res.* **2021**, *28*, 41576–41595. [CrossRef] [PubMed]
5. Li, S.; Wang, N.; Shen, J.; Sun, F. Pricing of water rights transactions for major water transfer projects considering water quantity and quality. *Environ. Dev. Sustain.* **2023**, *26*, 7735–7756. [CrossRef]
6. Cheng, K.; Wei, S.; Ren, Y.; Fu, Q. Optimal allocation of agricultural water resources under the background of China's agricultural water price reform—A case study of Heilongjiang province. *Appl. Math. Model.* **2021**, *97*, 636–649. [CrossRef]
7. Wang, Z.; Zhang, L.; Cheng, L.; Liu, K.; Wei, Y.-M. Basin-wide initial water rights allocation model considering both the quantity and quality of water. *Environ. Model. Assess.* **2020**, *25*, 581–589. [CrossRef]
8. Jia, S.; Sun, Y.; Svensson, J.; Mukherjee, M. Comparative analysis of water rights entitlements in India and China. *Water Policy* **2016**, *18*, 50–67. [CrossRef]
9. Xu, Y.J.; Zhu, X.T.; Wen, X.W. Fuzzy best-worst method and its application in initial water rights allocation. *Appl. Soft Comput.* **2021**, *101*, 107007. [CrossRef]
10. Zhou, J.L.; Xu, Q.Q.; Zhang, X.Y. Water Resources and Sustainability Assessment Based on Group AHP-PCA Method: A Case Study in the Jinsha River Basin. *Water* **2018**, *10*, 1880. [CrossRef]
11. Eras, J.J.C.; Fandiño, J.M.M.; Gutiérrez, A.S.; Bayona, J.G.R.; German, S.J.S. The inequality of electricity consumption in colombia. Projections and implications. *Energy* **2022**, *249*, 123711. [CrossRef]
12. Berbel, J.; Expósito, A. A decision model for stochastic optimization of seasonal irrigation-water allocation. *Agric. Water Manag.* **2022**, *262*, 107419. [CrossRef]
13. Xu, X.; Chen, Y.; Zhou, Y.; Liu, W.; Zhang, X.; Li, M. Sustainable management of agricultural water rights trading under uncertainty: An optimization-evaluation framework. *Agric. Water Manag.* **2023**, *280*, 108212. [CrossRef]
14. Wang, Y.B.; Liu, D.; Cao, X.C.; Yang, Z.Y.; Song, J.F.; Chen, D.Y.; Sun, S.K. Agricultural water rights trading and virtual water export compensation coupling model: A case study of an irrigation district in China. *Agric. Water Manag.* **2017**, *180*, 99–106. [CrossRef]

15. Li, K.; Xia, B.; Chen, Y.; Ding, N.; Wang, J. Environmental uncertainty, financing constraints and corporate investment: Evidence from China. *Pac. Basin Financ. J.* **2021**, *70*, 101665. [CrossRef]
16. Schoenenberger, L.; Schmid, A.; Tanase, R.; Beck, M.; Schwaninger, M. Structural analysis of system dynamics models. *Simul. Model. Pract. Theory* **2021**, *110*, 102333. [CrossRef]
17. Salehi, M. Global water shortage and potable water safety; Today's concern and tomorrow's crisis. *Environ. Int.* **2021**, *158*, 106936. [CrossRef] [PubMed]
18. Zheng, H.; Liu, Y.Y.; Zhao, J.S. Understanding water rights and water trading systems in China: A systematic framework. *Water Secur.* **2021**, *13*, 100094. [CrossRef]
19. Zhang, P.; Cai, Y.; Zhou, Y.; Tan, Q.; Li, B.; Li, B.; Jia, Q.; Yang, Z. Quantifying the water-energy-food nexus in Guangdong, Hong Kong, and Macao regions. *Sustain. Prod. Consum.* **2022**, *29*, 188–200. [CrossRef]
20. Li, X.; Engel, B.A.; Duan, P.; Sun, S.; Wang, Y. Developing an agricultural water pricing model considering both physical and virtual water: A case study of an irrigation district in China. *J. Clean. Prod.* **2022**, *368*, 133043. [CrossRef]
21. Zhang, Y.; Ge, M.; Zhang, Q.; Xue, S.; Wei, F.; Sun, H. What did irrigation modernization in China bring to the evolution of water-energy-greenhouse gas emissions? *Agric. Water Manag.* **2023**, *282*, 108283. [CrossRef]
22. Zhao, F.; Wu, Y.; Ma, S.; Lei, X.; Liao, W. Increased Water Use Efficiency in China and Its Drivers during 2000–2016. *Ecosystems* **2022**, *25*, 1476–1492. [CrossRef]
23. Kreinovich, V.; Kosheleva, O.; Shahbazova, S.N. Why Triangular and Trapezoid Membership Functions: A Simple Explanation. *Recent Dev. Fuzzy Log. Fuzzy Sets* **2020**, *391*, 25–31.
24. Kangmennaang, J.; Elliott, S.J. Linking water (in)security and wellbeing in low-and middle-income countries. *Water Security* **2021**, *13*, 100089.
25. Qian, X.L. Research on the coordinated development model of marine ecological environment protection and economic sustainable development. *J. Sea Res.* **2023**, *193*, 102377. [CrossRef]
26. Xin, Y.; Wang, D.; Zhang, L.; Ma, Y.; Chen, X.; Wang, H.; Wang, H.; Wang, K.; Long, H.; Chai, H.; et al. Cooperative analysis of infrastructure perfection and residents' living standards in poverty-stricken counties in Qinghai Province. *Environ. Dev. Sustain.* **2022**, *24*, 3687–3703. [CrossRef]
27. Ge, L.; Xie, G.; Zhang, C.; Li, S.; Qi, Y.; Cao, S.; He, T. An Evaluation of China's Water Footprint. *Water Resour. Manag.* **2011**, *25*, 2633–2647. [CrossRef]
28. Cai, J.; Xie, R.; Wang, S.; Deng, Y.; Sun, D. Patterns and driving forces of the agricultural water footprint of Chinese cities. *Sci. Total Environ.* **2022**, *843*, 156725. [CrossRef] [PubMed]
29. Wang, S.; Bai, X.; Zhang, X.; Reis, S.; Chen, D.; Xu, J.; Gu, B. Urbanization can benefit agricultural production with large-scale farming in China. *Nat. Food* **2021**, *2*, 183–191. [CrossRef]
30. Shu, H.; Xiong, P. The Gini coefficient structure and its application for the evaluation of regional balance development in China. *J. Clean. Prod.* **2018**, *199*, 668–686. [CrossRef]
31. Nicholson, S.R.; Rorrer, N.A.; Uekert, T.; Avery, G.; Carpenter, A.C.; Beckham, G.T. Manufacturing energy and greenhouse gas emissions associated with united states consumption of organic petrochemicals. *ACS Sustain. Chem. Eng.* **2023**, *11*, 2198–2208. [CrossRef]
32. Huang, G.; Hoekstra, A.Y.; Krol, M.S.; Jägermeyr, J.; Galindo, A.; Yu, C.; Wang, R. Water-saving agriculture can deliver deep water cuts for China. *Resour. Conserv. Recycl.* **2020**, *154*, 104578. [CrossRef]
33. Chen, Z.L.; Ma, T.H.; Hao, X.Z. Copula change point detection knowledge: The dynamic connection between international crude oil and China's nonferrous metal market. *J. Innov. Knowl.* **2022**, *7*, 100180. [CrossRef]
34. Lin, G.; Palopoli, M.; Dadwal, V. From causal loop diagrams to system dynamics models in a data-rich ecosystem. In *Leveraging Data Science for Global Health*; Springer: Cham, Switzerland, 2020; pp. 77–98.
35. Yao, X.X.; Ding, F.Q.; Luo, C. Time series prediction based on high-order intuitionistic fuzzy cognitive maps with variational mode decomposition. *Soft Comput. A Fusion Found. Methodol. Appl.* **2022**, *26*, 189–201.
36. Zadeh, L.A. Information and control. *Fuzzy Sets* **1965**, *8*, 338–353.
37. Atannassov, K. Intuitionistic fuzzy sets. *Fuzzy Sets Syst.* **1986**, *20*, 87–96. [CrossRef]
38. Zhang, Q.I.; Liu, F.; Fan, C.; Xie, W. Fuzzy numbers intuitionistic fuzzy descriptor systems. *Inf. Sci.* **2018**, *469*, 44–59. [CrossRef]
39. Pietrucha-Urbanik, K.; Rak, J. Water, Resources, and Resilience: Insights from Diverse Environmental Studies. *Water* **2023**, *15*, 3965. [CrossRef]
40. Valis, D.; Zak, L.; Walek, A. Selected mathematical functions used for operation data information. In *Safety, Reliability and Risk Analysis: Beyond the Horizon*; CRC Press-Taylor & Francis Group: Boca Raton, FL, USA, 2014; pp. 1303–1308.
41. Ma, X.; Zhang, S.; Mu, Q. How Do Residents Respond to Price under Increasing Block Tariffs? Evidence from Experiments in Urban Residential Water Demand in Beijing. *Water Resour. Manag.* **2014**, *28*, 4895–4909. [CrossRef]
42. Ziolkowska, J.R. Shadow price of water for irrigation—A case of the High Plains. *Agric. Water Manag.* **2015**, *153*, 20–31. [CrossRef]

water

MDPI

Article

Technical–Economic Feasibility of a New Method of Adsorbent Materials and Advanced Oxidation Techniques to Remove Emerging Pollutants in Treated Wastewater

Víctor Fabregat * and Juana María Pagán *

Department of Engineering and Innovation, Regenera Energy, C. Molina de Segura, 8, 30007 Murcia, Spain
* Correspondence: vfabregat@regeneraenergy.es (V.F.); jmpagan@regeneraenergy.es (J.M.P.); Tel.: +34-69-3367-275 (V.F.)

Abstract: The focus on emerging contaminants (ECs) in wastewater has intensified due to the considerable risks they present to human health and wildlife. This paper presents the results of the technical–economic assessment of the Clean Up solution, carried out in the framework of the project entitled "Validation of Adsorbent Materials and Advanced Oxidation Techniques to Remove Emerging Pollutants in Treated Wastewater". The viability of the Clean Up system is evaluated by being applied as an advanced treatment system for treated urban wastewater, that is, for the elimination of pathogens and emerging pollutants (EPs), while considering the established quality criteria by current regulations. In this sense, it is a technology that has been successfully validated at an experimental level, and that offers similar removal performance compared to that of the most efficient alternatives available on the market. The technical–economic assessment has been conducted through a systematic process. Initially, the estimation involved the calculation of treatment costs for the Clean Up system when applied at an industrial scale. Subsequently, the treatment costs were estimated for the most favorable technological alternative to the Clean Up system from a technical–economic standpoint, also applied at an industrial scale, within identical scenarios and conditions as those assumed for the Clean Up system. The final step involved a comprehensive comparison of treatment costs between both alternatives, implemented uniformly under analogous conditions and assumed similar performance across all cases.

Keywords: emerging contaminants; urban wastewater

1. Introduction

Integrated into the term "contaminants of emerging concern, CECs", the term "emerging pollutants, EPs" can include all active pharmacological compounds (PhACs), personal care products (PCPs), endocrine disruptors (EDCs), herbicides and pesticides, together with all their derived metabolization compounds [1]. According to the NORMAN network, there are more than 1000 of these substances that have been identified in the European aquatic environment [2,3]. One of the works that can be cited to reveal the extensive number of compounds that are included under the term of EPs in wastewater, is the one carried out by Comero et al. [4], where they analyzed the concentration of 156 organic compounds in the effluent of 90 European WWTPs. The results demonstrated the presence of 125 substances, in concentrations from ng/L to mg/L. The compounds with the highest mean concentrations were the artificial sweeteners acesulfame (2.5 mg/L) and sucralose (12.9 μg/L), benzotrols (221 μg/L), several flame retardants and pharmaceutical compounds such as carbamazepine (4669 ng/L), diclofenac (174 ng/L) and codeine (826 ng/L).

One of the main concerns associated with emerging pollutants is the poor performance in the removal of some of them by the technologies that are currently used in the treatment of urban wastewater [5]. This is because these facilities are designed to eliminate other conventional pollutants required by current regulations (Directive 91/271/EEC). Technologies used in water reclamation have the same problem, as they are not designed for EP removal, but for achieving a certain degree of quality in the reclaimed water to be reused that fits the level of quality required for each intended use (urban, industrial, agriculture, etc.). In this case, the referring legislation is Regulation (EU) 202/741 and Real Decreto 1620/2007, in Spain. The inefficiency in the elimination of EPs of the urban wastewater treatment and water reclamation systems that have been used until now causes the presence of some of these pollutants in the aquatic environment and/or in the reclaimed waters used in irrigation. This can entail several consequences, both in relation to environmental terms and public health. In this sense, the following aspects should be highlighted [4,6–10]: (i) human toxicity and ecotoxicity, (ii) presence and persistence, (iii) absorption by crops and (iv) effect on crops.

There are many challenges related to non-regulated pollutants whose effects are not fully understood. For instance, there is a threat linked to antibiotic-resistant bacteria, whose living environments are domestic wastewaters. These bacteria and their genes are even present in the reclaimed wastewater [3,11,12]. Therefore, there is an evident urgency to control and remove the pollutants that allow these bacteria and genes to proliferate in the WWTPs. As commented, the presence of EPs in treated waters discharged into water bodies or in reclaimed waters used in agriculture may carry a risk to human health or the environment. This has fostered the development of specific regulations for their control of water resources. Firstly, reference should be made to Directive 2013/39/EU, regarding priority substances in the field of water policy. This modifies the Directive 2008/105/CE, mentioned above, and establishes the EQS, defined as Maximum Allowable Concentrations (MAC), for a total of 45 compounds classified as priority substances, priority dangerous substances or other pollutants, in continental surface waters. This list is extended using the Commission Implementing Decision (EU) 2018/840, which establishes a watch list of substances for union-wide monitoring in the field of water policy. On the other hand, the European Commission is promoting the reuse of wastewater and, in this way, it has just developed Regulation (EU) 2020/741 on minimum requirements for water reuse. This regulation defines the microbiological and physicochemical parameters that must be measured in reclaimed water, and their associated MAC and monitoring frequency. That regulation does not establish, for the moment, limits for EPs in reclaimed water. However, the surveillance of some EPs such as personal care products, pharmaceuticals, drugs, etc., in irrigation water, has been established with a view to defining these limits in the near future. Another aspect to highlight of this regulation is that it establishes a series of obligations for water reclaiming plant operators, in addition to complying with the quality required for reclaimed water. In particular, the establishment of a risk management plan for reclaimed water is mandatory, in consultation with relevant stakeholders, such as wastewater providers, or end users, to address potential additional hazards.

EPs can be considered organic compounds, with medium or low biodegradability for which, in general, the biological treatments of WWTPs are not effective. Currently, there is a large number of works focused on the removal of EPs [13,14], that is, the development of water treatment processes for reducing and even eliminating the presence of said pollutants in treated water, obtaining higher quality water in the effluent of WWTPs. The most relevant ones are (i) adsorption processes, (ii) membrane processes, (iii) advanced oxidation (AOPs) and a combination of systems among others [15,16]. Within AOP processes, the most common use is combinations of ozone, hydrogen peroxide and UV radiation, with or without the use of catalysts [17,18].

The results of the different works carried out in recent years on the elimination of EPs in WWTPs have concluded, almost in a generalized way, that the most efficient technologies, both from a technical and economic point of view, are ozonation [19,20] and Powdered activated carbon (PAC) [21,22], both applied in WWTPs that already have advanced treatments for suspended solids and nutrients removal. These treatments must also include a final filtration stage, after O_3/PAC stage. That last stage would be a gravity sand filter, including biofilm formation, in the case of the O_3. In the case of PAC, they could be used as sand filters, microscreens, cloth filters or even membranes of microfiltration/ultrafiltration (MF/UF). Both processes are already being implemented at an industrial scale in WWTPs to avoid the incoming of emerging compounds into water bodies. In general, they offer similar EP removal performance (around 80%) at very similar costs (somewhat higher in the case of PAC treatment).

In this scenario, the Clean Up Project [23] aims to develop and validate a technology for the removal of EPs that presents as an alternative on a technical and economic level to the aforementioned treatments [24–28]. The EPs and pathogens contained in the treated wastewater have become a very important issue to consider in order to maintain the quality of the waterbodies and also reuse water without people, animals and ecosystems facing any risk. However, its removal is not guaranteed in the current WWTPs when conventional treatments are applied. This is because conventional secondary (e.g., activated sludge process) and tertiary such as nutrient removal, filtration and disinfection treatments in WWTPs are not effective in the removal of most EPs entering WWTPs [29]. A wide range of advanced treatment methods have been investigated for the removal of EPs from wastewater, including consolidated (activated carbon adsorption, ozonation and membrane filtration) and not intensively implemented treatments, such as advanced oxidation processes. The technologies that have been shown to be the most effective are oxidation (ozonation, particularly) and adsorption (PAC, particularly). Meanwhile, membranes have the inherent problem of the concentrate stream, which is why they cannot compete with the previously indicated methods. The Clean Up solution is based on the combination of these two technologies (adsorption and oxidation), but with an innovative approach that enables obtaining a treatment that can compete in efficiency with the aforementioned technologies. In previous research works, the Clean Up solution technology is described in detail [30–35]. This research proceeds to conduct the technical–economic feasibility study of the Clean Up technology.

In summary, the Clean Up process is designed to treat the effluent from WWTPs, removing pathogens and EPs, among other compounds, in the EPs case, with yields higher than 80%. The treated water can thus be discharged into water bodies without risk, or be used in agriculture, since a priori it would comply with the quality levels defined by the related regulation. Although the main stages of treatment for the removal of EPs are adsorption and oxidation, the treatment includes additional stages, whose mission is to ensure the correct functioning of the main stages. The stages that make up the Clean Up System and its operation are described below. (i) Ultrafiltration (UF), first of all, the effluent coming from the WWTP is pre-treated to remove the suspended solids and colloids that it could still contain, reducing that way its turbidity, *as* those compounds can negatively affect the following treatment stages. The selected technology is ultrafiltration due to the high quality of the produced permeate and its compactness. (ii) Adsorption (Ad), the permeate of the UF, with a flow rate of 5 m^3/h, goes then to the adsorption stage, where it passes through a column filled with the adsorbent material in an upward flow and fluidized bed regime, and then the EPs retained in the material. The adsorbent material is a non-soluble polymer of β-cyclodextrins (βCDs) cross-linked with DABCO (1,4-Diazabicyclo [2.2.2] octane) and BDE (1,4 butanediol diglycidyl ether). This material has been selected based on extensive laboratory tests in which the adsorbent potential of different types of CDs, native or modified, has been evaluated with a series of EPs, whose presence in treated wastewater was previously verified. (iii) Photocatalysis (Ph), the effluent from the adsorption stage may still contain residual amounts of organic pollutants or EPs with low adsorption rates due to the selectivity of the material. For that reason, the treatment includes a final stage of photocatalysis for oxidizing these compounds, so that the removal performance of the adsorption–photocatalysis system reaches at least 80% for the EPs. In the present project, this technique uses TiO_2 as a catalyst since it is non-toxic, low cost, and has high chemical stability and superior photoelectronic properties [36]. (iv) Desorption

(Ds), like any adsorbent, CDs have a maximum adsorption capacity, so that when this is reached, the EPs pass through the column without being retained. At that time, the column is regenerated by passing a desorbing agent (NaCl solution) that drags the adsorbed EPs out of it, producing a concentrate of EPs that must be subsequently treated. In this way, the column is ready to be used in a new adsorption cycle. Based on laboratory tests carried out, it has been determined that the NaCl solution meets the requirements of a desorbing agent for this application. (v) Pulsed light (PL), the concentrate of EPs in NaCl solution produced in the desorption stage is then treated in an advanced oxidation process, looking for the Eps' destruction using direct photo-oxidation. This technique uses huge spectrum light pulses at high intensity, short duration and high frequency, producing a high-power light with a moderate consumption of electrical energy. The possibility of adding H_2O_2 to promote the production of OH· radicals and increase the performance of removing refractory compounds is also considered.

Figure 1 shows the process flow chart. The effluent from the WWTP containing EPs is firstly treated by UF in order to remove those components that can unnecessarily exhaust the adsorbent (β-CD) in the column. Microbiological parameters (*E. coli*, *C. perfringens* and *C. perfringen* spores) are removed in the pre-treatment step by the ceramic ultrafiltration membrane (0.4 μm), and for the following sampling points the values are maintained at <10 cfu/100 mL. In any case, and given that photocatalysis has a disinfection capacity, wastewater disinfection is enhanced by this last treatment step. The permeate passes then to the adsorption, the second stage, through the fluidized bed of cyclodextrin's polymer, where most of the EPs are retained. After that, the water is treated by photocatalysis with TiO_2 for the removal of the remainder of EPs (third stage). The desorption process consists of making a NaCl solution pass through the bed of exhausted cyclodextrins. That solution drags the EPs from the polymer producing a concentrate which is afterwards treated by another advanced oxidation technique: pulsed light.

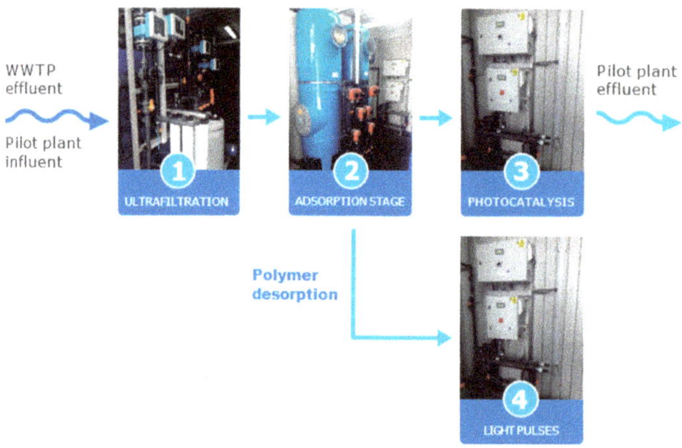

Figure 1. Experimental scheme of the modular pilot plant.

In addition, it is important to mention that the energy required by the Clean Up system is supplied by photovoltaic panels, covering the whole energy demand of the solution, as explained in Section 2.2. Therefore, the project Life Clean Up aims not only to use innovative processes in order to remove a wide range of EPs from urban wastewater at an industrial scale, but is also expected to be energy self-sufficient by implementing a solar panel system.

2. Methodology and Calculation of Treatment Costs

2.1. Application Scenarios for Clean Up Technology

When implementing the treatment system described in the previous point at an industrial scale, the primary application scenario to consider is the treatment of WWTP effluents for removing EPs and pathogens. The technology could be applied both to produce an effluent that could be discharged into water bodies and to produce reclaimed water that could be used in agriculture. Although there is no legal reference to the maximum allowable concentration of EPs, neither in the water that is discharged into water bodies nor in the reclaimed water used in agriculture, in both cases an effluent containing less than 20% of the initial concentration of EPs would be obtained. The application of this technology in these two scenarios could be carried out both in current and new WWTP projects. The two application cases are described in more detail below.

Urban wastewater treatment: the solution would be applied in WWTPs that discharge treated water into water bodies, as almost all facilities in Europe do. In addition, these WWTPs may or may not already have advanced treatments for nutrients and suspended solids removal, which divides this scenario into two possible sub-scenarios. In any case, the conventional technologies used in WWTPs have not allowed us to successfully remove EPs yet. This, along with the concern due to the increasing presence of EPs in the water cycle, has led to the development of various technological alternatives for the treatment of these wastewaters, some of them in the industrial implementation phase. These alternatives are basically ozonation and PAC, in which both cases are combined with the filtration stages, with which it is possible to achieve EP removal efficiencies above 80%. Obviously, the application of these treatments supposes an increase in the cost of wastewater treatment, which in this case is around 30%. The Clean Up process is presented as an alternative solution to those mentioned above, by allowing higher than 80% EPs removal, logically together with an increase in the cost of wastewater treatment. As this removal yield is similar to those of the alternatives mentioned above, it would be necessary to develop a competitive process in terms of treatment costs. In order to properly compare the costs of the different technologies, these costs should be obtained in all cases for the same EP removal performance. This is the assumption that is adopted in the present technical–economic study.

Urban wastewater reclamation. In this case, the Clean Up solution would be applied in WWTPs to produce reclaimed water from secondary effluent, suitable to be reused in agriculture, according to the current regulation (Regulation (EU) 2020/741). This case is especially relevant in water-stressed regions, such as the Mediterranean Basin. As in the previous case, two sub-scenarios would emerge depending on whether the WWTP already has or not an advanced treatment for nutrients and suspended solids removal. It has to be pointed out that the Clean Up system, besides the EPs removal, will act as advanced or tertiary treatment, removing BOD, suspended solids and pathogens, providing water suitable for irrigation. In this case, the situation is the same that was found in the previous case: water reclamation technologies commonly used are not efficient against EPs, except nanofiltration (NF) and reverse osmosis (RO). In any case, these membrane technologies are only used when the water has a high salinity, as they are the only viable alternative, but not with the aim to remove EPs, since in this case, these compounds would only be concentrated in a waste stream, which should be finally treated with a destructive technique. The technologies that have been defined as suitable in the previous point could also be suitable for reclaiming wastewater. That would be possible by implementing a final stage of UV disinfection, as the water produced by the filtration stages carried out after the O_3/PAC treatment would have very low values of particles and organic matter, but could also have a residual microbiological charge. Due to the low turbidity of the filtered water, the proper disinfection technology would consist of a UV irradiation and a final maintenance chlorination. This is the treatment scheme assumed in the present technical–economic study, as the alternative to the Clean Up system in water reclamation. The Clean Up solution would be suitable for water reclamation, as said before, without any additional stage. Anyway, in this case, it would be also necessary to implement the final chlorination step, and that has been assumed in the current study. On the other hand, it could also be considered the substitution of the UF stage of the Clean Up system by other advanced, less expensive treatments for suspended solids removal, such as direct filtration through sand, microscreens, textile filters, etc. Assuming similar performance for all the technical alternatives, the Clean Up solution will be advantageous if the cost of water reclamation that it entails is lower than that of the contemplated alternatives. In water reclamation, the economic comparison of the Clean Up system with the alternatives O_3/PAC would be more advantageous for Clean Up than in the previous scenario (wastewater treatment for discharge) because the Clean Up solution would be suitable for producing reclaimed water, while the alternatives should be modified for including a final stage of UV disinfection. On the other hand, the increase in the wastewater treatment costs, in the water reclamation scenario, would not be held by the beneficiaries of the sanitation and water treatment service, as it is in the first scenario, but by the end users of the reclaimed water, who are usually farmers. In this sense, the current cost of reclaimed water for agricultural use can be a reference to assess the economic viability of the removal of EPs, in the context of water reclamation.

Along with the urban wastewater treatment/reclamation, there could be another scenario considered, in which the system would be applied for the treatment of industrial wastewaters containing refractory or toxic organic compounds, such as effluents from the pharmaceutical industry, for example. This study does not consider that potential application.

2.2. *Energy Production by Photovoltaic Panels*

Among the characteristics of the Clean Up system, the generation of electricity on site, using photovoltaic panels, in order to power the treatment plant, is highlighted. This is intended to reduce the operating costs of said treatment system, since, currently, the costs of setting up a photovoltaic plant and producing electricity with it, which is defined as LCOE (levelized cost of electricity), can be, under certain conditions, lower than the cost of consuming the electricity from the grid. For this reason, in the industrial implementation of the considered treatment system, the inclusion of a photovoltaic plant is also considered as an option, so that the cost of treatment including this option can be calculated. To determine a priori if the inclusion of the photovoltaic (PV) system is economically efficient, the LCOE is determined as a function of the capacity of the PV plant, which will depend on the treatment capacity of the plant with Clean Up technology, and for a specific geographical location, since that last aspect will determine the energy production capacity as a function of the m^2 of installed panels.

Information sources from IRENA (International Renewable Energy Agency) [37] and the application of the JRC Photovoltaic Information System (PVGIS) of the European Commission have been used in order to specify the parameters that are considered for calculating the LCOE in two locations and based on the installed power of the PV plant. The results of the costs calculated using these sources have been checked with our own information coming from real PV plants. Table 1 shows the information used as input in the application PVGIS. It has been supposed to be an installed peak PV power of 1 kWp, in order to later extrapolate the results to the desired PV plant power.

Table 1. Input data used in PVGIS application for calculating the energy production based on the installed PV power.

Locations	Murcia	Bari
Latitude/longitude	37.995, −1.170	41.121, 16.860
Solar radiation database	PVGIS-SARAH	
PV technology	Crystalline silicon	
Installed peak PV power, kWp	1	
System loss, %	14	
Mounting	Fixed	
Position	Free standing	
Azimuth	0°	
Slope	35°	

Table 2 shows the results obtained using PVGIS for the two considered locations and the calculated average.

Table 2. Performance of the PV system (1 kWp) obtained for the two considered locations and calculated average.

Location	Murcia	Bari	Average
Yearly PV energy production, kWh	1635	1480	1558
Yearly in-plane irradiation, kWh/m^2	2099	1895	1997
Year-to-year variability, kWh	45	58	52
Total loss, %	−22.1	−21.9	−22.0

For the cost calculation, the following considerations are used: (i) operational specific costs—40,000 EUR per installed MW and year; (ii) investment specific costs—in this case, cost varies based on the installed PV power (this variation is reflected in Table 3); and (iii) investment financing conditions—investment lifetime of 25 years, and a financing interest of 7% is fixed.

Table 3. Specific investment costs as a function of the installed peak PV power.

Installed peak PV power, kWp	100	1000	10,000	100,000
Specific investment cost, EUR/kWp	1500	1000	750	700

The results of the LCOE calculation in the indicated location and depending on the installed peak PV power are presented in Table 4.

Table 4. Costs of the PV facility based on the installed peak PV power.

Installed peak PV power, kWp	100	1000	10,000	100,000
Yearly PV energy production, kWh	155,750	1,557,500	15,575,000	155,750,000
Operational costs, EUR/year	4000	40,000	400,000	4,000,000
Operational costs, EUR/kWh	0.03			
Investment, EUR	150,000	1,000,000	7,500,000	70,000,000
Repayment fee	0.086			
Capital costs, EUR/year	12,872	85,811	643,579	6,006,736
Capital costs, EUR/kWh	0.08	0.06	0.04	0.04
Total costs (LCOE), EUR/kWh	0.11	0.08	0.07	0.06

Only in the cases where the PV power to install entails a LCOE lower than the considered price of consumed electricity from the grid (0.12 EUR/kWh), a PV plant installation, associated with a water treatment plant, is considered for cost calculation. In addition, it must be considered that in these cases, the consumed electricity will not completely come from PV panels. Alternatively, it could come from the grid, depending on the time of the day. Therefore, the criterion followed to size the PV plant is that it is able to supply all the energy that the treatment plant needs in the month of maximum PV production is maximum, which in this case is July. In this month, during daylight there will be an energy surplus, that is, energy not consumed by the treatment plant, which will be supplied to the grid. That energy will be similar to the energy consumed at night, so the energy balance will be null. However, the energy supplied to the grid and the one consumed by the treatment plant will not mean a null economic balance, as the assumed price of grid electricity (0.12 EUR/kWh) will be higher than the benefit obtained when supplying energy, similar to the estimated LCOE. During the rest of the months, the energy consumption of the treatment plant will be higher than the energy produced by the PV plant. In that case, it is assumed that all the consumed energy will be taken from the grid, and all the produced energy will be supplied to the grid at a price similar to LCOE. This assumption does not exactly reflect the reality, as part of the electricity consumed by the treatment plant proceeds from the PV panels, and another part proceeds from the grid. In any case, this assumption has been reached because it facilitates calculations and because the difference with respect to calculating it as indicated is negligible, as it has been verified in an exploratory calculation carried out.

2.3. Technical Performance Evaluation

Previously, the treatment scheme of the Clean Up solution has been described at a basic level, as well as the forecasted application for this solution, once commercially developed. This section describes the issues related to the industrial implementation in a WWTP of the mentioned process, and particularly, the operational conditions, consumptions and performances that could be expected from said system are defined. This information is necessary for estimating the treatment costs of the considered technology and comparing it with the costs of the technical existing alternatives in the forecasted application scenarios. To estimate the performance of the Clean Up system at an industrial scale, the application scenarios have been considered: application in WWTPs that have an advanced treatment or not, and that aim to discharge treated water into water bodies or reclaim it to be used in agriculture. In addition, a treatment capacity between 1000 and 100,000 m^3/d has been considered. Due to the limitation of the Clean Up system's treatment capacity to 1000 m^3/d, as obtained in previous studies [35], a linear trend has been considered for the following orders of magnitude (10 units and 100 units of Life Clean Up in parallel).

The treatment system whose performance is intended to be calculated will have particular results, depending on the previously said application scenarios and, therefore, also particular costs. Regarding the calculation parameters used for sizing these systems, the operational conditions, consumptions and performances that could be expected from each considered system are defined below. For setting up these data, the values of 1000 m^3 for Case A are those obtained experimentally in the pilot plant. To conduct a more comprehensive study, not limited solely to the characteristics of the WWTP where the pilot plant has been located, other scenarios (Cases B, C, D, A′ and B′) have been considered. To facilitate a detailed analysis, the data required for these scenarios, which could not be obtained from the pilot plant, have been supplemented with bibliographic data [17–31,38–52].

Case A. The system is applied in a WWTP that does not have any advanced treatment for removing suspended solids after its secondary settlers, and where the treated water is discharged into a water body. The objective in this case is to limit the presence of EPs in the mentioned water body. The treatment system is composed then by all the elements included in the pilot plant; that is, a first stage of microfiltration followed by ultrafiltration for removing the suspended and colloidal solids, followed by the adsorption with cyclodextrins stage for EPs removal, and a final stage of photocatalysis for the degradation of the remaining organic pollutants. Below, the manner in which the implementation at the industrial level of the different stages that compose this treatment would be carried out, and the considerations that have been completed for estimating the treatment costs of the mentioned system are defined.

Direct filtration and ultrafiltration stage. The pilot plant includes a UF system with ceramic membranes, preceded by cartridge filtration (MF). This combined treatment is used to limit the amount of undissolved solids that reach the adsorption stage. If these solids were not removed by membranes, they could be retained or adsorbed on the adsorbent material, reducing the EP adsorption capacity and/or increasing the need for cleaning or regeneration operations of the adsorbent bed. To implement this system in a WWTP, the MF stage would be carried out by a direct filtration system using microscreens or cloth filters, technologies with filtration grades among 10–40 µm, which are well known and used in tertiary treatments in WWTPs. After that, the UF would be carried out, but in this case, using polymeric hollow-fiber membranes, instead of ceramic tubular membranes, as the former are cheaper than the latter, and very well known and validated in advanced treatments in WWTPs. This is the system proposed for the implementation of the technology in a WWTP and the calculation of costs. In the case of the MF a direct filtration system calculated as an average of microscreens and cloth filters used in tertiary treatment is assumed. Then, the considered calculation parameters are the following: (i) TSS in secondary effluent—15 mg/L; (ii) recovery—98%. The remaining 2% of water is used in cleaning operations and is then led to the inlet of the WWTP, as its total suspended solids (TSS) concentration is similar to that of the WWTP influent (checked in results chapter): (iii) TSS removal performance—60%; and (iv) electrical consumption—0.007 kWh/m^3. In the case of the UF, a system with polymeric hollow fiber membranes would be adopted, operating in dead-end mode. Hydraulic and chemical cleanings are carried out using permeate, so a permeate tank sized for storing enough amount of water to achieve these operations is necessary. The considered calculation parameters for UF are the following: (i) recovery—85%. The retentate stream, produced in membrane cleaning, is directed to the inlet of the WWTP: (ii) TSS removal performance—98% and (iii) electrical consumption—0.25 kWh/m^3. Both in the case of MF and UF, the concentrated streams produced in cleaning operations are directed to the inlet of the WWTP. For this reason, the MF stage is sized considering the increase in the treatment capacity that these two recirculated volumes suppose, and for the UF, the followed procedure is similar, but considering only the concentrate stream generated in said operation.

Adsorption—desorption stage. In the pilot plant, the adsorption operation is carried out by passing the UF permeate through a column filter with an upward flow direction. Within this column is the adsorbent material, which is fluidized when the permeate passes through. The used adsorbent is β-CDs cross-linked with DABCO and BDE. Once the adsorbent is exhausted, the same can be regenerated by passing through the column a regenerant solution. The regenerant passes also in an upward flow and fluidizes the adsorbent, carrying away the previously adsorbed compounds, leaving the column free to be used again in a new adsorption cycle. The NaCl solution is subsequently treated using a pulsed light system to eliminate dragged compounds. This treatment will be described later. The pilot plant has two adsorption columns, so that continuous operation can be ensured, as one is always in operation, and the other one is in the regeneration or waiting phase. Finally, it must be said that the regeneration of CDs cannot be completed indefinitely, since CDs, just like any adsorbent, reduce their adsorption performance as regeneration cycles are added, so there comes a time when it is necessary to replace them. After the industrial implementation of the adsorption—desorption stage, the operation of that process in a WWTP would be similar to that of the one described above for the pilot plant. The design of the operation is carried out based on the results obtained through the design and operation of the pilot plant, except where specified. Next, the data used in the sizing of the adsorption process are shown. (i) EPs average concentration in UF effluent: 4.79 µg/L. It is the sum of the concentration of all the different EPs measured in this stream and averaged along a complete adsorption cycle; that is, until the exhaustion of the

CDs: (ii) EPs average concentration in adsorption stage effluent—3.44 µg/L; (iii) amount of CDs as a function of the water flow to treat—9.5 kg/m^3/d; (iv) adsorption performance of CDs—4.24 m^3/kg CDs; (v) number of regeneration cycles until replacement of the CDs—10 cycles; (vi) electrical consumption in adsorption step—0.06 kWh/m^3; (vii) volume of regenerant solution as a function of the used amount of CDs—0.75 L/kg CDs; (viii) averaged value between 0.5 and 1 l/kg; (ix) it is assumed that when the CDs have to be replaced, the regenerant solution is also replaced; and (x) electrical consumption in desorption step: 0.04 kWh/m^3.

Photocatalysis stage. The pilot plant includes two photocatalysis (PH) reactors. The technology of the used reactors consists basically of monobloc vessels made of TiO_2, which include UV lamps, arranged parallel to the longitudinal axis of the vessel. Depending on the section of the vessel, one or more UV lamps are installed. In the case of the pilot plant, each vessel includes one lamp of 105 W, and the two PH reactors can be operated in series or parallel, since the contact time does not change. For the industrial implementation, the process would be similar to the one carried out in a pilot plant but working with higher capacity reactors and/or with several reactors in parallel, since this is a modular technology with commercially available units with treatment capacity from 1 to 1000 m^3/h. The design of the operation is carried out based on the results obtained in the design and operation of the pilot plant. Next, the data used in the sizing of the photocatalysis are showed: (i) EPs average concentration in adsorption stage effluent—3.44 µg/L; (ii) EPs average concentration in PH stage effluent—0.90 µg/L; and (iii) electrical consumption—1.7 kWh/m^3.

Pulsed light stage. In the pilot plant, after each regeneration step, the regenerant volume is treated by an advanced oxidation process based on irradiating with pulsed light (PL). The pulsed light system uses a xenon lamp which generates light flashes with a polychromatic emission spectrum. The volume contained in the regenerant tank is continuously circulated to the pulsed light treatment device, which is adapted to work in continuous mode, and returned to the tank, until the contact time is high enough to ensure the removal of the concentrated EPs, leaving the regenerant available for the next desorption cycle. Regarding industrial implementation, a pulsed light system for continuous treatment mode must be developed or found, since what is present in the pilot plant is an adaptation of a discontinuous treatment system, for this purpose. The design of the operation is based on the results obtained through the design and operation of the pilot plant. Next, data used in the sizing of the pulsed light system are shown: (i) EPs removal rate—0.25 mg EPs/(l·h); (ii) information about the installed equipment of pulsed light—lamp with the power of 3000 W, 500 J of energy per pulse and 3 Hz of pulse frequency; and (iii) applied power—1 kW/m^3/h. The value taken from the design of the pilot plant, which has a lamp of 3 kW of power, was installed in a plant with a treatment capacity of 3 m^3/h. Table 5 includes the results obtained for Case A.

Table 5. Results obtained in Case A sizing.

WWTP Influent, m^3/d	1000	10,000	100,000
Direct filtration stage			
Filtration influent, m^3/d	1200	12,005	120,048
Filtration effluent, m^3/d	1176	11,765	117,647
TSS in filtration effluent, mg/L		6.1	
Wastewater flow (from filter cleaning), m^3/d	24	240	2401
TSS in wastewater from filter cleaning, mg/L		450	
Electrical consumption, kWh/d	8	84	840
Ultrafiltration stage			
Ultrafiltration influent, m^3/d	1176	11,765	117,647
TSS in ultrafiltration influent, mg/L		6.1	
Ultrafiltration effluent, m^3/d	1000	10,000	100,000
Wastewater flow (from membranes cleaning), m^3/d	176	1765	17,647
TSS in wastewater from membrane cleaning, mg/L		40	
Electrical consumption, kWh/d	294	2941	29,412
CDs adsorption stage			
CDs adsorption influent, m^3/d	1000	10,000	100,000
EPs removal performance, %		28	
Required amount of CDs, ton	9.5	95	950
Volume of water treated per adsorption cycle, m^3	40,280	402,800	4,028,000
Time to complete 1 adsorption cycle, d		40	
Time until replacement of exhausted CDs, d		403	

Table 5. *Cont.*

Amount of adsorbed EPs until the replacement of exhausted CDs, kg	0.54	5.4	54.4
Equivalent CDs dose, mg/L		24	
Equivalent CDs consumption, kg/d	24	236	2358
Maximum adsorption capacity of EPs, mgEPs/gCDs		0.0057	
Electrical consumption, kWh/d	60	600	6000
WWTP influent, m^3/d	1000	10,000	100,000
Photocatalysis stage			
Photocatalysis influent, m^3/d	1000	10,000	100,000
EPs removal performance, %		74	
EPs removal performance (CDs + PH), %		81	
Electrical consumption, kWh/d	1700	17,000	170,000
CDs regeneration stage			
Required amount of regenerant solution, m^3	7.1	71	713
Equivalent consumption of regenerant solution, L/d	18	177	1769
Equivalent electrical consumption, kWh/d	0.001	0.007	0.071
Pulsed light stage			
Regenerant to treat per adsorption cycle, m^3	7.1	71.3	713
EPs concentration in regenerant solution to recover, mg/L		8.0	
EPs to remove in PL system per adsorption cycle, kg EPs	0.05	0.5	5.4
Rate of EPs removal, g EPs/h	1.8	17.8	178.1
Required time for regenerating the solution in PL, d		1.3	
Installed PL power, kW	42	417	4167
Equivalent electrical consumption, kWh/d	16	158	1579
Photovoltaic plant			
Electrical consumption of treatment plant, MWh/year	759	7586	75,858
Installed peak PV power, kWp	389	3893	38,929
Production cost (LCOE), EUR/kWh	0.093	0.077	0.063
PV plant installation (YES/NO)	YES	YES	YES
PV plant production, MWh/year	606	6063	60,632
Net cost of consumed electricity (averaged), EUR/kWh	0.108	0.101	0.095

Case B. The system is applied in a WWTP which does not have any advanced treatment for removing suspended solids after its secondary treatment, and where the aim is to reclaim water for being used in agriculture, including the removal of EPs in the water reclamation process. As said, the Clean Up system can produce reclaimed water suitable for irrigation, with the only inclusion of a final step, after disinfection, with the aim to maintain a minimum residual oxidant in the reclaimed water. So, the treatment system is similar to Case A, but includes that final chlorination step (NaClO dosing) to maintain this minimum residual. The calculation parameters used are similar to the previous case, and the final disinfection stage is described below.

Chlorination stage. Composed of chlorination by NaClO dosing in a contact reactor. It should not be forgotten that disinfection is achieved by the previous photocatalysis stage and that chlorination is carried out to maintain an oxidizing residual downstream of the WWTP. The objective is to reach the quality parameters set up by the current regulation

(Regulation (EU) 2020/741) regarding the presence of pathogens in reclaimed water. The calculation parameters used are the following: (i) NaClO dose—3 gCl_2/m^3. Table 6 includes the results obtained for Case B.

Table 6. Results obtained in Case B sizing.

WWTP Influent, m^3/d	1000	10,000	100,000
Direct filtration stage			
Filtration influent, m^3/d	1200	12,005	120,048
Filtration effluent, m^3/d		1176	
TSS in filtration effluent, mg/L		6.1	
Wastewater flow (from filter cleaning), m^3/d	24	240	2401
TSS in wastewater from filter cleaning, mg/L		450	
Electrical consumption, kWh/d	8	84	840
Ultrafiltration stage			
Ultrafiltration influent, m^3/d	1176	11,765	117,647
TSS in ultrafiltration influent, mg/L		6.1	
Ultrafiltration effluent, m^3/d	1000	10,000	100,000
Wastewater flow (from membranes cleaning), m^3/d	176	1765	17,647
TSS in wastewater from membrane cleaning, mg/L		40	
Electrical consumption, kWh/d	294	2941	29,412
CDs adsorption stage			
CDs adsorption influent, m^3/d	1000	10,000	100,000
EPs removal performance, %		28	
Required amount of CDs, ton	9.5	95	950
Volume of water treated per adsorption cycle, m^3	40,280	402,800	4,028,000
Time to complete 1 adsorption cycle, d		40	
Time until replacement of exhausted CDs, d		403	
Amount of adsorbed EPs until the replacement of exhausted CDs, kg	0.54	5.4	54.4
Equivalent CDs dose, mg/L		24	
Equivalent CDs consumption, kg/d	24	236	2358
Maximum adsorption capacity of EPs, mgEPs/gCDs		0.0057	
Electrical consumption, kWh/d	60	600	6000
Photocatalysis stage			
Photocatalysis influent, m^3/d	1000	10,000	100,000
EPs removal performance, %		74	
EPs removal performance (CDs + PH), %		81	
Electrical consumption, kWh/d	1700	17,000	170,000
Chlorination stage			
Disinfection influent, m^3/d	1000	10,000	100,000
NaClO consumption (50% solution), kg/d	13	126	1261
CDs regeneration stage			
Required amount of regenerant solution, m^3	7.1	71	713

Table 6. *Cont.*

Equivalent consumption of regenerant solution, L/d	18	177	1769
Equivalent electrical consumption, kWh/d	0.001	0.007	0.071
WWTP influent, m^3/d	1000	10,000	100,000
Pulsed light stage			
Regenerant to treat per adsorption cycle, m^3	7.1	71.3	713
EPs concentration in regenerant solution to recover, mg/L		8.0	
EPs to remove in PL system per adsorption cycle, kg EPs	0.05	0.5	5.4
Rate of EPs removal, g EPs/h	1.8	17.8	178.1
Required time for regenerating the solution in PL, d		1.3	
Installed PL power, kW	42	417	4167
Equivalent electrical consumption, kWh/d	16	158	1579
Photovoltaic plant			
Electrical consumption of treatment plant, MWh/year	759	7586	75,858
Installed peak PV power, kWp	389	3893	38,929
Production cost (LCOE), EUR/kWh	0.093	0.077	0.063
PV plant installation (YES/NO)	YES	YES	YES
PV plant production, MWh/year	606	6063	60,632
Net cost of consumed electricity (averaged), EUR/kWh	0.108	0.101	0.095

Case C. The system is applied in a WWTP, which already has an advanced treatment for removing suspended solids after the secondary treatment and where the treated water is discharged into a water body. The treatment system is similar to Case A but excludes the first stage consisting of direct filtration + ultrafiltration because that treatment is supposed to be carried out by the current facilities. As in Case A, the objective is to limit the presence of EPs in the mentioned water body.

Case D. The system applied in a WWTP, which already has a tertiary treatment for reclaiming water, but does not have a special treatment for EPs removal. The objective is to implement only the adsorption with CDs followed by photocatalysis stages, using them along with the rest of current tertiary treatment stages, for reclaiming water. The treatment is similar to Case B but excludes the first stage consisting of direct filtration + ultrafiltration because that treatment is supposed to be carried out by the current facilities. Therefore, new facilities are similar to those of Case C. Table 7 includes the results obtained for Cases C and D. The data regarding the operation of the existing reclamation facilities are not included.

Table 7. Results obtained in Cases C and D sizing.

WWTP Influent, m^3/d	1000	10,000	100,000
CDs adsorption stage			
CDs adsorption influent, m^3/d	1000	10,000	100,000
EPs removal performance, %			28
Required amount of CDs, ton	9.5	95	950
Volume of water treated per adsorption cycle, m^3	40,280	402,800	4,028,000
Time to complete 1 adsorption cycle, d		40	
Time until replacement of exhausted CDs, d	403		

Table 7. *Cont.*

WWTP influent, m^3/d	1000	10,000	100,000
CDs adsorption stage			
Amount of adsorbed EPs until the replacement of exhausted CDs, kg	0.54	5.4	54.4
Equivalent CDs dose, mg/L		24	
Equivalent CDs consumption, kg/d	24	236	2358
Maximum adsorption capacity of EPs, mgEPs/gCDs		0.0057	
Electrical consumption, kWh/d	60	600	6000
Photocatalysis stage			
Photocatalysis influent, m^3/d	1000	10,000	100,000
EPs removal performance, %		74	
EPs removal performance (CDs + PH), %		81	
Electrical consumption, kWh/d	1700	17,000	170,000
CDs regeneration stage			
Required amount of regenerant solution, m^3	7.1	71	713
Equivalent consumption of regenerant solution, L/d	18	177	1769
Equivalent electrical consumption, kWh/d	0.001	0.007	0.071
Pulsed light stage			
Regenerant to treat per adsorption cycle, m^3	7.1	71.3	713
EPs concentration in regenerant solution to recover, mg/L		8.0	
EPs to remove in PL system per adsorption cycle, kg EPs	0.05	0.5	5.4
Rate of EPs removal, g EPs/h	1.8	17.8	178.1
Required time for regenerating the solution in PL, d		1.3	
Installed PL power, kW	42	417	4167
Equivalent electrical consumption, kWh/d	16	158	1579
Photovoltaic plant			
Electrical consumption of treatment plant, MWh/year	648	6482	64,816
Installed peak PV power, kWp	333	3326	33,263
Production cost (LCOE), EUR/kWh	0.094	0.078	0.064
PV plant installation (YES/NO)	YES	YES	YES
PV Plant production, MWh/year	518	5181	51,806
Net cost of consumed electricity (averaged), EUR/kWh	0.109	0.101	0.095

Cases A and B assume that the WWTP does not have any tertiary treatment for the removal of suspended solids and turbidity, so this treatment must be included as a first step by the Clean Up system, so that the subsequent stages of EPs removal and disinfection may work properly. The proposed treatment in these cases is direct filtration (microfiltration) followed by ultrafiltration, which is similar to the one included at the Clean Up pilot plant. It must be considered that the UF is an expensive treatment, as compared to other tertiary treatments, both at an operational level and investment level. Thus, the use of UF as a treatment stage of the Clean Up system could not be justified in a technical–economic term, both if the objective is to discharge the treated effluent into the water bodies or whether it serves to reclaim water. It must be noted that in the field of water reclamation, the UF is only used in those cases in which high-quality water is required, along with total removal of Escherichia coli (residential urban use or cooling towers, for example), but in most expected uses for reclaimed water, such as agriculture, urban services or industrial processes, the required quality can be obtained through a physicochemical stage (P&C), followed by direct filtration (sand filters, microscreens or cloth filters) and a final disinfection stage with UV radiation, or simply through direct filtration followed by UV disinfection [53]. In fact, the treatment technology which has been considered an alternative to the Clean Up system, which is later compared to the Clean Up in economic terms, also needs a first stage for suspended solids and turbidity removal, for optimizing the later EPs removal and disinfection stages. However, it has been found that this tertiary treatment can be carried out by technologies such as the ones indicated in previous paragraphs. Finally, the selected tertiary treatment depends on the quality of the secondary effluent and the quality required for the treated water, according to its forecasted use or following treatment stages. Thus, depending on the concentration and characteristics of the particles and colloids in the secondary effluent, it is possible that these indicated technologies can ensure the proper performance of the adsorption stage, not necessarily the use of a UF stage. For this reason, additional study cases are now proposed, so that the possible technical scenarios are reflected. These cases are named A′ and B′, as they would be applied in the same scenario cases as Cases A and B, but substituting now the microfiltration + ultrafiltration stage for conventional tertiary treatment.

Case A′. The system is similar to Case A; that is, it is applied in a WWTP, which does not have any advanced treatment for removing suspended solids after its secondary settlers, and where the treated water is discharged into a water body. The objective is to limit the presence of EPs in the mentioned water body. The treatment system is composed then by all the elements included in the pilot plant with the exception of the micro and ultrafiltration stages. These are substituted by a direct filtration stage, as explained below.

Direct filtration stage. This stage is designed for treating the water coming from the secondary settlers, with the aim of limiting the number of undissolved solids that reach the adsorption stage. There are different treatment trains for reaching this objective, depending basically on the quality of the secondary effluent. In this case, it is assumed that the quality of the secondary effluent is high enough to require only a direct filtration stage as a tertiary treatment. This direct filtration system is calculated as an average of microscreens, cloth filters and sand filters (open and closed), all commonly used in tertiary treatments. Then, the considered calculation parameters are the following: (i) TSS in secondary effluent—15 mg/L; (ii) recovery—98% (the remaining 2% of water is used in cleaning operations and is after led to the inlet of the WWTP, as its TSS concentration is similar to that of the WWTP influent; (iii) TSS removal performance—55%; and (iv) electrical consumption—0.15 kWh/m^3.

The concentrate produced in cleaning operations is directed to the inlet of the WWTP. For this reason, the direct filtration stage is sized considering the treatment capacity increase that this recirculated volume supposes. Table 8 includes the results obtained for Case A′.

Table 8. Results obtained in Case A′ sizing.

WWTP Influent, m^3/d	**1000**	**10,000**	**100,000**
Direct filtration stage			
Filtration influent, m^3/d	1020	10,204	102,041
Filtration effluent, m^3/d		1000	
TSS in filtration effluent, mg/L		6.9	
Wastewater flow (from filter cleaning), m^3/d	20	204	2041
TSS in wastewater from filter cleaning, mg/L		413	
Electrical consumption, kWh/d	153	1531	15,306
CDs adsorption stage			
CDs adsorption influent, m^3/d	1000	10,000	100,000

Table 8. *Cont.*

WWTP Influent, m^3/d	1000	10,000	100,000
EPs removal performance, %		28	
Required amount of CDs, ton		9.5	
Volume of water treated per adsorption cycle, m^3	40,280	402,800	4,028,000
Time to complete 1 adsorption cycle, d		40	
Time until replacement of exhausted CDs, d		403	
Amount of adsorbed EPs until the replacement of exhausted CDs, kg	0.54	5.4	54.4
Equivalent CDs dose, mg/L		24	
Equivalent CDs consumption, kg/d		24	
Maximum adsorption capacity of EPs, mgEPs/gCDs		0.0057	
Electrical consumption, kWh/d	60	600	6000
Photocatalysis stage			
Photocatalysis influent, m^3/d	1000	10,000	100,000
EPs removal performance, %		74	
EPs removal performance (CDs + PH), %		81	
Electrical consumption, kWh/d	1700	17,000	170,000
CDs regeneration stage			
Required amount of regenerant solution, m^3		7.1	
Equivalent consumption of regenerant solution, L/d	18	177	1769
Equivalent electrical consumption, kWh/d	0.001	0.007	0.071
WWTP influent, m^3/d		1000	
Pulsed light stage			
Regenerant to treat per adsorption cycle, m^3	7.1	71.3	713
EPs concentration in regenerant solution to recover, mg/L		8.0	
EPs to remove in PL system per adsorption cycle, kg EPs	0.05	0.5	5.4
Rate of EPs removal, g EPs/h	1.8	17.8	178.1
Required time for regenerating the solution in PL, d		1.3	
Installed PL power, kW	42	417	4167
Equivalent electrical consumption, kWh/d	16	158	1579
Photovoltaic plant			
Electrical consumption of treatment plant, MWh/year	704	7040	70,403
Installed peak PV power, kWp	361	3613	36,130
Production cost (LCOE), EUR/kWh	0.094	0.077	0.063
PV plant installation (YES/NO)	YES	YES	YES
PV Plant production, MWh/year	563	5627	56,272
Net cost of consumed electricity (averaged), EUR/kWh	0.108	0.101	0.095

Case B′. The system is similar to Case B; that is, it is applied in a WWTP that does not have any advanced treatment for removing suspended solids after its secondary treatment, and where the aim is to reclaim water for being used in agriculture, including the removal of EPs in the water reclamation process. The treatment system is composed of all the elements included in the pilot plant with the exception of the micro and ultrafiltration stages. These are substituted by a direct filtration stage, as has been explained in Case A′. Additionally, the system includes a final chlorination step (NaClO dosing) to maintain a minimum residual oxidant in the reclaimed water. Table 9 includes the results obtained for Case B′.

Table 9. Results obtained in Case B′ sizing.

WWTP Influent, m^3/d	**1000**	**10,000**	**100,000**
Direct filtration stage			
Filtration influent, m^3/d	1020	10,204	102,041
Filtration effluent, m^3/d		1000	
TSS in filtration effluent, mg/L		6.9	
Wastewater flow (from filter cleaning), m^3/d	20	204	2041
TSS in wastewater from filter cleaning, mg/L		413	
Electrical consumption, kWh/d	153	1531	15,306
CDs adsorption stage			
CDs adsorption influent, m^3/d	1000	10,000	100,000
EPs removal performance, %		28	
Required amount of CDs, ton		9.5	
Volume of water treated per adsorption cycle, m^3	40,280	402,800	4,028,000
Time to complete 1 adsorption cycle, d		40	
Time until replacement of exhausted CDs, d		403	
Amount of adsorbed EPs until the replacement of exhausted CDs, kg	0.54	5.4	54.4
Equivalent CDs dose, mg/L		24	
WWTP influent, m^3/d		1000	
CDs adsorption stage			
Equivalent CDs consumption, kg/d	24	236	2358
Maximum adsorption capacity of EPs, mgEPs/gCDs		0.0057	
Electrical consumption, kWh/d	60	600	6000
Photocatalysis stage			
Photocatalysis influent, m^3/d		1000	
EPs removal performance, %		74	
EPs removal performance (CDs + PH), %		81	
Electrical consumption, kWh/d		1700	
Chlorination stage			
Disinfection influent, m^3/d	1000	10,000	100,000
NaClO consumption (50% solution), kg/d		13	
CDs regeneration stage			
Required amount of regenerant solution, m^3	7.1	71	713
Equivalent consumption of regenerant solution, L/d		18	
Equivalent electrical consumption, kWh/d	0.001	0.007	0.071
Pulsed light stage			
Regenerant to treat per adsorption cycle, m^3		7.1	

Table 9. *Cont.*

WWTP Influent, m^3/d	1000	10,000	100,000
EPs concentration in regenerant solution to recover, mg/L		8.0	
EPs to remove in PL system per adsorption cycle, kg EPs	0.05	0.5	5.4
Rate of EPs removal, g EPs/h	1.8	17.8	178.1
Required time for regenerating the solution in PL, d		1.3	
Installed PL power, kW	42	417	4167
Equivalent electrical consumption, kWh/d	16	158	1579
Photovoltaic plant			
Electrical consumption of treatment plant, MWh/year	704	7040	70,403
Installed peak PV power, kWp	361	3613	36,130

2.4. Capital Costs

Once the different treatments considered are sized, the following step is the calculation of the corresponding treatment costs. The necessary investment depends on the studied case, as the considered technologies may vary from case to case. For part of the assessed technologies (adsorption on cyclodextrins, photocatalysis and pulsed light), no industrial plant that can serve as a reference exists, so it is difficult to define the investment cost of these technologies at that scale. The only reference available is the cost estimation of the project's pilot plant, which can be seen in Table 10.

Table 10. Cost estimation of the Clean Up pilot plant.

Item	Cost, EUR
Pilot plant materials	37,906
Pulsed light system	53,496
Civil work	9520
Photovoltaic plant	32,732
Photocatalysis equipment	8461
Total	142,115

Using these data, a methodology for estimating the investment costs as a function of the treatment capacity of the facilities has been established, within the range assessed in the study (from 1000 to 100,000 m^3/d). For the cost estimation of the pilot plant (Table 10), the following points must be considered: (i) in the cases where the treatment plant does not include treatment of MF + UF (cases C, D, A′ and B′); (ii) in the cases where the treatment plant includes a final step for chlorination (cases B and B′), the investment costs for said step included in Table 11 are considered; and (iii) in the cases where a first stage of direct filtration, as tertiary treatment, is included, it is calculated as an average of microscreens, cloth filters and sand filters (cases A′ and B′), and the investment costs for that step included in Table 11 are considered.

The investment calculated in each case from the data in Table 10, and the aspects indicated in the previous point is increased a 30% for auxiliary materials, assembly and installation. The result corresponds to the material execution of the project in each case. From the obtained material execution, the benefit rate and general expenses are added in all cases, obtaining the cost basis, that is, the investment cost excluding VAT tax. From the cost basis and considering the treatment capacity of the pilot plant (3 m^3/h) as a reference, the investment (cost basis) of 1000 m^3/d is calculated using the rule of 6.10. This rule has its origin in the relationship between the increase in equipment cost and the increase in capacity [54]. As a general rule, this can be used for estimating the cost associated with a capacity from the cost of the same facility but with other capacities, with an error not higher than 20%. Once the investment cost of the 1000 m^3/d plant is known for all the foreseen cases, those of the 10,000 and 100,000 m^3/d are also calculated, considering this a variation in investment costs with respect to the treatment capacity for said interval that is similar to that of other conventional tertiary treatment technologies.

Table 11. Information considered for capital cost calculation.

WWTP Influent, m^3/d		1000	10,000	100,000
Investment costs EUR/m^3/d	Final chlorination (Cases B and B′)	45	41	37
	Direct filtration (Cases A′ and B′)	125	175	50
Benefit rate, % [1]			6	
General expenses rate, % [1]			13	
VAT, %			21	
Investment lifetime, years			20	
Financing interest, %			5	

Note: [1] Applied over material execution.

Table 11 gathers all the information considered for the calculation of the capital costs, based on the studied cases and the treatment capacity of the facilities. For the investment costs of the final chlorination and direct filtration stages, several references have been revised: [43,49,51,55–61].

Tables 12–16 show the results of the capital costs calculation. Capital costs are calculated based on the basis values, as it has been assumed that the investment would be carried out by the public sector.

Table 12. Capital costs calculated for Case A.

WWTP Influent, m^3/d	1000	10,000	100,000
Investment costs EUR/m^3/d	821	423	284
Investment, EUR	992,874	5,114,805	34,385,246
Investment (basis), EUR	820,557	4,227,112	28,417,558
Material execution, EUR	689,268	3,550,774	23,870,749
Capital costs, EUR/year	65,844	339,194	2,280,298
Capital costs, EUR/m^3	0.18	0.09	0.06

Table 13. Capital costs calculated for Case B.

WWTP Influent, m^3/d	1000	10,000	100,000
Investment costs EUR/m^3/d	866	464	321
Investment, EUR	1,047,324	5,610,905	38,862,246
Investment (basis), EUR	865,557	4,637,112	32,117,558
Material execution, EUR	727,068	3,895,174	26,978,749
Capital costs, EUR/year	69,455	372,094	2,577,196
Capital costs, EUR/m^3	0.19	0.10	0.07

It is assumed that the overall objective of the investments is to achieve significant removals of micropollutants in the WWTP, whatever the destination of the treated water is, as a response to a risk to human health. For that reason, it is considered that the investment is undertaken by the public sector, as said. However, it should not be forgotten that part of the investment has the objective of removing pathogens, as a necessary step for reclaiming water, as can be seen in cases B and B′. In those cases, the additional treatments to the ones that are considered for the EP removal can be paid for by the end users of the reclaimed waters. For doing so, a price for reclaimed water that defrays the capital and operational cost of that disinfection stage can be fixed, maintaining a null benefit, as it is a public service. This situation is assumed, but not included in the costs analysis, since it would be similar in all the studied cases (Clean Up system and alternatives), so it would not affect the results of the economic analysis.

Table 14. Capital costs calculated for Cases C&D.

WWTP Influent, m^3/d	**1000**	**10,000**	**100,000**
Investment costs EUR/m^3/d	593	305	205
Investment, EUR	717,502	3,696,223	24,848,560
Investment (basis), EUR	592,977	3,054,730	20,536,000
Material execution, EUR	498,101	2,565,973	17,250,240
Capital costs, EUR/year	47,582	245,119	1,647,862
Capital costs, EUR/m^3	0.13	0.07	0.05

Table 15. Capital costs calculated for Case A′.

WWTP Influent, m^3/d	**1000**	**10,000**	**100,000**
Investment costs EUR/m^3/d	718	380	255
Investment, EUR	868,752	4,603,723	30,898,560
Investment (basis), EUR	717,977	3,804,730	25,536,000
Material execution, EUR	603,101	3,195,973	21,450,240
Capital costs, EUR/year	57,612	305,301	2,049,075
Capital costs, EUR/m^3	0.16	0.08	0.06

Table 16. Capital costs calculated for Case B′.

WWTP Influent, m^3/d	**1000**	**10,000**	**100,000**
Investment costs EUR/m^3/d	763	421	292
Investment, EUR	923,202	5,099,823	35,375,560
Investment (basis), EUR	762,977	4,214,730	29,236,000
Material execution, EUR	640,901	3,540,373	24,558,240
Capital costs, EUR/year	61,223	338,201	2,345,972
Capital costs, EUR/m^3	0.17	0.09	0.06

2.5. Operational Costs

Below it is included all the information that has been used for carrying out the operational cost calculation, for each considered case. For that, the results obtained in the sizing of the different cases have been used (Tables 5–9), as well as information coming from real tertiary treatment facilities, regarding prices (chemicals, electricity cost, etc.), labor costs, maintenance costs, etc. The chemicals and costs considered in the study are the following: (i) membrane cleaning chemicals (applied in cases A and B) a cost of EUR 0.03 per m^3 treated in the ultrafiltration system is set up; (ii) β-Cyclodextrins (applied in all cases), considering all these factors a price of 5 EUR/kg is set up for βCDs; (iii) regenerant solution (applied in all cases), a price of 1 EUR/kg is set up; (iv) hypochlorite solution (cases B and B′), a price of 0.55 EUR/kg, assuming a 50% solution; and (v) the net energy cost is averaged for each case and included in Tables 5–9. Table 17 sums up that information.

Table 17. Averaged net costs of consumed electricity.

WWTP Influent, m^3/d		1000	10,000	100,000
Net cost of consumed electricity (averaged), EUR/kWh	Case A	0.108	0.101	0.095
	Case B			
	Cases C and D	0.109		
	Case A′	0.108		
	Case B′			

Labor costs depend on the treatment stages that every proposed case includes, and the treatment capacity of the facility. For the calculation, only labor costs associated with the operation of the new facilities are considered. Table 18 includes the considered labor costs.

Table 18. Calculated labor costs for Cases A, B, C, D, A′ and B′.

WWTP Influent, m^3/d		1000	10,000	100.000
Labor costs, EUR/year	Case A Case B	15,000	55,000	250,000
	Cases C and D	12,000	44,000	200,000
	Case A′ Case B′	15,000	55,000	250,000

Maintenance and conservation costs are assumed to be a yearly cost equivalent to 2% of the material execution of the investment. Regarding equipment replacement costs, it is assumed that it will be necessary to replace electro-mechanical equipment in the midterm of the investment lifetime, for which a cost equivalent to 30% of the material execution of the initial investment is applied. It is also assumed that this cost is distributed linearly throughout the investment lifetime, without considering any discount rate. Additionally, a cost due to the replacement of the photocatalysis and pulse light lamps is applied. For this concept, a cost of EUR 0.015 per m^3 treated in the photocatalysis system is set up. Administrative and analysis costs include all the additional costs not previously mentioned, as derived from the analytic control of waters or administrative expenses. It is supposed to be 3% of the operational costs (Table 19).

Table 19. Calculated administrative and analysis costs for Cases A, B, C, D, A′ and B′.

WWTP Influent, m^3/d		1000	10,000	100,000
Administrative and analysis costs, EUR/year	Case A	5800	50,000	460,000
	Case B	5900	51,000	470,000
	Cases C and D	4800	41,000	380,000
	Case A′	5100	44,000	410,000
	Case B′	5300	45,000	420,000

Tables 20–24 include the results of the operational costs calculation, depending on each studied case and the treatment capacity of the plant. These costs come only from the new treatment stages to be implemented, and they are referred to as the m^3 of produced water.

Table 20. Operational costs calculated for Case A.

WWTP Influent, m^3/d		1000	10,000	100,000
Chemicals	EUR/year EUR/m^3	62,381 0.17	623,812 0.17	6,238,117 0.17

Table 20. *Cont.*

WWTP Influent, m^3/d		1000	10,000	100,000
Electrical consumption	EUR/year EUR/m^3	81,992 0.22	764,108 0.21	7,182,144 0.20
Labor	EUR/year EUR/m^3	15,000 0.041	55,000 0.015	250,000 0.007
Maintenance and conservation	EUR/year EUR/m^3	13,785 0.038	71,015 0.019	477,415 0.013
Equipment replacement	EUR/year EUR/m^3	15,814 0.043	108,012 0.030	905,561 0.025
Administrative and analysis costs	EUR/year EUR/m^3	5800 0.016	50,000 0.014	460,000 0.013
Operational costs	EUR/year EUR/m^3	194,773 0.53	1,671,947 0.46	15,513,238 0.43

Table 21. Operational costs calculated for Case B.

WWTP Influent, m^3/d		1000	10,000	100,000
Chemicals	EUR/year EUR/m^3	64,913 0.178	649,127 0.178	6,491,267 0.178
Electrical consumption	EUR/year EUR/m^3	81,992 0.22	764,108 0.21	7,182,144 0.20
Labor	EUR/year EUR/m^3	15,000 0.041	55,000 0.015	250,000 0.007
Maintenance and conservation	EUR/year EUR/m^3	14,541 0.040	77,903 0.021	539,575 0.015
Equipment replacement	EUR/year EUR/m^3	16,381 0.045	113,178 0.031	952,181 0.026
Administrative and analysis costs	EUR/year EUR/m^3	5900 0.016	51,000 0.014	470,000 0.013
Operational costs	EUR/year EUR/m^3	198,727 0.80	1,710,316 0.73	15,885,167 0.69

Table 22. Operational costs calculated for Cases C&D.

WWTP Influent, m^3/d		1000	10,000	100,000
Chemicals	EUR/year EUR/m^3	49,499 0.136	494,988 0.136	4,949,882 0.136
Electrical consumption	EUR/year EUR/m^3	70,419 0.19	655,854 0.18	6,161,121 0.17
Labor	EUR/year EUR/m^3	12,000 0.033	44,000 0.012	200,000 0.005
Maintenance and conservation	EUR/year EUR/m^3	9962 0.027	51,319 0.014	345,005 0.009
Equipment replacement	EUR/year EUR/m^3	12,947 0.035	93,240 0.026	806,254 0.022
Administrative and analysis costs	EUR/year EUR/m^3	4800 0.013	41,000 0.011	380,000 0.010
Operational costs	EUR/year EUR/m^3	159,626 0.44	1,380,401 0.38	12,842,262 0.35

Table 23. Operational costs calculated for Case A′.

WWTP Influent, m^3/d		1000	10,000	100,000
Chemicals	EUR/year EUR/m^3	49,499 0.136	494,988 0.136	4,949,882 0.136
Electrical consumption	EUR/year EUR/m^3	76,282 0.21	710,683 0.19	6,678,185 0.18
Labor	EUR/year EUR/m^3	15,000 0.041	55,000 0.015	250,000 0.007
Maintenance and conservation	EUR/year EUR/m^3	12,062 0.033	63,919 0.018	429,005 0.012
Equipment replacement	EUR/year EUR/m^3	14,522 0.040	102,690 0.028	869,254 0.024
Administrative and analysis costs	EUR/year EUR/m^3	5100 0.014	44,000 0.012	410,000 0.011
Operational costs	EUR/year EUR/m^3	172,464 0.47	1,471,280 0.40	13,586,326 0.37

Table 24. Operational costs calculated for Case B′.

WWTP Influent, m^3/d		1000	10,000	100,000
Chemicals	EUR/year EUR/m^3	52,030 0.143	520,303 0.143	5,203,031 0.143
Electrical consumption	EUR/year EUR/m^3	76,281 0.21	710,683 0.19	6,678,183 0.18
Labor	EUR/year EUR/m^3	15,000 0.041	55,000 0.015	250,000 0.007
Maintenance and conservation	EUR/year EUR/m^3	12,818 0.035	70,807 0.019	491,165 0.013
Equipment replacement	EUR/year EUR/m^3	15,089 0.041	107,856 0.030	915,874 0.025
Administrative and analysis costs	EUR/year EUR/m^3	5300 0.015	45,000 0.012	420,000 0.012
Operational costs	EUR/year EUR/m^3	176,518 0.48	1,509,649 0.41	13,958,252 0.38

2.6. Total Costs

Table 25 includes the calculated costs for all cases. Several potential regressions have been fitted from the obtained results, which can be seen in Figure 2.

Table 25. Total costs calculated for all the studied cases (A, B, C, D, A′ and B′).

	WWTP Influent, m^3/d	1000	10,000	100,000
Case A	Capital costs, EUR/m^3 Operation costs, EUR/m^3	0.18 0.53	0.09 0.46	0.06 0.43
	Total costs, EUR/m^3	0.71	0.55	0.49
Case B	Capital costs, EUR/m^3	0.19	0.10	0.07
	Operation costs, EUR/m^3	0.54	0.47	0.44
	Total costs, EUR/m^3	0.73	0.57	0.51

Table 25. *Cont.*

WWTP Influent, m³/d		1000	10,000	100,000
Cases C and D	Capital costs, EUR/m³	0.13	0.07	0.05
	Operation costs, EUR/m³	0.44	0.38	0.35
	Total costs, EUR/m³	0.57	0.45	0.40
Case A′	Capital costs, EUR/m³	0.16	0.08	0.06
	Operation costs, EUR/m³	0.47	0.40	0.37
	Total costs, EUR/m³	0.63	0.49	0.43
Case B′	Capital costs, EUR/m³	0.17	0.09	0.06
	Operation costs, EUR/m³	0.48	0.41	0.38
	Total costs, EUR/m³	0.65	0.51	0.45

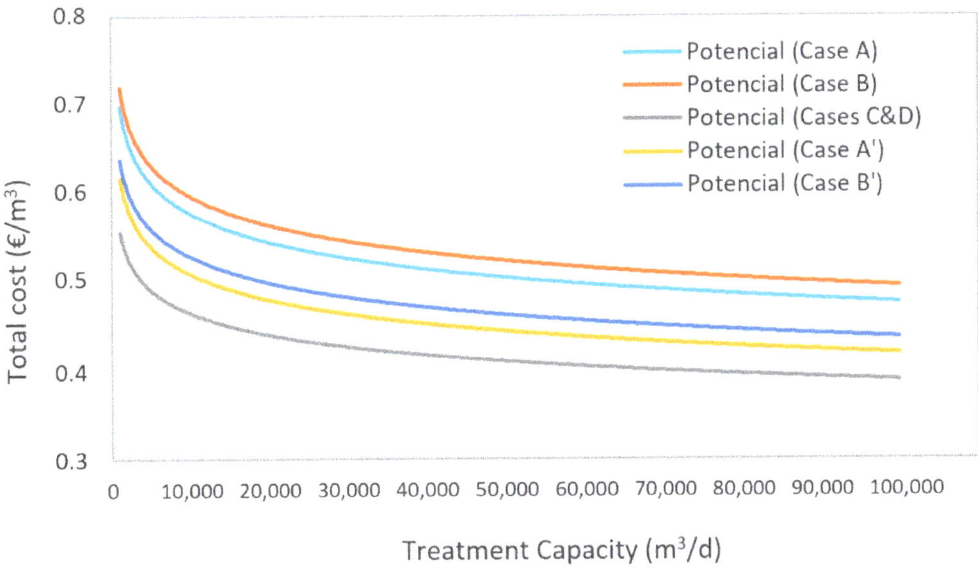

Figure 2. Total costs of all the studied cases. Data fitted to a potential regression.

The previous results clearly show that, for all the foreseen scenarios, the sum of the costs of chemicals and electrical consumption exceeds 73% of the operational costs and 54% of the total costs. Focusing on the analysis of these two operational costs, it can be determined which operations of all those that integrate into the water treatment system outweigh these costs. The values are averages calculated considering all the scenarios where these operations take place, as well as the different treatment capacities considered. Averages have been calculated instead of using values for each case separately because the variation in these costs for the different cases and capacities is not significant, so Figure 3 can represent all the studied cases. Particularly, it must be pointed out that filtration only applies in cases A′ and B′, and chlorination only in B and B′.

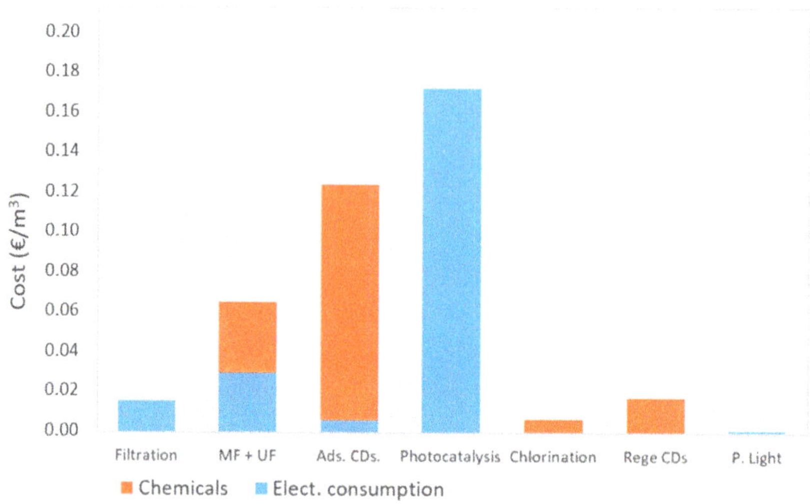

Cost (€/m3)	Filtration	MF + UF	Ads. CDs.	Photocat.	Chlorinat.	Rege CDs	P. Light
Elec. Consumption	0.016	0.029	0.006	0.172	< 0.001	< 0.001	0.001
Chemicals	< 0.001	0.036	0.118	0.001	0.007	0.017	< 0.001

Figure 3. Averaged treatment cost by treatment operation.

3. Results of Economic Feasibility Analysis

In this section, the procedures followed to calculate the treatment costs of the considered technical alternative to the Clean Up system are described, as well as the obtained results. Then, the technical–economic viability of the Clean Up solution is determined through the comparison between its treatment costs and the ones for the technical alternatives.

3.1. Treatment Costs of Technical Alternatives

The technical alternatives to the Clean Up solution, both from a technical and economic point of view, the most efficient ones are ozonation and PAC. These treatments must be applied in WWTPs that already have advanced treatments for nutrients and suspended solids removal so that this is effective. On the other hand, these treatments must also include a final filtration stage, after the O_3/PAC stage. That last stage can be a gravity sand filter including biofilm formation, in the case of the O_3. In the case of PAC, they could be used in sand filters, microscreens, cloth filters or even membranes of MF or UF. The efficiency of these two treatments is proven, so both are already being implemented at an industrial scale in WWTPs to avoid the incoming of micropollutants into water bodies. For this reason, these treatments and not others have been considered in principle as technical alternatives to the Clean Up treatment. In general, they offer similar EP removal performance (around 80%). Anyway, only the O_3 option has been finally considered as an alternative to Clean Up, finding the same application scenarios for both technologies. The PAC option has been discarded due to several disadvantages that emerge when compared to O_3. Summing up, PAC application entails the presence of exhausted PAC with EPs in the produced sewage sludge, which can limit its use in agriculture. Above this, the treatment with PAC is in general terms more expensive than the O_3 one. So, only the O_3 treatment is considered to be compared to the Clean Up treatment.

To estimate the treatment costs of the O_3 system, the same scenarios indicated previously for the Clean Up case have been considered, that is, application in WWTPs that either have an advanced treatment or not, and the aim to discharge treated water into water bodies or reclaim it to be used in agriculture. In addition, as in the Clean Up case, a treatment capacity between 1000 and 100,000 m^3/d has been considered. The treatment system, whose costs are intended to be calculated, will have particular characteristics, depending on the application scenario and, therefore, also particular costs. Regarding the calculation parameters used for sizing these systems, the operational conditions, consumptions and performances that could be expected from said systems are described below. For setting up these data, general information obtained from various bibliographic sources is used. This information is later specified, in every case where it is used.

Case A*. The system is applied in a WWTP that does not have any advanced treatment for removing suspended solids after its secondary settlers, and where the treated water is discharged into a water body. Then, the objective is to limit the presence of EPs in the mentioned water body. The treatment system is composed of a first stage of tertiary treatment (filtration) for suspended solids removal, followed by the ozonation contact reactor and a final stage of high-rate biofiltration using inert media (sand). Below, it is described how the implementation at the industrial level of the different stages that compose this treatment would be completed, as well as the considerations that have been carried out for estimating the treatment costs of the mentioned system. The sources that have been consulted to define the previous design parameters are the following: [21–30,37,39,41–51,58,60,62,63].

In addition, this information has been verified with available data from real tertiary treatment facilities.

Direct filtration stage. This stage is designed for treating the water coming from secondary settlers, providing water with a concentration of both, suspended solids and dissolved organic carbon (DOC), lower than 10 ppm. There are different treatment trains for aiming this objective, depending basically on the quality of the secondary effluent. These systems are mainly composed of physicochemical and filtration treatments. In this case, it is assumed that the level of quality of the secondary effluent is high enough to only require a direct filtration stage as a tertiary treatment. This direct filtration system is calculated as an average of microscreens, cloth filters and sand filters (open and closed) all commonly used in tertiary treatments. Then, the considered calculation parameters are the following: (i) TSS in secondary effluent—15 mg/L; (ii) recovery—98%; (iii) TSS removal performance—55%; and (iv) electrical consumption—0.15 kWh/m^3. Both in the case of direct filtration and biofiltration stages, the concentrate produced in cleaning operations is directed to the inlet of the WWTP. For this reason, the direct filtration stage is sized considering the increase in the treatment capacity that these two recirculated volumes suppose, and for the biofiltration, the followed procedure is similar, but considering only the recirculate stream generated in said operation.

Ozonation stage. This stage is designed to oxidize the remaining organic matter present in the direct filtration effluent, including the micropollutants. The treatment supposes a micropollutant removal higher than 80%. These compounds are mainly mineralized to CO_2 and H_2O, being the remaining ones degraded to oxidation by-products, which are less toxic and more biodegradable, so they are removed in the final biofiltration stage. For sizing the ozonation stage, the considered calculation parameters are the following: (i) DOC in secondary effluent—7.5 mg/L; (ii) O_3 dose—5 mg/L; (iii) electrical consumption for ozone generation 12.5 kWh/kgO_3; (iv) electrical consumption for water pumping 0.03 kWh/m^3; and (v) EPs removal performance—80% (ozonation + biofiltration).

Biofiltration stage. In this stage, the ozonation by-products and residual organic compounds are removed. It is a slow gravity filtration through an inert granular media (sand), in which the organic compounds are removed by the biofilm that grows over the surface of the media. That biofilm grows in the upper zone of the filter, where the sand is in contact with oxygenated water. The biofilters are cleaned regularly, and the wastewater produced in said operation goes to the WWTP inlet. The calculation parameters used for biofiltration sizing are the following: (i) recovery—98%; (ii) TSS removal performance—60%; (iii) EPs removal performance—80% (ozonation + biofiltration); and (iv) electrical consumption—0.05 kWh/m^3. Table 26 includes the results obtained for Case A*.

Table 26. Results obtained in Case A* sizing.

WWTP Influent, m^3/d	1000	10,000	100,000
Direct filtration stage			
Filtration influent, m^3/d	1041	10,412	104,123
Filtration effluent, m^3/d			
TSS in filtration effluent, mg/L		6.9	
Wastewater flow (from filter cleaning), m^3/d	21	208	2082
TSS in wastewater from filter cleaning, mg/L		412	
Electrical consumption, kWh/d	156	1562	15,618
WWTP influent, m^3/d	1000	10,000	100,000
Ozonation stage			
Ozonation influent, m^3/d	1020	10,204	102,041
TSS in ozonation influent, mg/L			
Electrical consumption, kWh/d		94	
Biofiltration stage			
Biofiltration influent, m^3/d		1020	
TSS in biofiltration influent, mg/L		6.9	
Biofiltration effluent, m^3/d		1000	
TSS in biofiltration effluent, mg/L		2.8	
Wastewater flow (from filter cleaning), m^3/d		20	
TSS in wastewater from filter cleaning, mg/L		207	
Electrical consumption, kWh/d		51	
Photovoltaic plant			
Electrical consumption of treatment plant, MWh/year		110	
Installed peak PV power, kWp		56.5	
Production cost (LCOE), EUR/kWh		0.110	
PV plant installation (YES/NO)	YES	YES	YES
PV Plant production, MWh/year		88	
Net cost of consumed electricity (averaged), EUR/kWh	0.115	0.107	0.100

Case B*. The system is applied in a WWTP that does not have any advanced treatment for removing suspended solids after its secondary settlers, and where the aim is to reclaim water to be used in agriculture, including the removal of EPs in the water reclamation process. The treatment system is similar to Case A*, but includes a final stage consisting of UV disinfection, and a final chlorination step (NaClO dosing) to maintain a minimum residual in the reclaimed water. The calculation parameters used are similar to the previous case, and for the final disinfection stage, they are described below:

Disinfection stage. The stage is composed of irradiation by UV lamps and the subsequent stage of chlorination by NaClO dosing in a contact reactor. The objective is to reach the quality parameters set up by the current regulation (Regulation (EU) 2020/741) regarding the presence of pathogens in reclaimed water. The calculation parameters used are the following: (i) electrical consumption of 0.06 kWh/m^3 (it includes the UV lamps and the rest of the equipment) and (ii) NaClO dose of 3 gCl_2/m^3. Table 27 includes the results obtained for Case B*.

Table 27. Results obtained in Case B* sizing.

WWTP Influent, m³/d	1000	10,000	100,000
	Direct filtration stage		
Filtration influent, m^3/d	1041	10,412	104,123
Filtration effluent, m^3/d			
TSS in filtration effluent, mg/L		6.9	
Wastewater flow (from filter cleaning), m^3/d		21	
TSS in wastewater from filter cleaning, mg/L		412	
Electrical consumption, kWh/d		156	
	Ozonation stage		
Ozonation influent, m^3/d		1020	
TSS in ozonation influent, mg/L		6.9	
Electrical consumption, kWh/d		94	
	Biofiltration stage		
Biofiltration influent, m^3/d		1020	
TSS in biofiltration influent, mg/L		6.9	
Biofiltration effluent, m^3/d		1000	
TSS in biofiltration effluent, mg/L		2.8	
Wastewater flow (from filter cleaning), m^3/d	20	204	2041
TSS in wastewater from filter cleaning, mg/L		207	
Electrical consumption, kWh/d	51	510	5102
	Disinfection stage		
Disinfection influent, m^3/d	1000	10,000	100,000
TSS in biofiltration effluent, mg/L	2.8		
NaClO consumption (50% solution), kg/d	13	126	1261
Electrical consumption, kWh/d	60	600	6000
	Photovoltaic plant		
Electrical consumption of treatment plant, MWh/year	132	1320	13,198
Installed peak PV power, kWp	67.7	677.3	6773.0
Production cost (LCOE), EUR/kWh	0.108	0.089	0.073
PV plant installation (YES/NO)	YES	YES	YES
PV plant production, MWh/year	105	1055	10,549
Net cost of consumed electricity (averaged), EUR/kWh	0.115	0.106	0.099

Case C*. The system is applied in a WWTP that already has an advanced treatment for removing suspended solids after its secondary settlers, and where the treated water is discharged into a water body. The treatment system is similar to Case A*, but excluding the first stage consisting of direct filtration, because that treatment is supposed to be carried out by the current facilities. As of Case A*, the objective is to limit the presence of EPs in the mentioned water body.

Case D*. The system applied in a WWTP that already has a tertiary treatment for reclaiming water, but the same does not have a special treatment for EP removal. The objective is to implement only the ozonation and biofiltration stages, using them along with the rest of the current tertiary treatment stages, for reclaiming water. The treatment is similar to Case B*, but excluding the direct filtration and final disinfection stages, because that treatment is supposed to be carried out by the current facilities. Therefore, new facilities are similar to that of Case C*. Table 28 includes the results obtained for Cases C* and D*. The data regarding the operation of the existing reclamation facilities are not included.

Table 28. Results obtained in Cases C* and D* sizing.

WWTP Influent, m^3/d	1000	10,000	100,000
Ozonation stage			
Ozonation influent, m^3/d	1020	10,204	102,041
TSS in ozonation influent, mg/L			
Electrical consumption, kWh/d		94	
Biofiltration stage			
Biofiltration influent, m^3/d		1020	
TSS in biofiltration influent, mg/L		6.9	
Biofiltration effluent, m^3/d		1000	
TSS in biofiltration effluent, mg/L		2.8	
Wastewater flow (from filter cleaning), m^3/d		20	
TSS in wastewater from filter cleaning, mg/L		207	
Electrical consumption, kWh/d		51	
Photovoltaic plant			
Electrical consumption of treatment plant, MWh/year		53	
Installed peak PV power, kWp		27.2	
Production cost (LCOE), EUR/kWh		0.117	
PV plant installation (YES/NO)	YES	YES	YES
PV plant production, MWh/year		42	
Net cost of consumed electricity (averaged), EUR/kWh	0.119	0.109	0.102

Once the different treatments considered are sized, the following step is the calculation of the corresponding treatment costs. Parameters and factors used for cost calculation and the obtained results are shown below. This work is divided into two sections: capital costs and operational costs.

Capital costs. The necessary investment depends on the studied case. Table 29 gathers all the information considered for the calculation of capital costs, based on the studied case and the treatment capacity of the facilities. For defining the investment costs, several references have been revised [43,49,51,55–61]:

Tables 30–32 show the results of the capital costs calculation, for Cases A*, B* and C*&D*, respectively. Capital costs are calculated based on the basis values (values excluding VAT), as it has been assumed that the investment would be carried out by the public sector.

Operational costs. All the information that has been used for carrying out the operational cost calculation for each considered case is included below. For doing so, the same information sources previously indicated have been used for the capital costs calculation, as well as information coming from real treatment facilities. (i) Chemicals cost is only applied in Case B*, as it is the only case for which it is necessary to implement new equipment for disinfection. The cost is due to the NaClO consumption, which is used for assuring a chlorine residual concentration in treated waters. The price set up for hypochlorite is 0.55 EUR/kg, assuming a 50% solution. (ii) Energy costs for each case depend on the consumption of electrical energy and the grade of the implementation of the PV system.

The net cost of consumed electricity is averaged for each case and included in Tables 26–28. Table 33 summarizes that information.

Table 29. Information considered for capital cost calculation for Cases A*, B*, C* and D*.

WWTP Influent, m³/d		**1000**	**10,000**	**100,000**
Investment costs, EUR/m³/d	Case A*	1145	595	400
Investment costs, EUR/m³/d	Case B*	1275	670	455
Investment costs, EUR/m³/d	Cases C* and D*	1020	520	350
Benefit rate, % [1]		6		
General expenses rate, % [1]		13		
VAT, %		21		
Investment lifetime, years		20		
Financing interest, %		5		

Note: [1] Applied over material execution.

Table 30. Capital costs calculated for Case A*.

WWTP Influent, m³/d	**1000**	**10,000**	**100,000**
Investment, EUR	1,275,000	6,700,000	45,500,000
Investment (basis), EUR	1,053,719	5,537,190	37,603,306
Material execution, EUR	885,124	4,651,240	31,586,777
Capital costs, EUR/year	84,553	444,318	3,017,387
Capital costs, EUR/m³	0.23	0.12	0.08

Table 31. Capital costs calculated for Case B*.

WWTP Influent, m³/d	**1000**	**10,000**	**100,000**
Investment, EUR	1,145,000	5,950,000	40,000,000
Investment (basis), EUR	946,281	4,917,355	33,057,851
Material execution, EUR	794,876	4,130,579	27,768,595
Capital costs, EUR/year	75,932	394,581	2,652,648
Capital costs, EUR/m³	0.21	0.11	0.07

Table 32. Capital costs calculated for Cases C* and D*.

WWTP Influent, m³/d	**1000**	**10,000**	**100,000**
Investment, EUR	1,020,000	5,200,000	35,000,000
Investment (basis), EUR	842,975	4,297,521	28,925,620
Material execution, EUR	708,099	3,609,917	24,297,521
Capital costs, EUR/year	67,643	344,844	2,321,067
Capital costs, EUR/m³	0.19	0.09	0.06

Table 33. Averaged net costs of consumed electricity for Cases A*, B*, C* and D*.

WWTP Influent, m³/d		**1000**	**10,000**	**100,000**
Net cost of consumed electricity (averaged), EUR/kWh	Case A*	0.115	0.107	0.100
	Case B*	0.115	0.106	0.099
	Cases C* and D*	0.119	0.109	0.102

Labor costs depend on the treatment stages that every proposed case includes, and the treatment capacity of the facility. For the calculation, only labor costs associated with the operation of the new facilities are considered. Table 34 includes the considered labor costs.

Table 34. Calculated labor costs for Cases A*, B*, C* and D*.

WWTP Influent, m^3/d		**1000**	**10,000**	**100,000**
Labor costs, EUR/year	Case A*	15,000	55,000	250,000
	Case B*			
	Cases C* and D*	12,000	44,000	200,000

Maintenance and conservation costs are assumed to be a yearly cost equivalent to 2% of the material execution of the investment. It is assumed that regarding equipment replacement costs in the midterm of the investment lifetime, it is necessary to replace electro-mechanical equipment, for which a cost equivalent to 30% of the material execution of the initial investment is applied. It is also assumed that this cost is distributed linearly throughout the investment lifetime, without considering any discount rate. In addition, for the option that entails the implementation of a disinfection stage (case B*), a cost due to the replacement of the UV lamps of EUR 0.01 per treated m3 is assumed to take place. Finally, administrative and analysis costs include all the additional costs not previously mentioned, as derived from the analytic control of waters or administrative expenses. It is supposed to be 3% of the operational costs (Table 35).

Table 35. Calculated administrative and analysis costs for Cases A*, B*, C* and D*.

WWTP Influent, m^3/d		**1000**	**10,000**	**100,000**
Administrative and analysis costs, EUR/year	Case A*	1700	9900	72,000
	Case B*	2100	13,000	102,000
	Cases C* and D*	1350	7000	50,000

Tables 36–38 include the results of the operational costs calculation, depending on each studied case and the treatment capacity of the plant. These costs come only from the new treatment stages to implement, and they refer to the m^3 of produced water.

Table 36. Operational costs calculated for Case A*.

WWTP Influent, m^3/d		**1000**	**10,000**	**100,000**
Electrical consumption	EUR/year	12,711	117,563	1,097,160
	EUR/m^3	0.035	0.032	0.030
Labor	EUR/year	15,000	55,000	250,000
	EUR/m^3	0.041	0.015	0.007
Maintenance and conservation	EUR/year	15,898	82,612	555,372
	EUR/m^3	0.044	0.023	0.015
Equipment replacement	EUR/year	11,923	61,959	416,529
	EUR/m^3	0.033	0.017	0.011
Administrative and analysis costs	EUR/year	1700	9900	72,000
	EUR/m^3	0.005	0.003	0.002
Operational costs	EUR/year	57,231	327,034	2,391,061
	EUR/m^3	0.16	0.09	0.07

Table 37. Operational costs calculated for Case B*.

WWTP Influent, m³/d		1000	10,000	100,000
Chemicals	EUR/year	2531	25,315	253,149
	EUR/m³	0.007	0.007	0.007
Electrical consumption	EUR/year	15,141	140,142	1,308,772
	EUR/m³	0.041	0.038	0.036
Labor	EUR/year	15,000	55,000	250,000
	EUR/m³	0.041	0.015	0.007
Maintenance and conservation	EUR/year	17,702	93,025	631,736
	EUR/m³	0.048	0.025	0.017
WWTP influent, m³/d	1000	10,000	100,000	
Equipment replacement	EUR/year	16,927	106,269	838,802
	EUR/m³	0.046	0.029	0.023
Administrative and analysis costs	EUR/year	2100	13,000	102,000
	EUR/m³	0.006	0.004	0.003
Operational costs	EUR/year	69,402	432,750	3,384,459

Table 38. Operational costs calculated for Cases C*&D*.

WWTP Influent, m³/d		1000	10,000	100,000
Electrical consumption	EUR/year	6294	58,043	540,174
	EUR/m³	0.017	0.016	0.015
Labor	EUR/year	12,000	44,000	200,000
	EUR/m³	0.033	0.012	0.005
Maintenance and conservation	EUR/year	14,162	72,198	485,950
	EUR/m³	0.039	0.020	0.013
Equipment replacement	EUR/year	10,621	54,149	364,463
	EUR/m³	0.029	0.015	0.010
Administrative and analysis costs	EUR/year	1350	7000	50,000
	EUR/m³	0.004	0.002	0.001
Operational costs	EUR/year	44,427	235,390	1,640,587
	EUR/m³	0.12	0.06	0.04

Total costs. Table 39 includes the calculated costs for cases A, B and C&D, respectively.

Table 39. Total costs calculated for all the studied Cases A*, B*, C* and D*.

WWTP Influent, m³/d		1000	10,000	100,000
Case A*	Capital costs, EUR/m³	0.21	0.11	0.07
	Operation costs, EUR/m³	0.16	0.09	0.07
	Total costs, EUR/m³	0.36	0.20	0.14
Case B*	Capital costs, EUR/m³	0.23	0.12	0.08
	Operation costs, EUR/m³	0.19	0.12	0.09
	Total costs, EUR/m³	0.42	0.24	0.18
Cases C* and D*	Capital costs, EUR/m³	0.19	0.09	0.06
	Operation costs, EUR/m³	0.12	0.06	0.04
	Total costs, EUR/m³	0.31	0.16	0.11

3.2. Comparative Cost Study

Once the treatment costs of both the Clean Up system and the proposed alternative have been analyzed, and for all the contemplated scenarios, the comparison of the costs of both systems allows us to know whether the Clean Up solution is competitive compared to the alternative in each scenario or not. In this sense, when comparing Tables 25 and 39, it is observed that in all cases, the total costs of the Clean Up solution are higher than those of the alternatives discussed in previous sections. A more detailed analysis of the results shows that, although the investment costs of the Clean Up system are lower than those of the alternative in all scenarios, the operational costs are much higher. Focusing the analysis on the operational costs of the Clean Up system, it is observed that the factors with the most influence are the electrical consumption of the photocatalytic stage, the chemicals used in the adsorption stage (cyclodextrins and regenerating solution), and the micro + ultrafiltration stage, as indicated in Figure 4.

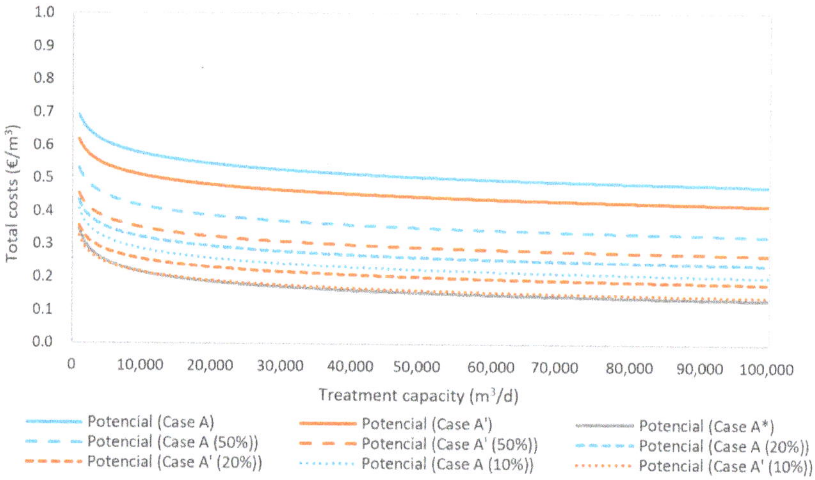

Figure 4. Total costs of Clean Up system and considered alternative for implementation in WWTPs without advanced treatment and discharge of treated water into water bodies.

Considering that the proposed alternative has already been demonstrated and optimized, and is being implemented on a full scale in many WWTPs in Europe, especially in Switzerland, and that, on the other hand, the Clean Up solution is a recent development, and therefore its operating costs could be optimized, a comparative study of costs between both technologies is then considered in which the variation in the costs of the Clean Up system is taken into account as a function of these commented factors, namely, the energy consumption of photocatalysis, acquisition cost of chemicals used in the adsorption stage, and the MF + UF stage. In this way, it is possible to know, for each scenario, the conditions that should exist for the Clean Up solution to be economically competitive compared to the proposed alternative. Thus, the following graphs show, for each of the contemplated scenarios, and depending on the treatment capacity of the facility, the total costs of the Clean Up solution compared to those of the alternatives considered. In the case of Clean-up costs, these are presented as a function of the percentage of reduction in the cost of electricity consumption for photocatalysis and the purchase price of the chemicals used in adsorption–regeneration operations.

Scenario 1: Application in WWTPs without advanced treatment for the removal of suspended solids, which discharge the treated water into water bodies. In this scenario, both the Clean Up system (Cases A and A'), as well as the alternative (Case A*) would be implemented in the WWTP with the aim of limiting the presence of EPs in said water bodies. It is convenient to remember the difference between the two considered cases of the Clean

Up implementation (Case A and A′). While Case A includes a microfiltration followed by an ultrafiltration stage, as an advanced treatment for the elimination of suspended solids, turbidity and pathogenic microorganisms, Case A′ includes instead a direct filtration process similar to the one used in the majority of WWTPs that includes advanced treatment, as it is assumed that this treatment is sufficient to give a proper degree of removal of suspended solids. This system is proposed as an alternative to Case A, given the high cost involved in the UF stage. Figure 4 shows the graphs with the total costs calculated and adjusted to a potential relationship in all cases. The dashed lines represent different cases in which it has been assumed that the costs of the factors indicated above are reduced by a certain percentage. For example, the curve "Case A (50%)" represents the costs of applying the Clean Up system, including the MF + UF stage, and in which it has been assumed that both the electrical consumption of the photocatalysis stage and the cost of the chemicals used in the adsorption–regeneration stage is reduced by 50%.

According to the results obtained for this scenario, the Clean Up solution would only be economically competitive not including a UF stage, but rather another direct filtration treatment similar to those used in most WWTPs that have advanced treatment, and if the electricity consumption of the photocatalysis and the acquisition costs of the chemicals of the adsorption–desorption stage were reduced to approximately 10% or less of the costs considered for the calculation of Cases A and A′. This would imply the need to achieve an electrical consumption of 0.17 kWh/m^3 or less, and costs of 0.5 EUR/kg for the CDs and 0.1 EUR/kg for the regenerating solution.

Scenario 2: Application in WWTPs without advanced treatment for removal of suspended solids, which discharge the treated water into water bodies, but intend to reclaim water. In this scenario, both the Clean Up system (Cases B and B′), as well as the alternative (case B*), would be implemented in the WWTP with the aim of limiting the presence of EPs in reclaimed water. Figure 5 includes the graphs with the total costs calculated, and adjusted to a potential relationship in all cases.

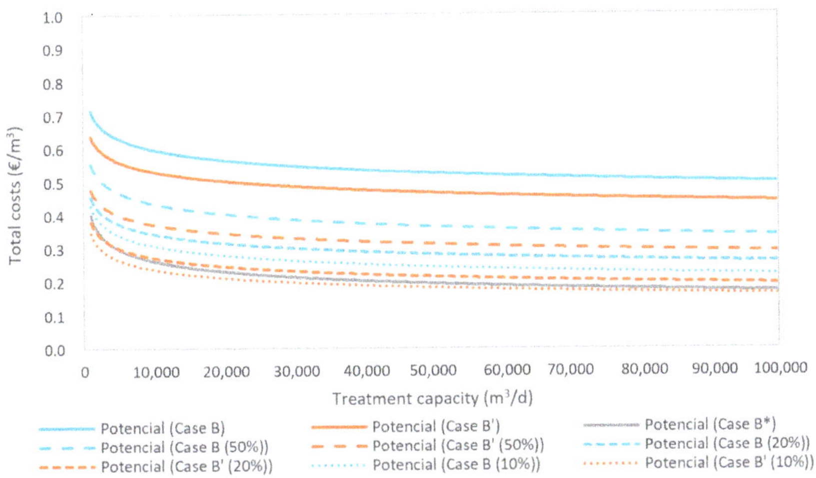

Figure 5. Total costs of Clean Up system and considered alternative for implementation in WWTPs without advanced treatment, which discharge the treated water into water bodies, and which intend to reclaim water.

In this scenario, the Clean Up solution would be economically competitive not including a UF stage, but rather another direct filtration treatment, as in the previous case, and if the electricity consumption of the photocatalysis and the acquisition costs of the chemicals of the adsorption–desorption stage were reduced to approximately 12% or less of the costs considered for the calculation of Cases B and B′. This would imply the need to achieve an electrical consumption of 0.20 kWh/m^3 or less, and costs of 0.6 EUR/kg for the CDs and 0.12 EUR/kg for the regenerating solution. The results are slightly better for the Clean Up case than in the previous scenario because said system is valid for obtaining reclaimed water, with the simple addition of a final chlorination stage, while with the proposed alternative it would be necessary to apply a final stage of UV disinfection and final chlorination.

Scenario 3: Application in WWTPs that already have an advanced treatment for the removal of suspended solids and the UV disinfection stage, and intend to discharge treated water into water bodies or to reclaim water. In this scenario, both the Clean Up system (Cases C and D′), as well as the alternative (case C* and D*), would be implemented in the WWTP with the aim of limiting the presence of EPs in discharged or reclaimed water. Cases C and C* refer to a situation in which it is intended to discharge the treated water into water bodies, while D and D* are intended to reclaim water. Figure 6 includes the graphs with the total costs calculated, and adjusted to a potential relationship in all cases.

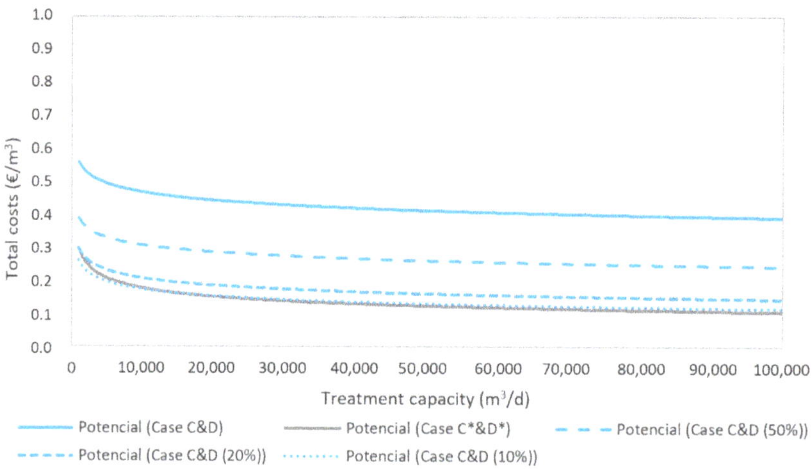

Figure 6. Total costs of Clean Up system and considered alternative for implementation in WWTPs that already have advanced treatment for suspended solids removal and UV disinfection stage and which intend to discharge treated water into water bodies or to reclaim water.

According to the results obtained for this scenario, the Clean Up solution would only be economically competitive if the electricity consumption of the photocatalysis and the acquisition costs of the chemicals of the adsorption–desorption stage were reduced to approximately 10% or less of the costs considered for the calculation of Cases A and A′. Like the first scenario, this would imply the need to achieve an electrical consumption of 0.17 kWh/m^3 or less, and costs of 0.5 EUR/kg for the CDs and 0.1 EUR/kg for the regenerating solution.

4. Conclusions

The present report describes the results of the technical–economic assessment of the Clean Up solution. From a technical point of view, the viability of the Clean Up system is evaluated by being applied as an advanced treatment system for treated urban wastewater, for the elimination of pathogens and emerging pollutants (EPs), considering the established quality criteria by current regulations. In this sense, it is a technology that has been successfully validated at an experimental level, and that offers similar removal performance to those of the most efficient alternatives available on the market.

The technical–economic assessment of the Clean Up solution has been based on the following steps: (i) Estimation of the treatment costs of the Clean Up system, applied at an industrial level. For said estimation, it has been considered both data obtained in the experimental phase of the project carried out with a pilot plant and general information obtained from various technical bibliographic sources. (ii) Estimation of the treatment costs of the most advantageous technological alternative to the Clean Up system from the technical–economic point of view, applied at an industrial scale, and in the same scenario and conditions as those assumed for the Clean Up system. This alternative is based on an ozonation treatment followed by a biological filtration stage (slow sand filters with biofilm formation in upper layers). It has already been validated at a technical and economical level and is being implemented at an industrial scale in several European countries, as a way to limit the presence of EPs in WWTP effluents. To carry out the estimation, information from industrial facilities that operate in the same application with the aforementioned technology has been taken. (iii) Comparison of the treatment costs of both alternatives, applied in all cases under similar conditions and assuming similar performance. Treatment costs are considered as the sum of operating and capital costs. On the other hand, for the proper comparison of the costs of both technologies, a similar EP removal performance has been assumed in both cases, specifically, yields of EP removal higher than 80% and figures that have been experimentally validated in each case.

Both in the case of the Clean Up solution and the proposed alternative, costs have been estimated for the same application scenarios. Firstly, the treatment capacity of the facility has been considered as a factor influencing costs. Thus, the costs have been estimated for an interval between 1000 and 100,000 m^3/d of treatment capacity. On the other hand, it has also been considered as a factor whether or not the WWTP has a tertiary treatment for the removal of the suspended solids that remain in the secondary effluent, since this stage is necessary for the proper operation of the process, both in the case of the Clean Up system, as in the proposed alternative. Finally, whether the objective of the WWTP is to discharge the treated water into water bodies or to reclaim water for using it in agriculture, has also been considered.

Regarding the obtained results, although the treatment costs of the Clean Up system are competitive and are in line with those of most water reclamation treatments, they are higher than those of the proposed alternative. Specifically, they vary between 0.73 and 0.40 EUR/m^3 depending on the factors indicated in the previous paragraph, while in the case of ozonation + biological filtration, they vary between 0.42 and 0.11 EUR/m^3. Regarding the investment costs, they have been estimated lower in the case of the Clean Up alternative. Specifically, they could vary between 0.19 and 0.05 EUR/m^3, while in the ozonation + biological filtration case, they could vary between 0.23 and 0.06 EUR/m^3, depending on the factors previously pointed out. On the other hand, the operation costs are higher in the case of the Clean Up system (0.54–0.35 EUR/m^3) as compared with the raised alternative (0.19–0.04 EUR/m^3). Focusing the analysis on the operational costs of the Clean Up system, it can be observed that the operational factors with the most influence are the electrical consumption of the photocatalysis stage, the chemicals used in the adsorption stage (cyclodextrins and regenerating solution), and the consumptions associated with the micro + ultrafiltration stage. Considering that the proposed alternative has already been demonstrated and optimized, and is being implemented on a full scale, and that on the other hand, the Clean Up solution is of recent development, and therefore its operating costs could be optimized, a comparative study of costs between both technologies is then considered in which the variation in the costs of the Clean Up system is taken into account as a function of these commented factors.

This analysis has been carried out for each of the considered scenarios in order to determine in each case the conditions that should exist for the Clean Up solution to be economically competitive compared to the proposed alternative. Considering the application in WWTPs without advanced treatment for removal of suspended solids, which currently discharge the treated water into water bodies, the Clean Up solution would only be economically competitive not including a UF stage, but rather another direct filtration treatment similar to those used in most WWTPs that include advanced treatment. And, if the electricity consumption of the photocatalysis and the acquisition costs of the chemicals of the adsorption–desorption stage were reduced to approximately 10% or less of the costs considered for the cost estimation. This would imply the need to achieve an electrical consumption of 0.17 kWh/m^3 or less, and costs of 0.5 EUR/kg for the CDs and 0.1 EUR/kg for the regenerating solution (sodium chloride, NaCl). On the other hand, considering the application in WWTP without advanced treatment for removal of suspended solids, which currently discharge the treated water into water bodies, but intend to reclaim water, the Clean Up solution would be economically competitive not including a UF stage, but rather another direct filtration treatment, as in the previous case, and if the electricity consumption of the photocatalysis and the acquisition costs of the chemicals of the adsorption–desorption stage were reduced to approximately 12% or less of the costs considered for the cost estimation. This would imply the need to achieve an electrical consumption of 0.20 kWh/m^3 or less, and costs of 0.6 EUR/kg for the CDs and 0.12 EUR/kg for the regenerating solution (NaCl). The results are slightly better for the Clean Up case than in the previous scenario because the said system is valid for obtaining reclaimed water, with the simple addition of a final chlorination stage, for assuring the presence of a residual oxidant in the treated water, while regarding the proposed alternative, it would be necessary to apply a final stage of UV disinfection and final chlorination. Finally, we consider the application in WWTPs, which already have advanced treatment for the removal of suspended solids, and the UV disinfection stage, which intends to discharge treated water into water bodies or to reclaim water. According to the results obtained for this scenario, the Clean Up solution would only be economically competitive if the electricity consumption of the photocatalysis and the acquisition costs of the chemicals of the adsorption–desorption stage were reduced to approximately 10% or less of the costs considered for the cost estimation. Like the first scenario, this would imply the need to achieve an electrical consumption of 0.17 kWh/m^3 or less, and costs of 0.5 EUR/kg for the CDs and 0.1 EUR/kg for the regenerating solution (NaCl).

Bearing in mind that the Clean Up system is designed for tertiary or advanced wastewater treatment, an objective of transferability to other sectors is set as a polishing stage as a way to increase the degree of treatment of the effluents generated in the industrial wastewater treatment plants (IWWTP), thus opening up the possibility for their reuse. Knowing that the difference between the Clean Up system and conventional tertiary treatments is that with the former, it is possible to remove EPs, its application as a polishing stage in the treatment of industrial wastewaters would make sense in those cases in which the IWWTP's effluents to be treated may contain this type of compounds because they have not been efficiently removed in the existing industrial wastewater treatments. Then, the Clean Up system would be applied with the aim of reclaiming water, also avoiding the presence of these pollutants in the reclaimed water. The water treatment industry and the agri-food sector are identified as a potential target for the transfer of Clean Up technology. The agri-food sector's wastewater, similar in quality and quantity to municipal wastewater, necessitates additional treatment stages for effluent discharged directly into water bodies, highlighting the Clean Up technology's efficacy in removing persistent pollutants common in certain agri-food sub-sectors. Moreover, this sector presents a substantial market for wastewater treatment and reclamation, especially for agricultural reuse. Most companies already comply with legal discharge requirements, positioning water reclamation as a feasible advancement. On the other hand, the waste management sector, particularly those managing biodegradable wastewater with potential synthetic pollutants, like chemical toilets, also emerges as a key area for applying Clean Up technology, enhancing water treatment to meet discharge standards into natural water bodies. Due to the treatment flow limitation of the Clean Up system to 1000 m^3/d and the requirement to consider parallel units for scaling up the daily treatment capacity, it is determined that the most suitable scenarios for the commercial implementation of the Clean Up system are in WWTPs with a small flow or in the previously described industries (also typically with small flows), which do not necessitate an excessive number of Clean Up units.

Supplementary Materials: The following supporting information can be downloaded at: https://www.mdpi.com/article/10.3390/w16060814/s1.

Author Contributions: Methodology, J.M.P.; Formal analysis, V.F.; Investigation, V.F.; Data curation, J.M.P.; Writing—original draft, J.M.P.; Writing—review & editing, V.F.; Project administration, V.F. All authors have read and agreed to the published version of the manuscript.

Funding: This research was funded by the European Commission, Grant Agreement LIFE16ENV/ES/000169, "Validation of Adsorbent Materials and Advanced Oxidation Techniques to Remove Emerging Pollutants in Treated Wastewater", Life Clean Up.

Data Availability Statement: The original contributions presented in the study are included in the article/Supplementary Material, further inquiries can be directed to the corresponding authors.

Acknowledgments: The authors wish to express their gratitude to CETENMA for their collaboration in the execution of economic analyses and to David Campos and Paula Sanchez for their participation in the drafting of this report.

Conflicts of Interest: The authors declare that the research was conducted in the absence of any or financial no-financial aspect that could be construed as a potential conflict of interest.

References

1. Vasilachi, I.C.; Asiminicesei, D.M.; Fertu, D.I.; Gavrilescu, M. Occurrence and Fate of Emerging Pollutants in Water Environment and Options for Their Removal. *Water* **2021**, *13*, 181. [CrossRef]
2. NORMAN Network, Emerging Substances List. Available online: https://www.norman-network.net/ (accessed on 5 March 2024).
3. Dulio, V.; van Bavel, B.; Bronrström-Lundén, E.; Harmsen, J.; Hollender, J.; Schalabach, M.; Slobodnick, J.; Thomas, J.; Koschorreck, J. Emerging pollutants in the EU: 10 years of NORMAN in support of environmental policies and regulations. *Environ. Sci. Eur.* **2018**, *30*, 5. [CrossRef]
4. Comero, S.; Loos, R.; Carvalho, R.; Anto, D.C.; Locoro, G.; Tavazzi, S.; Gawlik, B.M. EU-wide monitoring survey on emerging polar organic contaminants in wastewater treatment plant effluents. *Water Res.* **2013**, *47*, 6475–6487. [CrossRef]
5. Morin-Crini, N.; Lichtfouse, E.; Fourmentin, M.; Lado Ribeiro, A.R.; Noutsopoulos, C.; Mapelli, F.; Fenyvesi, E.; Adeodato Vieira, M.G.; Picos-Corrales, L.A.; Moreno-Piraján, J.C.; et al. Removal of emerging contaminants from wastewater using advanced treatments. A review. *Environ. Chem. Lett.* **2022**, *20*, 1333–1375. [CrossRef]
6. Sophia, A.C.; Lima, E. Removal of emerging contaminants from the environment by adsorption. *Ecotoxicol. Environ. Saf.* **2018**, *150*, 1–17. [CrossRef]
7. Bernabeu, A.; Vercher, R.F.; Santos-Juanes, L.; Simón, P.J.; Lardín, C.; Martínez, M.A.; Vicente, J.A.; González, R.; Llosá, C.; Arques, A.; et al. Solar photocatalysis as a tertiary treatment to remove emerging pollutants from wastewater treatment plant effluents. *Catal. Today* **2011**, *161*, 235–240. [CrossRef]
8. Christou, A.; Agüera, A.; Bayona, J.M.; Cytryn, E.; Fotopoulos, V.; Lambropoulou, D.; Manaia, C.M.; Costas, M.; Revitt, M.; Schröder, P.; et al. The potential implications of reclaimed wastewater reuse for irrigation on the agricultural environment: The knowns and unknowns of the fate of antibiotic resistant bacteria and resistance genes. A review. *Water Res.* **2017**, *123*, 448–467. [CrossRef] [PubMed]
9. Calderón-Preciado, D.; Matamoros, V.; Savé, V.; Muñoz, P.; Biel, C.; Bayona, J.M. Uptake of microcontaminants by crops irrigated with reclaimed water and groundwater under real field greenhouse conditions. *Environ. Sci. Pollut. Res.* **2013**, *20*, 3629–3638. [CrossRef]
10. Krzeminski, P.; Tomei, M.C.; Karaolia, P.; Langenhoff, A.; Almeida, C.M.; Felis, E.; Gritten, F.; Andersen, H.R.; Fernandes, T.; Manaia, C.M.; et al. Performance of secondary wastewater treatment methods for the removal of contaminants of emerging concern implicated in crop uptake and antibiotic resistance spread: A review. *Sci. Total Environ.* **2019**, *648*, 1052–1081. [CrossRef]
11. Rusiñol, M.; Hundesa, S.; Cárdenas-Youngs, Y.; Fernández-Bravo, A.; Pérez-Cataluña, A.; Moreno-Mesonero, L.; Moreno, Y.; Calvo, M.; Alonso, J.L.; Figueras, M.J.; et al. Microbiological contamination of conventional and reclaimed irrigation water: Evaluation and management measures. *Sci. Total Environ.* **2020**, *710*, 136298. [CrossRef] [PubMed]
12. Shi, Q.; Chen, Z.; Yan, H.; Xu, M.; Cao, K.F.; Mao, Y.; Chen, X.; Hu, H.Y. Identification of significant live bacterial community shifts in different reclaimed waters during ozone and chlorine disinfection. *Sci. Total Environ.* **2023**, *896*, 165199. [CrossRef]
13. Mahmood, T.; Momin, S.; Ali, R.; Naeem, A.; Khan, A. Technologies for Removal of Emerging Contaminants from Wastewater. In *Wastewater Treatment*, 1st ed.; Muharrem Ince, Olcay Kaplan Ince; IntechOpen: London, UK, 2022. [CrossRef]
14. Ahmed, S.; Mofijur, M.; Nuzhat, S.; Chowdhury, A.T.; Rafa, N.; Uddin, M.A.; Inayat, A.; Mahlia, T.; Ong, H.C.; Chia, W.Y.; et al. Recent developments in physical, biological, chemical and hybrid treatment techniques for removing emerging contaminants from wastewater. *J. Hazard. Mater.* **2021**, *416*, 125912. [CrossRef] [PubMed]
15. Kashif Shahid, M.; Kashif, A.; Fuwad, A.; Choi, Y. Current advances in treatment technologies for removal of emerging contaminants from water—A critical review. *Coord. Chem. Rev.* **2021**, *442*, 213993. [CrossRef]

16. Kalmakhanova, M.S.; Diaz de Tuesta, J.L.; Malakar, A.; Gomes, H.T.; Snow, D.D. Wastewater Treatment in Central Asia: Treatment Alternatives for Safe Water Reuse. *Sustainability* **2023**, *15*, 14949. [CrossRef]
17. Bracamontes-Ruelas, A.R.; Ordaz-Díaz, L.A.; Bailón-Salas, A.M.; Ríos-Saucedo, J.C.; Reyes-Vidal, Y.; Reynoso-Cuevas, L. Emerging Pollutants in Wastewater, Advanced Oxidation Processes as an Alternative Treatment and Perspectives. *Processes* **2022**, *10*, 1041. [CrossRef]
18. Bracamontes-Ruelas, A.R.; Reyes-Vidal, Y.; Irigoyen-Campuzano, J.R.; Reynoso-Cuevas, L. Simultaneous Oxidation of Emerging Pollutants in Real Wastewater by the Advanced Fenton Oxidation Process. *Catalysts* **2023**, *13*, 748. [CrossRef]
19. Guo, Y.; Zhao, E.; Wang, J.; Zhang, X.; Huang, H.; Yu, G.; Wang, Y. Comparison of emerging contaminant abatement by conventional ozonation, catalytic ozonation, O_3/H_2O_2 and electro-proxone processes. *J. Hazard. Mater.* **2020**, *389*, 121829. [CrossRef]
20. Fraiese, A.; Naddeo, V.; Uyguner-Demirel, C.S.; Prado, M.; Cesaro, A.; Zarra, T.; Liu, H.; Belgiorno, V.; Ballesteros, F., Jr. Removal of Emerging Contaminants in Wastewater by Sonolysis, Photocatalysis and Ozonation. *Glob. NEST J.* **2018**, *21*, 98–105. [CrossRef]
21. García, L.; Leyva-Díaz, J.C.; Díaz, E.; Ordóñez, S. A review of the adsorption-biological hybrid processes for the abatement of emerging pollutants: Removal efficiencies, physicochemical analysis, and economic evaluation. *Sci. Total Environ.* **2021**, *780*, 146554. [CrossRef]
22. Dong, Y.; Yuan, H.; Ge, D.; Zhu, N. A novel conditioning approach for amelioration of sludge dewaterability using activated carbon strengthening electrochemical oxidation and realized mechanism. *Water Res.* **2022**, *220*, 118704. [CrossRef]
23. Life Clean Up. Available online: https://www.lifecleanup.eu/ (accessed on 5 March 2024).
24. Gubitosa, J.; Mongiovi, C.; Romita, R.; Cosma, P.; Nuzzo, S.; Rizzi, V.; Fini, P. Removal of Emerging Contaminants from Water Using Cyclodextrin-Based Polymers and Advanced Oxidation Processes: The Case of Carbamazepine. *Processes* **2022**, *10*, 1703. [CrossRef]
25. Gómez-Morte, T.; Gómez-López, V.; Lucas-Abellán, C.; Martínez-Alcalá, I.; Ayuso, M.; Martínez-López, S.; Montemurro, N.; Pérez, S.; Barceló, D.; Fini, P.; et al. Removal and toxicity evaluation of a diverse group of drugs from water by a cyclodextrin polymer/pulsed light system. *J. Hazard. Mater.* **2021**, *402*, 123504. [CrossRef] [PubMed]
26. Rizzi, V.; Romanazzi, F.; Gubitosa, J.; Fini, P.; Romita, R.; Agostiano, A.; Petrella, A.; Cosma, P. Chitosan Film as Eco-Friendly and Recyclable Bio-Adsorbent to Remove/Recover Diclofenac, Ketoprofen, and Their Mixture from Wastewater. *Biomolecules* **2019**, *9*, 571. [CrossRef]
27. Rizzi, V.; Gubitosa, J.; Fini, P.; Romita, R.; Nuzzo, S.; Cosma, P. Chitosan Biopolymer from Crab Shell as Recyclable Film to Remove/Recover in Batch Ketoprofen from Water: Understanding the Factors Affecting the Adsorption Process. *Materials* **2019**, *12*, 3810. [CrossRef] [PubMed]
28. Rizzi, V.; Gubitosa, J.; Fini, P.; Romita, R.; Agostiano, A.; Nuzzo, S.; Cosma, P. Commercial bentonite clay as low-cost and recyclable "natural" adsorbent for the Carbendazim removal/recover from water: Overview on the adsorption process and preliminary photodegradation considerations. *Colloids Surf. A Physicochem. Eng. Asp.* **2020**, *602*, 125060. [CrossRef]
29. Rizzi, V.; Gubitosa, J.; Fini, P.; Romita, R.; Nuzzo, S.; Gabaldón, J.A.; Fortea, M.I.; Gómez, T.; Cosma, P. Chitosan film as recyclable adsorbent membrane to remove/recover hazardous pharmaceutical pollutants from water: The case of the emerging pollutant Furosemide. *J. Environ. Sci. Health-Toxic/Hazard. Subst. Environ. Eng.* **2021**, *56*, 145–156. [CrossRef] [PubMed]
30. Rizzo, L.; Malato, S.; Antakyali, D.; Beretsou, V.G.; Dolic, M.B.; Gernjak, W.; Ribeiro, A. Consolidated vs new advanced treatment methods for the removal of contaminants of emerging concern from urban wastewater. *Sci. Total Environ.* **2019**, *655*, 986–1008. [CrossRef]
31. Romita, R.; Rizzi, V.; Semeraro, P.; Gubitosa, J.; Gabaldón, J.A.; Fortea, M.I.; Gómez, V.M.; Cosma, P.; Fini, P. Operational parameters affecting the atrazine removal from water by using cyclodextrin based polymers as efficient adsorbents for cleaner technologies. *Environ. Technol. Innov.* **2019**, *16*, 100454. [CrossRef]
32. Rizzi, V.; Gubitosa, J.; Fini, P.; Petrella, A.; Romita, R.; Agostiano, A.; Cosma, P. A "classic" material for capture and detoxification of emergent contaminants for water purification: The case of tetracycline. *Environ. Technol. Innov.* **2020**, *19*, 100812. [CrossRef]
33. Rizzi, V.; Gubitosa, J.; Signorile, R.; Fini, P.; Cecone, C.; Matencio, A.; Trotta, F.; Cosma, P. Cyclodextrin nanosponges as adsorbent material to remove hazardous pollutants from water: The case of ciprofloxacin. *J. Chem. Eng.* **2021**, *411*, 128514. [CrossRef]
34. Romita, R.; Rizzi, V.; Gubitosa, J.; Gabaldón, J.A.; Fortea, M.I.; Gómez, T.; Gómez, V.M.; Fini, P.; Cosma, P. Cyclodextrin polymers and salts: An Eco-Friendly combination to modulate the removal of sulfamethoxazole from water and its release. *Chemosphere* **2021**, *283*, 131238. [CrossRef] [PubMed]
35. Rizzi, V.; Romita, R.; Gómez, V.M.; Gubitosa, J.; Gabaldón, J.A.; Fortea, M.I.; Gómez, T.; Cosma, P.; Fini, P. The synergistic action of cyclodextrin-based adsorbent and advanced oxidation processes for sulfamethoxazole removal from water. *Int. J. Environ. Sci. Technol.* **2022**, *19*, 10663–10676. [CrossRef]
36. Landy, D.; Mallard, I.; Ponchel, A.; Monflier, E.; Fourmentin, S. Remediation technologies using cyclodextrins: An overview. *Environ. Chem. Lett.* **2012**, *10*, 225–237. [CrossRef]
37. IRENA. *Renewable Power Generation Costs in 2019*; International Renewable Energy Agency: Abu Dhabi, United Arab Emirates, 2020.
38. Rodríguez-Narváez, O.M.; Peralta, J.M.; Goonetilleke, A.; Bandala, E. Treatment technologies for emerging contaminants in water: A review. *J. Chem. Eng.* **2017**, *323*, 361–380. [CrossRef]
39. Sornalingam, K.; McDonagh, A.; Zhou, J.L. Photodegradation of estrogenic endocrine disrupting steroidal hormones in aqueous systems: Progress and future challenges. *Sci. Total Environ.* **2016**, *550*, 209–224. [CrossRef]

40. Tuerk, J.; Sayder, B.; Boergers, A.; Vits, H.; Kiffmeyer, T.K.; Kabasci, S. Efficiency, costs and benefits of AOPs for removal of pharmaceuticals from the water cycle. *Water Sci. Technol.* **2010**, *61*, 985–993. [CrossRef]
41. Kanakaraju, D.; Glass, B.D.; Oelgemöller, M. Advanced oxidation process-mediated removal of pharmaceuticals from water: A review. *J. Environ. Manag.* **2018**, *219*, 189–207. [CrossRef]
42. Zhang, Y.; Wang, J.; Cui, H.; Gao, S.; Ye, L.; Li, Z.; Nie, S.; Han, J.; Wang, A.; Liang, B. Environmental occurrence, risk and removal strategies of pyrazolones: A critical review. *J. Hazard. Mater.* **2023**, *460*, 132471. [CrossRef]
43. Iglesias Esteban, R. La Reutilización de Efluentes Depurados en España. Retrospectiva, Desarrollo del Marco Normativo, Estudio de las Etcnologías de Regeneración Frente a los Biorreactores de Membrana y sus Costes en Función del uso. Ph.D. Thesis, Escuela Técnica Superior de Ingenieros Agrónomos (Universidad Politécnica de Madrid), Madrid, España, 2016.
44. Cooley, H. *Implications of Future Water Supply Sources for Energy Demand*; WateReuse Research Foundation: Alexandria, VA, USA, 2012.
45. Hardy, L.; Garrido, A.; Juana, L. Evaluation of Spain's Water-Energy Nexus. *Int. J. Water Resour. Dev.* **2012**, *28*, 151–170. [CrossRef]
46. IDAE. *Estudio de Prospectiva. Consumo Energético en el Sector del Agua*; Instituto para la Diversificación y Ahorro de la Energía: Madrid, Spain, 2010.
47. Lyons, E.; Zhang, P.; Benn, T.; Sharif, F.; Li, K.; Crittenden, J.; Costanza, M.; Chen, S. Life Cycle Assessment of three water supply systems: Importation, reclamation and desalination. *Water Sci. Technol. Water Supply* **2009**, *9*, 439–448. [CrossRef]
48. Sala, L. Balances energéticos del ciclo del agua y experiencias de reutilización planificada en municipios de la Costa Brava. In Proceedings of the Seminario Internacional Agua, Energía y Cambio Climático, Valencia, Spain, 29–31 October 2007.
49. Sanz, J.; Ferrer, C. The astidisk process for water reclamation: An experimental performance assessment. In Proceedings of the 6th IWA Specialist Conference on Wastewater Reclamation and Reuse for Sustainability, Amberes, Belgium, 9–12 October 2007.
50. Klein, G.; Krebs, M.; Hall, V.; O'Brien, T.; Blevins, B. *California's Water-Energy Relationship—Final Staff Report*; California Energy Commission: Sacramento, CA, USA, 2005.
51. Rougé, P. Evaluación técnica y económica de las tecnologías de regeneración de aguas. In Proceedings of the Technical Workshop: The Integration of Reclaimed Water in Water Resource Management, Lloret de Mar, Gerona, Spain, 19–20 October 2005.
52. Degremont, G. *Water Treatment Handbook*, 6th ed.; Intercept Ltd.: London, UK, 1991.
53. Ministerio de Medio Ambiente y Medio Rural y Marino. *Gobierno de España. Guía para la Aplicación del R.D. 1620/2007, por el que se Establece el Régimen Jurídico de la Rutilización de las Aguas Depuradas*; Ministerio de Medio Ambiente y Medio Rural y Marino. Gobierno de España: Madrid, Spain, 2010.
54. Tribe, M.A.; Alpine, R.L. Scale Economies and the "0.6 rule". *Eng. Costs Prod. Econ.* **1986**, *10*, 271–278. [CrossRef]
55. Mas, J. Análisis Coste/Beneficio Aplicado a los Procesos de Depuración y Reutilización. Master's Thesis, Universitario en Gestión Sostenible y Tecnologías del Agua (Universidad de Alicante), Alicante, Spain, 2016.
56. Villar-García, A. Reutilización de aguas regeneradas. Aproximación a los costes de producción y valoración de su uso. *Water Landsc.* **2016**, *8*, 70–79. [CrossRef]
57. Guo, T.; Englehardt, J.; Wu, T. Review of cost versus scale: Water and wastewater treatment and reuse processes. *Water Sci. Technol.* **2014**, *69*, 223–234. [CrossRef] [PubMed]
58. Plumlee, M.; Stanford, B.; Debroux, J.F.; Hopkins, C.; Snyder, S. Costs of advanced treatment in water reclamation. *Ozone Sci. Eng.* **2014**, *36*, 485–495. [CrossRef]
59. TRAGUA. *Tecnologías de Tratamiento de Aguas Para su Regeneración*; Programa Consolider Tragua: Madrid, Spain, 2014.
60. FOEN. *Micropollutants in Municipal Wastewaters. Processes for Advanced Removal in Wastewater Treatment Plants*; Federal Office for the Environment: Berna, Switzerland, 2012.
61. McGivney, W.; Kawamura, S. *Cost Estimating Manual for Water Treatment Facilities*, 1st ed.; John Wiley & Sons, Inc.: Hoboken, NJ, USA, 2008. [CrossRef]
62. Eggen, R.; Hollender, J.; Joss, A.; Schärer, M.; Stamm, C. Reducing the discharge of micropollutants in the aquatic environment: The benefits of upgrading wastewater treatment plants. *Environ. Sci. Technol.* **2014**, *48*, 7683–7689. [CrossRef]
63. Hollender, J.; Zimmerman, S.; Koepke, S.; Krauss, M.; McArdell, C.S.; Ort, C.; Singer, H.; von Gunten, U.; Siegrist, H. Elimination of organic micropollutants in a municipal wastewater treatment plant upgraded with a full-scale post-ozonation followed by sand filtration. *Environ. Sci. Technol.* **2009**, *43*, 7862–7869. [CrossRef]

water

MDPI

Article

Comprehensive Evaluation and Coupled Coordinated Development Study of Water–Economic–Ecological Systems in the Five Northwestern Provinces of China

Jiahao Shi [1,2], Huan Yang [1,2], Fuqiang Wang [1,2,*], Di Sun [1] and Yushan Run [1]

[1] North China University of Water Resources and Electric Power, Zhengzhou 450046, China; shijiahao@ncwu.edu.cn (J.S.); huanyang@ncwu.edu.cn (H.Y.); sundi730610@163.com (D.S.); rys197228@163.com (Y.R.)

[2] Key Laboratory of Conservation and Intensive Use of Water Resources in the Yellow River Basin of Henan Province, North China University of Water Resources and Electric Power, Zhengzhou 450046, China

* Correspondence: wangfuqiang@ncwu.edu.cn

Abstract: The five northwestern provinces face numerous challenges in sustainable development, particularly water scarcity, economic imbalances, and ecological degradation. This study aims to deeply assess the region's water resource conditions, the current status of economic development, and the health of the ecosystem while exploring the relationships and coupling mechanisms among them. Using the obstacle model, the research analyzes the primary barriers affecting these three significant factors in the region. The study further reveals a continually improving trend of coordinated development within the water–economic–ecological system in the five northwestern provinces of China, indicating that water usage per ten thousand GDP is the primary obstacle. This research enriches our understanding of the development in China's five northwestern provinces and provides a theoretical foundation for achieving sustainable development.

Keywords: five northwestern provinces; water–economic–ecological systems; analyzes the primary barriers

1. Introduction

Water resources, economic development, and ecosystems are three crucial aspects of regional sustainable development. As an integral part of China's western region, the five northwestern provinces and regions (Gansu, Ningxia, Qinghai, Shaanxi, and Xinjiang) possess abundant natural resources and unique geographical advantages [1]. However, the long-term impacts of natural conditions and human activities have led to increasingly prominent challenges in water supply–demand conflicts, imbalanced economic development, and ecosystem degradation, severely constraining the area's sustainable development [2].

Over the past few decades, the five northwestern provinces and regions have achieved significant development in industry, agriculture, and urbanization [3]. However, this development often comes at the cost of sacrificing the environment and ecosystems. Issues such as water scarcity, water pollution, land degradation, and deteriorating ecological conditions have become urgent and significant challenges to be addressed [4]. Moreover, with the increasing severity of global environmental problems, the region faces even more formidable tests in balancing economic growth and environmental protection [5].

Researchers have proposed various evaluation index systems to quantify the interactions between water resources, socio-economics, and ecosystems. These systems typically include indicators such as water resource availability, water use efficiency, economic development levels, social welfare, and ecosystem health. Through these indices, researchers can evaluate the degree of coupling and coordination in different regions and time periods.

To more accurately assess the relationships between water, socio-economics, and ecosystems, various mathematical models have been introduced by researchers. These models can predict based on historical data and can also be used to simulate the impact of different management strategies on the coupled system. There have been numerous empirical studies worldwide that analyze the coupling and coordination relationships of water, socio-economics, and ecosystems under different geographical, climatic, and economic conditions. These empirical findings provide valuable references for decision-makers, aiding them in formulating more rational water resource management strategies. Based on the research results of coupling and coordination evaluations, many scholars have proposed specific management strategies and policy recommendations. These suggestions aim to achieve sustainable utilization of water resources, promote healthy socio-economic development, and protect the integrity of ecosystems.

In summary, while significant progress has been made in research on the coupling and coordination evaluation of water, socio-economics, and ecosystems, there remain numerous challenges, such as accurately quantifying interactions between systems and developing more effective management strategies. Therefore, in-depth research on the comprehensive evaluation and coupling coordination of water resources and comprehensive consideration of sustainable development strategies, economic development, and ecosystems in the five northwestern provinces and regions is of great significance for formulating scientifically reasonable development strategies, promoting rational resource allocation, improving the ecological environment, and achieving sustainable development [6].

Firstly, this paper will conduct an in-depth evaluation of water resources in the five northwestern provinces and regions [7–10]. Water is the source of life, and in such arid areas, the scarcity of water resources is particularly pronounced. By studying the total water resources, the distribution pattern of water resources, and the utilization of water resources in each province and region, we can gain a comprehensive understanding of the current situation and challenges facing the water resources in the five northwestern provinces and regions. Special attention needs to be paid to the rationality and sustainability of water resource development and utilization, as well as the impact of water resources on the ecosystem, to ensure the reasonable distribution and efficient utilization of water resources [11–13]. Secondly, this research will conduct a comprehensive evaluation of economic development in the five northwestern provinces and regions. While the region has achieved rapid economic growth in the past few decades, imbalances in economic development still exist. Some provinces have made significant breakthroughs in economic development, while others lag behind. Therefore, it is necessary to analyze the economic structure, industrial layout, and driving factors of economic growth in different provinces and regions to find effective ways to promote coordinated economic development. In addition, this paper will also assess the state of ecosystems in the five northwestern provinces and regions. The degradation of the ecological environment has become a major factor constraining the region's sustainable development. We will focus on the integrity of natural ecosystems, the protection of biodiversity, and the stability of ecosystem functions. In-depth understanding of the threats and pressures on ecosystems will help formulate corresponding strategies for ecological protection and restoration to achieve a win-win situation for the economy and the ecosystem. Lastly, this research will focus on exploring the interrelationships and coupling mechanisms among water resources, economic development, and ecosystems in the five northwestern provinces and regions. These three aspects have close interconnections and feedback relationships. Economic development requires a considerable amount of water resources, while excessive exploitation and pollution of water resources can also negatively impact economic sustainable development and people's quality of life [14–16]. At the same time, ecosystem deterioration also affects water resources and the economy negatively [16,17]. Therefore, we need to find a path of coordinated development among water resources, economic development, and ecosystems and explore the feasibility of protecting the ecological environment while promoting economic growth [18].

In conclusion, this paper aims to conduct an in-depth analysis of the current situation of water resources, economic development, and ecosystems in the five northwestern provinces and regions, exploring their interrelationships and coupling mechanisms, and proposing corresponding development strategies and recommendations based on practical conditions. By comprehensively assessing the integrated development of water resources, economic development, and ecosystems and providing comprehensive consideration of the interaction between indicators, we hope to provide theoretical references and practical guidance for promoting the sustainable development of the five northwestern provinces and regions and enhancing the overall development level of China's western region.

2. Materials and Methods

2.1. Study Area

The five northwestern provinces of China are located in arid and semi-arid regions (Figure 1), facing significant challenges in water resources. The Yellow River Basin serves as a crucial water source for the region. However, years of excessive extraction and improper usage have resulted in reduced water flow and declining water quality in the Yellow River. Moreover, the impact of climate change has led to irregular rainfall patterns and exacerbating drought conditions. In regions like Ningxia and Xinjiang, where rivers are scarce, strict water conservation measures are essential to meet the demands of daily life and agriculture. To address water scarcity, the government has implemented various measures, including water resource allocation and transfer projects, integrated water management, and the promotion of water-saving technologies.

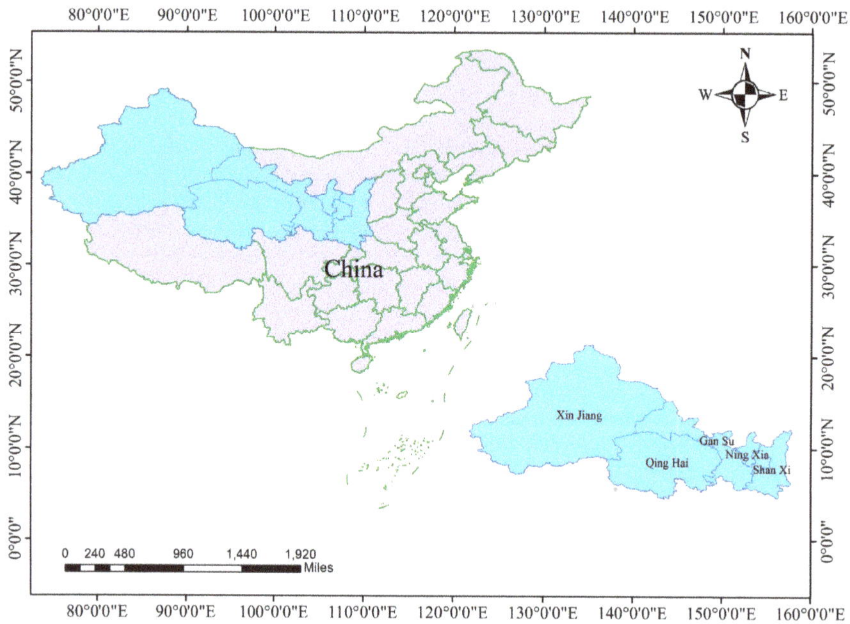

Figure 1. Overview map of the five northwestern provinces in China.

The five northwestern provinces have made remarkable progress in economic development, benefiting from government support and open policies that have provided new opportunities for industrial upgrading and growth. These provinces are actively developing their respective advantageous industries, fostering economic diversification. Shaanxi Province relies on its rich historical and cultural resources, actively promoting cultural tourism. Gansu Province has boosted economic growth through infrastructure development and the expansion of emerging industries. Qinghai Province is focused on developing green energy, tourism, and modern agriculture to build eco-friendly and livable cities. In

Ningxia and Xinjiang, the emphasis lies on energy, metallurgy, and chemical industries, while also increasing efforts to alleviate poverty and improve residents' income. However, striking a balance between economic development and resource conservation remains a challenge. The government needs to take effective measures to ensure the sustainability of economic growth while protecting the environment and people's well-being.

The five northwestern provinces possess unique natural landscapes and are significant ecological conservation areas in China. However, due to excessive exploitation and improper utilization, some regions are facing threats to their ecological environment. In grassland areas, overgrazing and grassland degradation have led to soil erosion and desertification, disrupting the ecological balance. Desertification is also becoming increasingly severe, with desert areas expanding and posing serious threats to neighboring regions. The government has recognized the urgency of ecological conservation and has implemented various measures, such as afforestation, returning farmland to forests and grasslands, and desertification control, to restore and protect the ecological environment.

In conclusion, as an essential geographic region in China, the five northwestern provinces face numerous challenges and opportunities. The government needs to increase investment and policy support to promote regional coordinated development, sustainable economic growth, and environmental protection. Strengthening international cooperation and learning from international best practices are of vital significance for solving the region's significant issues.

2.2. Coordinated Evaluation Index System for Coupling of Five Northwestern Provinces in China

In the process of constructing the index system, the indicators we choose follow the sustainable development strategy and the people-oriented principle and build a scientific evaluation index system. The principles for constructing the evaluation index system for the coupling coordination of water resources, socio-economic factors, and ecological environment in the five northwestern provinces are as follows.

Systematic Principle: The evaluation index system should comprehensively consider various factors such as water resources, socio-economic aspects, and the ecological environment, forming a systematic evaluation framework to ensure mutual interactions and coordination among these factors [19]. Scientific Principle: The selection and design of indicators should be based on scientific theories and empirical research, ensuring the accuracy and reliability of the indicators. This will provide scientific interpretability and comparability of the evaluation results [20–22].

Operability Principle: The evaluation indicators should be feasible for measurement and calculation in practical applications, facilitating assessment and comparison in real-world scenarios. Balancing Principle: The selection of indicators should strike a balance among different factors, avoiding excessive emphasis on one aspect at the expense of others [23]. This approach achieves the coordinated development of water resources, socio-economic factors, and the ecological environment. Sustainability Principle: The evaluation index system should consider the requirements of long-term sustainable development, ensuring that the evaluation results can reflect the system's evolution and changes. This guides decisions and management toward sustainability. Applicability Principle: The index system should be adjusted and optimized based on the actual conditions of the five northwestern provinces, adapting to the characteristics and needs of different regions, thus enhancing the applicability and effectiveness of the evaluation [24].

Participatory Principle: During the construction of the evaluation index system, the opinions and suggestions of various stakeholders should be fully considered, enhancing the participatory and democratic nature of the evaluation.

The principles for constructing the evaluation index system for coupling coordination encompass a comprehensive approach that balances relationships among different factors. The aim is to objectively and comprehensively reflect the status and development trends of water resources, socio-economic factors, and the ecological environment in the five northwestern provinces [25–28].

The evaluation framework of this study consists primarily of three criterion layers and sixteen indicator layers (Figure 2). These criterion layers encompass the water resources system, the socio-economic system, and the ecological environment system. Each of these systems incorporates relevant indicators, aiming to ensure the accuracy of the assessment for the coupling coordination of water resources, society, and ecology in the five northwestern provinces of China. The water resources system comprises six indicators: Per Capita Water Resource Quantity, Proportion of Groundwater Supply, Water Resource Development and Utilization Rate, Per Capita Domestic Water Consumption, Water Consumption per Ten Thousand Yuan of Industrial Value Added, and Effective Irrigation Water Use Coefficient for Farmland. The socio-economic system includes five indicators: Per Capita GDP, Water Consumption per Ten Thousand Yuan of GDP, Per Capita Industrial Output Value, Natural Population Growth Rate, and Per Capita Urban Road Area. The ecological environment system encompasses five indicators: Urban Green Coverage Rate, Proportion of Ecological Water Use, Wastewater Treatment Rate, Annual COD Emissions, and Proportion of Rivers with Water Quality Class III or Higher. These three criterion layers and sixteen indicator layers are interrelated, collectively forming the evaluation index system for the water resources, socio-economic, and ecological systems in the five northwestern provinces.

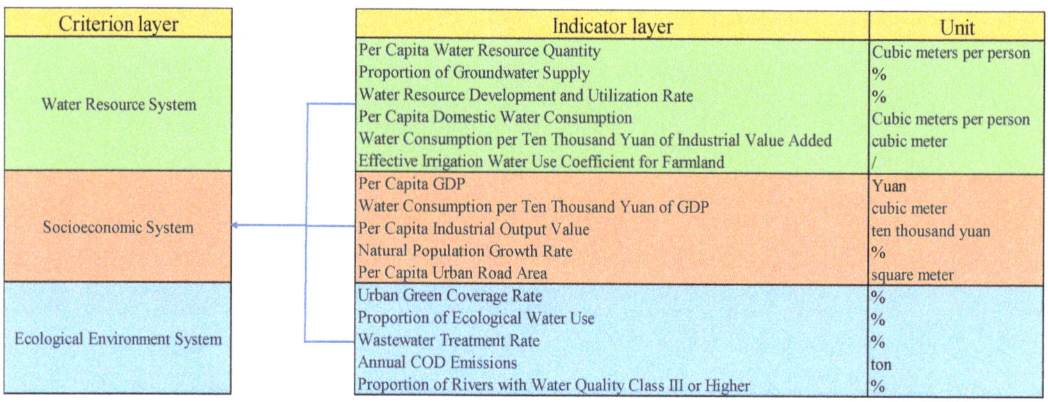

Figure 2. Evaluation framework for coupling coordination of water resources, socio-economic factors, and ecological systems in the five northwestern provinces.

2.3. The Weighting Method

$$x_{ij} = \left(x_{ij} - \overline{X_j}\right)/S_j$$

In the formula, x_{ij} is the original value of the evaluation index; $\overline{X_j}$ is the mean value of item j; and S_j is the standard deviation of indicator j.

Improved coefficient of variation (ICV):

$$V_i = \frac{\sigma_i}{\bar{i}}$$

$$w_i = \frac{w_i - c_i}{\sum_{i=1}^{n} w_i - c_i},\ i = 1, 2, \ldots, n$$

In the formula, $\bar{i}$ and σ_i represent the mean and standard deviation of the indicator. i_k and j_k represent the Eth sample values of indicators i and j, respectively, while $\bar{j}$ represents the average value of indicator j.

2.4. Three-Subsystem Comprehensive Evaluation Method

$$R_{WR} = \sum\nolimits_{j=1}^{m} W_{ij} \times X_{ij}$$

$$R_{ES} = \sum\nolimits_{j=1}^{m} W_{ij} \times X_{ij}$$

$$R_{EE} = \sum\nolimits_{j=1}^{m} W_{ij} \times X_{ij}$$

$$T = a \times R_{WR} + b \times R_{ES} + c \times R_{EE}$$

In the formula, R_{WR}, R_{ES}, and R_{EE} are the comprehensive evaluation indices of water resources, the economic society, and the ecological environment system, respectively; T is the comprehensive evaluation index of the three systems; and a, b, and c are the weights of each system, a = b = c = 1/3.

2.5. Evaluation Method of Coupling Coordination Degree

$$C = 3 \times \left\{ \frac{R_{ES} \times R_{EE} \times R_{WR}}{(R_{ES} + R_{EE} + R_{WR})^3} \right\}^{1/3}$$

$$D = \sqrt{C \times T}$$

In the formula, C is the coupling degree and D is the coupling coordination degree.

Classification of the CCI Index

The evaluation method we constructed comprehensively considers the interaction among the selected indicators. When calculating the weight of the indicators, we consider the comprehensive weight value of objective and subjective weights so as to consider the integrity of the overall structure of the evaluation system. After considering the multifaceted factors of water resources, socioeconomic development, and ecological environment in the five northwestern provinces of China, these regions can be categorized into six levels to depict the overall degree of coordination. The first level, "Maladjustment", encompasses areas such as Shaanxi, Gansu, Qinghai, Ningxia, and Xinjiang, characterized by scarce water resources, low socioeconomic development, and a fragile ecological environment, posing significant challenges to coordination. The subsequent level, "Borderline disorder", pertains to regions with limited socioeconomic development, despite facing water scarcity and gradual ecological degradation. Following this is the "Primary coordination" level, covering areas where water resources are relatively limited, but socioeconomic development is gradually improving and ecological environment protection is swiftly advancing. Progressing to the "Intermediate coordination" level, these areas exhibit efficient water resource utilization, ongoing socioeconomic development, and continuous enhancement of the ecological environment. The "Advanced coordination" level includes a few regions marked by abundant water resources, high socioeconomic prosperity, and excellent ecological conditions, showcasing a trend of balanced development. Finally, the top tier is "Quality coordination", encompassing regions with abundant water resources, highly developed socioeconomic status, and a favorable ecological environment. This multi-tiered classification system offers a nuanced reference for assessing and managing the water-resource, socioeconomic, and ecological coordination of the five northwestern provinces, guiding the formulation and implementation of sustainable development strategies. The classification criteria of this study are presented in Figure 3.

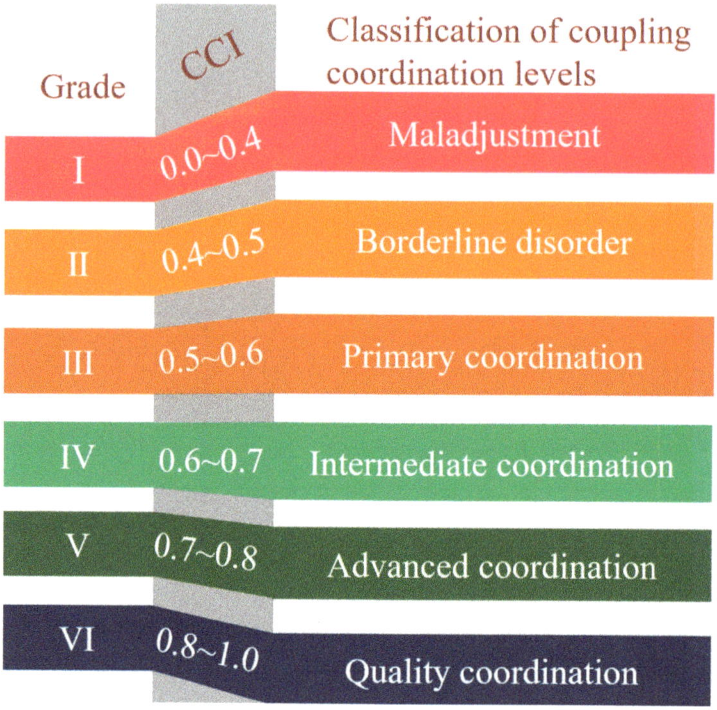

Figure 3. Classification criteria chart for the five northwestern provinces.

2.6. Coupling Coordination Degree Obstacle Factor Analysis

This study introduced the obstacle degree model, analyzed the obstacle factors of each index in the evaluation system, determined the main obstacles affecting the health of the water cycle, and formulated targeted improvement measures. The specific steps of obstacle factor analysis are as follows.

(1) Calculate the contribution degree F_j of the j evaluation indicator:

$$F_j = w_i^* \times w_i$$

In the formula, w_i^* represents the weight value of the corresponding criterion layer for the indicator.

(2) Calculate I_j, which represents the deviation degree.

$$I_j = 1 - x_{ij}$$

(3) Calculate P_j, which represents the obstacle degree of each evaluation index.

$$P_j = \frac{F_j I_j}{\sum_{j=1}^{n} F_j I_j}$$

3. Results

3.1. Coupling Coordination Results

3.1.1. Weight Calculation Results of the Evaluation Index System for Water Resources, Socio-Economic Factors, and Ecological Environment

Within the criteria layer, the highest-weighted criterion is the ecological environment system, with a weight value of 0.4856, while the weight values for the water resources system and the socioeconomic system are approximately equal, at 0.2492 and 0.2652, respectively. Within the indicator layer, the highest-weighted indicator is the proportion of rivers with water quality above Class III in the ecological environment system, with a weight value of 0.16617. Following this is the effective utilization coefficient of irrigation water in the water resources system, with a weight value of 0.15460. The indicator with the lowest weight value is the per capita water resources in the water resources system. The weight distribution diagram of the evaluation indicator system is shown in Figure 4.

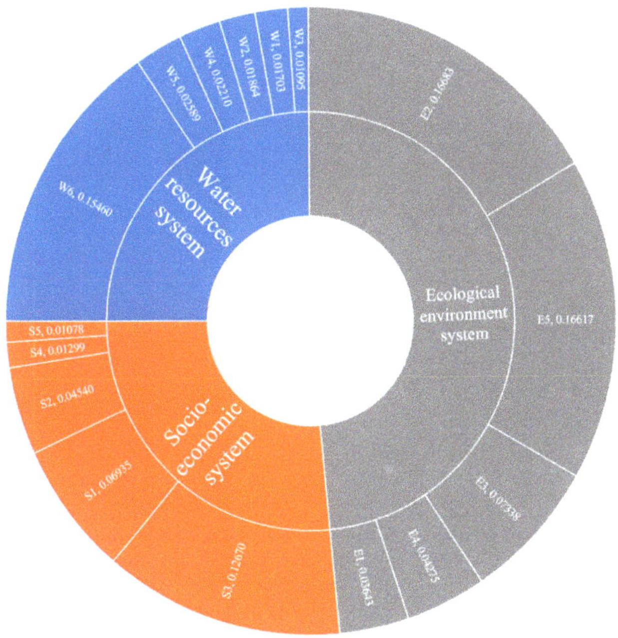

Figure 4. Weight distribution diagram of the evaluation indicator system.

3.1.2. CCI Temporal and Spatial Change Analysis

This study first conducts a comprehensive evaluation of water resources, the ecological environment, and socio-economic aspects in the five provinces and regions of northwestern China. The evaluation results indicate that, overall, the comprehensive evaluation scores of water resources, ecological environment, and socio-economic aspects in these five provinces and regions have been gradually improving.

Spatial analysis reveals that Xinjiang and Qinghai have higher scores in ecological environment and water resources, but lower scores in socio-economic aspects. This is primarily due to their significant industrial development, which has a considerable impact on their socio-economic indicators, while human activities have had a relatively lower negative impact on their ecological environment. On the other hand, Shaanxi, Gansu, and Ningxia have higher socio-economic scores, largely attributed to the substantial influence of human activities on their ecological environment.

In terms of the temporal aspect, the comprehensive scores for these five provinces and regions were relatively low before 2015. However, after 2015, with the introduction of various national policies, there has been a significant enhancement in the scores for all three criteria in these areas. The comprehensive evaluation results are depicted in Figure 5.

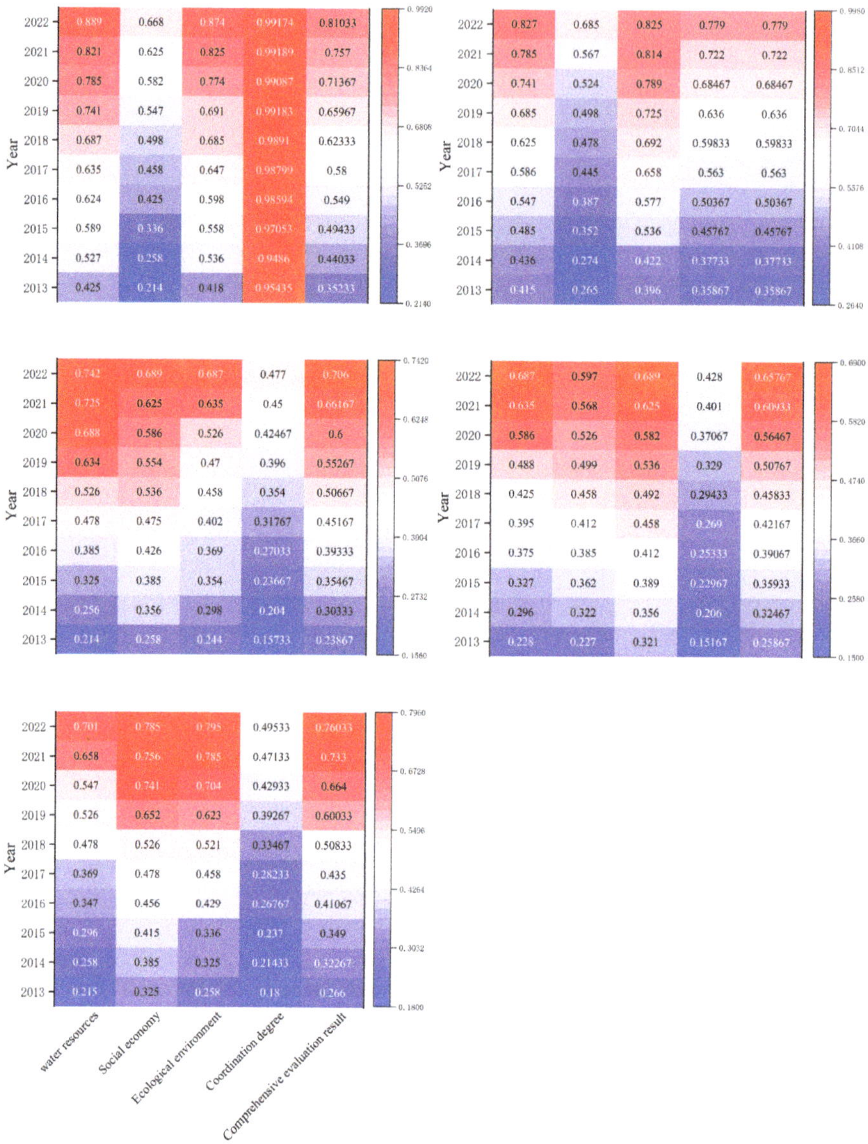

Figure 5. Evaluation results at the criterion level.

Based on the evaluation results at the criterion level and the corresponding calculation of coupling degrees, this study comprehensively analyzes the coupling coordination of water resources, socio-economic aspects, and the ecological environment in the five provinces and regions of northwestern China. In order to clearly depict the temporal and spatial variations of coupling coordination among these provinces and regions, this study employs ArcGIS maps (Figure 6) and bubble charts (Figure 7) to vividly illustrate the changing trends over time and space.

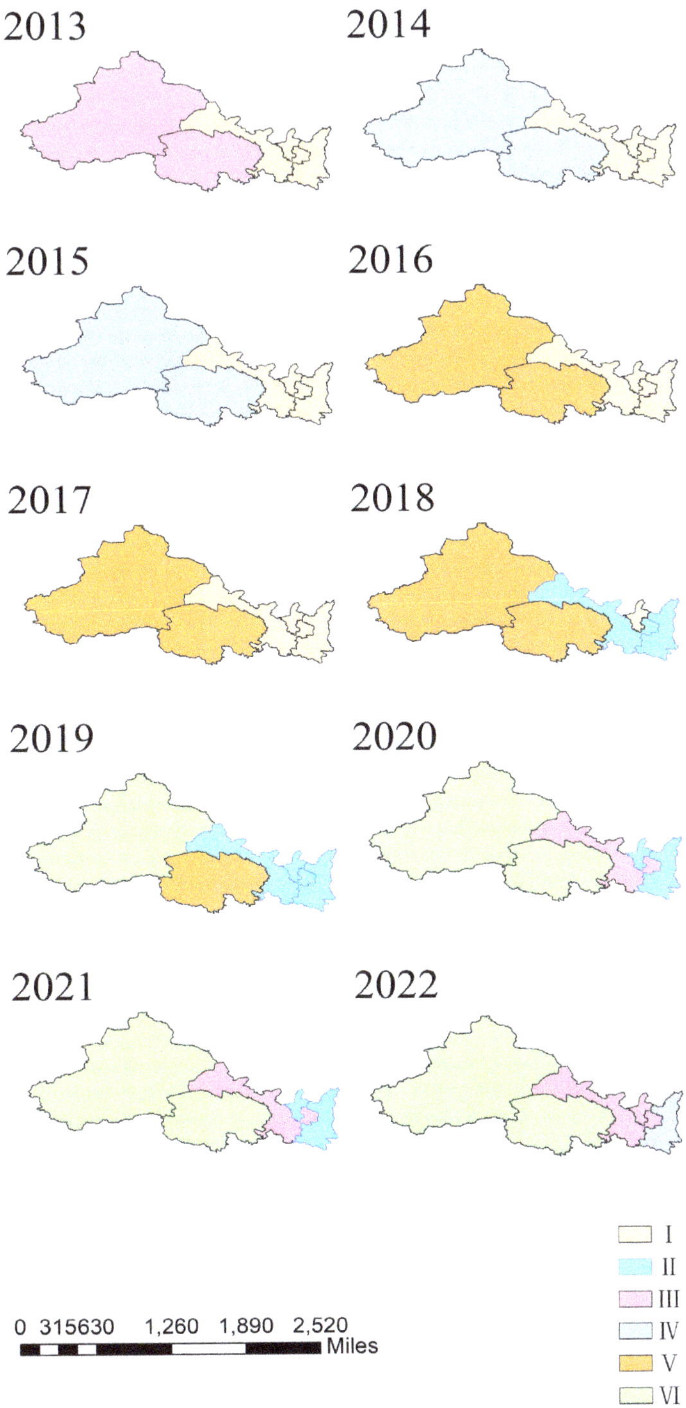

Figure 6. GIS map of the coupling coordination results.

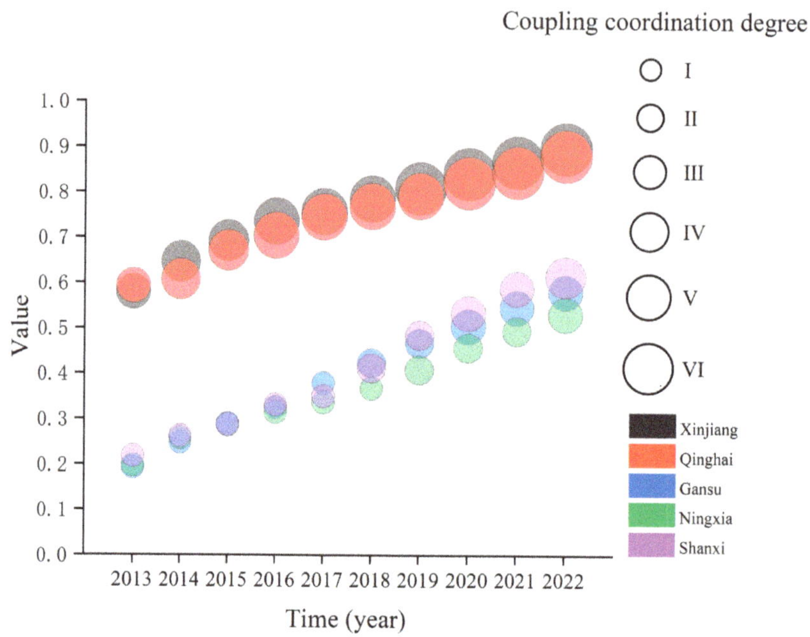

Figure 7. Bubble chart of the coupling coordination results.

In terms of spatial distribution, Xinjiang and Qinghai exhibit relatively higher levels of coupling coordination, while Shaanxi, Gansu, and Ningxia have comparatively lower levels. This disparity can be attributed to the lower impact of human activities on the natural environment in Xinjiang and Qinghai, leading to a milder influence, whereas Shaanxi, Gansu, and Ningxia experience more intensive human activities and consequently exert a higher impact on the natural environment. Despite these variations, the overall differences in coupling coordination across the five provinces and regions are not substantial, as they all demonstrate favorable degrees of coupling coordination.

Regarding the temporal aspect, all five provinces and regions are witnessing positive development over the years. Shaanxi, Gansu, and Ningxia have shown faster rates of improvement, with more pronounced trends. While Xinjiang and Qinghai display slower trends, they are still moving towards positive development trajectories.

3.1.3. Analysis of Factors Hindering Water Resources, Socio-Economic Factors and Ecological Environment in Five Northwestern Provinces of China

This study introduces the obstacle degree model to calculate the primary obstacles affecting the three major factors in five provinces and regions (Figure 8). From the calculated results, it is evident that the obstacle factor with the highest average obstacle degree is the water usage per 10,000 GDP yuan. This is mainly due to the rapid economic development and the fast-growing tourism industry in the five northwestern provinces and regions. The obstacle degrees for urban green coverage rate and water usage per 10,000 industrial values added are the lowest among the six major obstacle degrees, with values of 6.692 and 6.924, respectively. This indicates that urban greening and industrial water control in the five northwestern provinces and regions are well managed. The second-highest obstacle degree is for the ecological water usage ratio, which is 13.758, suggesting that the five provinces and regions should allocate more water for ecological purposes. The obstacle degrees for the proportion of rivers with water quality above Grade III and the effective utilization coefficient of agricultural irrigation water are 8.656 and 10.868, respectively, indicating that the five provinces and regions should optimize agricultural irrigation water usage and increase the proportion of rivers with water quality above Grade III.

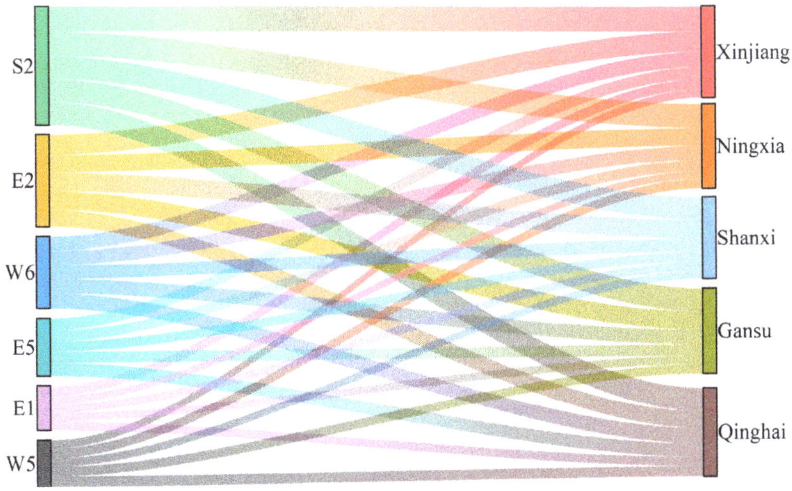

Figure 8. Analysis of primary obstacle factors.

4. Discussion and Policy Suggestion

4.1. Discussion

The comprehensive evaluation and coupled coordinated development study of water–economic–ecological systems in the five northwestern provinces of China holds significant implications for both regional and national sustainable development strategies. This research endeavor delves into the intricate interplay between water resources, economic activities, and ecological well-being, shedding light on the complex dynamics that underlie the region's socio-environmental landscape.

4.1.1. Integrated Resource Management and Sustainability

One of the pivotal insights gleaned from this study pertains to the importance of integrated resource management. By examining the interconnections between water availability, economic growth, and ecological integrity, the research underscores the necessity of adopting a holistic approach to ensure long-term sustainability.

4.1.2. Socio-Economic Implications

The findings of this study have profound socio-economic implications. The northwestern provinces of China have historically been characterized by their water scarcity and vulnerability to climate change impacts. The comprehensive evaluation showcases the potential trade-offs between economic growth and ecological health, emphasizing the need for balanced development strategies. This study thus equips policymakers and stakeholders with valuable insights to formulate effective policies that harmonize economic advancement with environmental preservation.

4.1.3. Policy Formulation and Governance

Effective governance and policy formulation emerge as critical aspects elucidated by this research. The study illuminates the challenges of achieving coupled coordinated development within water–economic–ecological systems. It underscores the necessity of cross-sectoral collaboration and innovative governance mechanisms to tackle the intricate challenges posed by resource scarcity and environmental stressors [17]. The insights garnered from this research can aid in the design of robust policy frameworks that foster sustainable growth while safeguarding ecological resilience.

4.1.4. Adaptation to Changing Conditions

The research also underscores the imperative of adaptive management in the face of changing conditions. With climate change exacerbating water scarcity and altering ecological dynamics, the northwestern provinces must embrace flexibility and resilience in their development paradigms. The study's comprehensive evaluation provides a baseline to monitor changes and adapt strategies accordingly, ensuring that developmental efforts remain aligned with the evolving socio-environmental context.

4.1.5. Knowledge Extension and Global Relevance

While this study focuses on the specific context of the five northwestern provinces of China, its insights reverberate globally. Water scarcity, economic growth, and ecological preservation constitute universal challenges [18]. The methodologies employed and lessons learned from this research can inspire similar assessments in other regions grappling with similar concerns. By disseminating these findings, the study contributes to a broader dialogue on sustainable development strategies across diverse geographical contexts.

4.2. Policy Suggestion

In recent years, the five provinces and regions in northwestern China have increasingly emphasized the coordinated development of water resources, socio-economic progress, and ecological environment, alongside their economic growth. To optimize the coupling coordination of water resources, socio-economic aspects, and the ecological environment, formulating corresponding policies becomes particularly crucial. Firstly, the government can enhance water resource management, promote efficient utilization and conservation of water resources, establish a water resource allocation system, and rationally distribute water resources to reduce wastage. Secondly, encouraging industrial structure upgrading and transformation can drive the economy towards green and low-carbon development, lessening pressure on the ecological environment. Additionally, intensifying environmental protection efforts, strictly controlling pollution emissions, advancing ecological restoration projects, and safeguarding the integrity of ecosystems are vital. Concurrently, strengthening research capabilities and fostering interdisciplinary collaboration can provide scientific evidence and technical support for policy formulation. Lastly, establishing a robust monitoring and assessment system to regularly evaluate coupling coordination and adjusting policy measures promptly ensures effective policy implementation and continuous improvement [19]. By implementing comprehensive strategies, the northwestern provinces and regions can achieve synergistic development of water resources, socio-economic aspects, and the ecological environment, ultimately realizing sustainable development goals.

5. Conclusions

In conclusion, the comprehensive evaluation and coupled coordinated development study of water–economic–ecological systems in China's five northwestern provinces significantly enriches our understanding of the intricate relationships shaping regional development. By examining the interdependencies between water, economy, and ecology, the study not only offers valuable insights for regional policymakers but also contributes to the broader discourse on achieving sustainable development within the constraints of a resource-constrained world. The study's emphasis on integrated resource management, socio-economic implications, governance considerations, adaptation strategies, and global relevance positions it as a seminal contribution to the field of sustainable development.

The comprehensive evaluation and coupled coordinated development analysis conducted in this study shed light on the dynamic changes within the water–economic–ecological systems of the five northwestern provinces of China, revealing two key trends:

(1) Positive Development Trend in the Comprehensive Evaluation of Three Subsystems: The comprehensive evaluation of the water, economic, and ecological subsystems demonstrates a positive developmental trajectory over the years. As time progresses, these provinces have exhibited improvements in various aspects of these subsystems. Effective water resource management has strengthened the sustainable supply of water. Additionally, economic growth has led to optimized resource utilization, curbing excessive exploitation of water resources. The comprehensive evaluation of the ecological subsystem indicates positive outcomes in ecosystem restoration and protection efforts, with biodiversity conservation and ecological functionality gradually recovering.

(2) Positive Development Trend in Coupled Coordinated Development Across the Five Provinces: The study also highlights the collaborative and coordinated development trend among the five provinces within their water–economic–ecological systems. Over time, the relationships between water, economy, and ecology in these provinces have become more interconnected. Scientific water resource utilization has provided a solid foundation for economic development while simultaneously emphasizing ecosystem protection to ensure sustainable resource utilization. Economic growth strategies increasingly prioritize eco-friendly development, resulting in a virtuous cycle of economic growth and ecological preservation. This trend of coordinated development contributes to ensuring sustainable water resource utilization, economic prosperity, and ecological health over the long term.

In summary, our study primarily focused on quantitative measures, but we understand the importance of integrating a human perspective into sustainable development research. The comprehensive evaluation and coupled coordinated development analysis of the water–economic–ecological systems in the five northwestern provinces of China highlight the positive achievements in sustainable development within these provinces. This not only offers valuable insights for regional decision-makers but also provides valuable experience for addressing similar challenges on a global scale. Furthermore, this study underscores the importance of comprehensive evaluation and coordinated development in resource-constrained settings, offering valuable lessons for future research endeavors with similar objectives. In future studies, we will consider how to incorporate qualitative analyses to provide a more comprehensive interpretation of sustainable development.

Author Contributions: Conceptualization, J.S. and F.W.; methodology, J.S.; software, H.Y.; validation, F.W., D.S. and Y.R.; formal analysis, J.S.; investigation, F.W.; resources, D.S.; data curation, F.W.; writing—original draft preparation, H.Y.; writing—review and editing, H.Y.; visualization, D.S.; supervision, J.S.; project administration, J.S.; funding acquisition, F.W. All authors have read and agreed to the published version of the manuscript.

Funding: It was jointly supported by the National Natural Science Foundation of China (52279014 and 52109085), the Key Research and Promotion Project of Henan Province (232102320257), and the Key Research and Development Project of Ningxia Hui Autonomous Region (2021BEG02012).

Data Availability Statement: Data will be made available on request.

Conflicts of Interest: The authors declare that they have no known competing financial interests or personal relationships that could have appeared to influence the work reported in this paper.

References

1. Zhang, H.; Sun, M.; Zhang, H.; Zhang, L.; Wang, Z. Spatial Distribution and Influencing Factors of Chinese Time-Honored Catering Brands in the Five Northwestern Provinces. *Sustainability* **2021**, *13*, 3755. [CrossRef]
2. Zhang, Z.; Jia, J.; Guo, Y.; Wu, B.; Chen, C. Scenario of carbon dioxide (CO_2) emission peaking and reduction path implication in five northwestern provinces of China by the low emissions analysis platform (LEAP) model. *Front. Energy Res.* **2022**, *10*, 983751. [CrossRef]
3. Wongchuig, S.; Espinoza, J.C.; Condom, T.; Junquas, C.; Sierra, J.P.; Fita, L.; Sörensson, A.; Polcher, J. Changes in the surface and atmospheric water budget due to projected Amazon deforestation: Lessons from a fully coupled model simulation. *J. Hydrol.* **2023**, *625*, 130082. [CrossRef]

4. Arlos, M.J.; Arnold, V.I.; Bumagat, J.S.; Zhou, J.; Cereno, K.M.; Deas, A.; Dai, K.; Ruecker, N.J.; Munkittrick, K.R. Combining chemical, bioanalytical and predictive tools to assess persistence, seasonality, and sporadic releases of organic micropollutants within the urban water cycle. *Water Res.* **2023**, *244*, 120454. [CrossRef] [PubMed]
5. Nakagawa, T. Numerical modeling on global-scale mantle water cycle and its impact on the sea-level change. *Earth Planet. Sci. Lett.* **2023**, *619*, 118312. [CrossRef]
6. Mohtar, W.H.M.W.; Razali, M.A.M.; Mazlan, M.A.; Rozaini, A.Z.A.; Mooralitharan, S.A.; Hamid, A.A.; Buyong, M.R. Rapid detection of ESKAPE and enteric bacteria using tapered dielectrophoresis and their presence in urban water cycle. *Process. Saf. Environ. Prot.* **2023**, *177*, 427–435. [CrossRef]
7. Zhou, F.; Zhang, W.; Jiang, A.; Peng, H.; Li, L.; Deng, L.; Sun, Y.; Wang, H. Spatial-temporal variation characteristics and coupling coordination of the "water resources—Water environment—Water ecology" carrying capacity in the Three Gorges Reservoir Area. *Ecol. Indic.* **2023**, *154*, 110874. [CrossRef]
8. Grigg, N. Water Resource Engineering: A Discipline or a Specialty and Why It Matters. *J. Hydraul. Eng.* **2023**, *149*, 13583. [CrossRef]
9. Liang, H.; Yu, L. Effects of reservoir system historical evolution on water system landscape patterns: The case of Changshou, China. *Environ. Sci. Pollut. Res. Int.* **2023**, 1–16. [CrossRef]
10. Su, C.; Wang, M.; Xie, X.; Han, Z.; Jiang, J.; Wang, Z.; Xiao, D. Natural and anthropogenic factors regulating fluoride enrichment in groundwater of the Nansi Lake Basin, Northern China. *Sci. Total. Environ.* **2023**, *904*, 166699. [CrossRef]
11. Ma, W.; Lian, J.; Rene, E.R.; Zhang, P.; Liu, X. Enhanced thyroxine removal from micro-polluted drinking water resources in a bio-electrochemical reactor amended with TiO2@GAC particles: Efficiency, mechanism and energy consumption. *Environ. Res.* **2023**, *237*, 116949. [CrossRef]
12. Bhaga, T.D.; Dube, T.; Shekede, M.D.; Shoko, C. Investigating the effectiveness of Landsat-8 OLI and Sentinel-2 MSI satellite data in monitoring the effects of drought on surface water resources in the Western Cape Province, South Africa. *Remote. Sens. Appl. Soc. Environ.* **2023**, *32*, 101037. [CrossRef]
13. Piao, J.; Nam, S.W.; Kim, Y.; Park, E. Enhancing groundwater management using aggregated-data analysis and segmented robust regression: A case study on spatiotemporal changes in water quality. *Sci. Total. Environ.* **2023**, *899*, 165981. [CrossRef] [PubMed]
14. Bresinsky, L.; Kordilla, J.; Hector, T.; Engelhardt, I.; Livshitz, Y.; Sauter, M. Managing climate change impacts on the Western Mountain Aquifer: Implications for Mediterranean karst groundwater resources. *J. Hydrol. X* **2023**, *20*, 100153. [CrossRef]
15. Deng, Y.; Shao, Z.; Dang, C.; Huang, X.; Zhuang, Q. The impact of policies on land cover and ecosystem services dynamics in the Poyang Lake Ecological Economic Zone, China. *Ecol. Indic.* **2023**, *156*, 111169. [CrossRef]
16. Hamdi Aya, A.; Abdulhameed Isam, M.; Mawlood Ibtihal, A. Application of Weap Model for Managing Water Resources in Iraq: A Review. *IOP Conf. Ser. Earth Environ. Sci.* **2023**, *1222*, 012032. [CrossRef]
17. Gidey, E.; Mhangara, P. An Application of Machine-Learning Model for Analyzing the Impact of Land-Use Change on Surface Water Resources in Gauteng Province, South Africa. *Remote. Sens.* **2023**, *15*, 4092. [CrossRef]
18. Meiyan, H.; Peijiang, Z.; Chaoqi, C. Study on coupling of typical elements in surface water and groundwater in the middle reaches of the Yangtze River, China. *J. Hydrol.* **2023**, *626*, 130298. [CrossRef]
19. Bakas, T.; Papadopoulos, C.; Latinopoulos, D.; Kagalou, I.; Akratos, C.; Angelidis, P.; Pliakas, F.-K.; Spiliotis, M. Supporting Participatory Management Planning for Catchment Operationalization with Intuitionistic Fuzzy Sets—A Study in Laspias River, Thrace, Greece. *Water* **2023**, *15*, 2928. [CrossRef]
20. Yoosefdoost, I.; Basirifard, M.; Álvarez-García, J.; Río-Rama, M.d.l.C.d. Increasing Agricultural Resilience through Combined Supply and Demand Management (Case Study: Karaj Reservoir Dam, Iran). *Agronomy* **2022**, *12*, 1997. [CrossRef]
21. Hoffmann, A.A.; Sgrò, C.M. Climate change and evolutionary adaptation. *Nature* **2011**, *470*, 479–485. [CrossRef] [PubMed]
22. Hernández-Bedolla, J.; Solera, A.; Paredes-Arquiola, J.; Pedro-Monzonís, M.; Andreu, J.; Sánchez-Quispe, S.T. The Assessment of Sustainability Indexes and Climate Change Im-pacts on Integrated Water Resource Management. *Water* **2017**, *9*, 13. [CrossRef]
23. Xin, Y.; Zhang, J.; Lu, T.; Wei, Y.; Shen, P. Response of prokaryotic, eukaryotic and algal communities to heavy rainfall in a reservoir supplied with reclaimed water. *J. Environ. Manag.* **2023**, *334*, 117394. [CrossRef] [PubMed]
24. Tang, Y.; Pan, Y.; Zhang, L.; Yi, H.; Gu, Y.; Sun, W. Efficient Monitoring of Total Suspended Matter in Urban Water Based on UAV Multi-spectral Images. *Water Resour. Manag.* **2023**, *37*, 2143–2160. [CrossRef]
25. Lv, C.; Xu, X.; Guo, X.; Feng, J.; Yan, D. Basin water ecological compensation interval accounting based on dual perspectives of supply and consumption: Taking Qingyi River Basin as an example. *J. Clean. Prod.* **2023**, *385*, 135610. [CrossRef]
26. Zhu, H.; Hu, X.-D.; Wu, P.-P.; Chen, W.-M.; Wu, S.-S.; Li, Z.-Q.; Zhu, L.; Xi, Y.-L.; Huang, R. Development and testing of the phytoplankton biological integrity index (P-IBI) in dry and wet seasons for Lake Gehu. *Ecol. Indic.* **2021**, *129*, 107882. [CrossRef]
27. Bu, J.; Li, C.; Wang, X.; Zhang, Y.; Yang, Z. Assessment and prediction of the water ecological carrying capacity in Changzhou city, China. *J. Clean. Prod.* **2020**, *277*, 123988. [CrossRef]
28. Li, J.; Zhao, M.; Han, Y.; Wei, J. Assessment on water cycle health in the Central Plains Urban cluster based on the DSWU NWU SWS NWS A—WCHI model. *Ecol. Indic.* **2023**, *157*. [CrossRef]

water

MDPI

Review

Barriers and Motivators of Household Water-Conservation Behavior: A Bibliometric and Systematic Literature Review

Carolina Sanchez [1], Carla Rodriguez-Sanchez [2] and Franco Sancho-Esper [2,*]

[1] Facultad de Ciencias Económicas, Universidad Católica de Córdoba, Córdoba X5016DHK, Argentina; csanchez@unc.edu.ar

[2] Department Marketing, Universidad de Alicante, San Vicente del Raspeig, 03690 Alicante, Spain; carla.rodriguez@ua.es

* Correspondence: franco.sancho@ua.es; Tel.: +34-965903400 (ext. 3169)

Abstract: Water scarcity, aggravated by growing demands, represents a significant challenge for humanity. Promoting household sustainable water-consumption behaviors has become vital. The Community-Based Social Marketing (CBSM) framework stands out among many strategies to promote water conservation. However, many interventions in this domain often neglect significant theoretical insights, leading to gaps in addressing key social and contextual drivers of behavior. This study conducts a systematic and bibliometric literature review aimed at identifying determinants underlying household water-conservation behaviors. This review encompasses 155 papers published from 1984 to early 2023. Our findings show that this is a highly multidisciplinary field of study with a marked increase in research attention discerned post-2010, particularly from water-stressed regions. Furthermore, our findings also reveal an often-overlooked integration of guiding theories and an over-reliance on self-reported measures in prior research. Factors such as attitude, perceived efficacy, emotions, and habits emerge as pivotal in understanding water conservation. However, while attitudes have been extensively analyzed in previous research, the other factors deserve greater attention from researchers. Inconsistencies in demographic predictors further hint at potential moderating roles. This paper offers valuable insights for designing effective household water-conservation interventions through a social marketing lens.

Keywords: barriers; motivators; water conservation; bibliometric; systematic; review

1. Introduction

Climate change intensifies water scarcity and associated hazards such as floods, rising sea levels, and droughts. Rising temperatures disrupt the water cycle, posing threats to sustainable development, biodiversity, and access to water [1]. Water scarcity, driven by escalating demand, is a critical global challenge [2]. Fostering sustainable water use requires urging individuals to adopt conservation behaviors. The Community-Based Social Marketing (CBSM) framework [3] is recognized as a highly effective tool for this purpose [4]. The CBSM emphasizes the need to address barriers and enhance motivating factors for effective behavioral change. However, social marketing often neglects theoretical insights and overlooks social and contextual factors affecting the target audience [5–7]. Additionally, interventions often overlook the distinction between internal and external factors influencing individuals [4]. A thorough analysis of these issues is vital to ensure the efficacy of water-conservation programs.

To assess barriers and motivators, social marketing employs two approaches: formative research and theory [4]. Formative research, also called consumer or audience research, employs methods such as interviews and focus groups to explore consumer insights and the factors that either encourage or hinder their behaviors [8]. However, criticism arises due to heavy reliance on self-reported methods and the use of a single research method, potentially limiting a complete understanding of the behavior [8,9]. In contrast, theory, such as a literature review, serves as a valuable research tool, bridging the theory-practice gap by summarizing empirical evidence and offering insights from various disciplinary perspectives [10].

Based on the above, this research aims to conduct a literature review to identify the determinants (barriers and motivators) previously used to explain water-conservation behavior at home. To do this, a systematic and bibliometric literature review to date is performed. By understanding these determinants, policymakers and social marketers can design tailored interventions and broaden the field of knowledge. Additionally, this study also examines prevalent theories, seeks to understand the evolution of the field of knowledge, and identifies potential future research directions.

This study has several contributions to the body of knowledge concerning household water conservation. Primarily, it pioneers an integrated approach by conducting both a bibliometric (quantitative) and systematic (qualitative) literature review to find the determinants of household water conservation. This synthesis fills a notable gap in the existing literature, as most prior studies (e.g., [11–14]) undertook either bibliometric or systematic reviews in isolation. Our approach not only minimizes potential researcher bias through a quantitative review but also offers a critical evaluation of the relevance of these determinants via qualitative analysis. Further, adopting a comprehensive lens, this research delineates both the internal factors (encompassing psychosocial and socio-demographic dimensions) and external (contextual) variables that explain water conservation and consumption patterns. This review also involves a great diversity of geographical, cultural, and social contexts, contributing to a comprehensive and empirically grounded understanding of the subject matter. Lastly, our in-depth analysis, coupled with a discerning discussion and ensuing conclusions, yields valuable managerial implications. These insights hold significant merit for social marketing professionals, offering them pragmatic strategies on how behavioral determinants can be effectively leveraged to craft campaigns that foster water-conservation behaviors.

2. Methodological Approach

The literature review in this research is based on two complementary methodologies: a bibliometric analysis and a systematic analysis. The bibliometric analysis offers a quantitative perspective, providing an objective assessment of the field's status through an exhaustive evaluation of published research, thus enhancing rigor and minimizing potential researcher bias [15]. This approach enables extracting and visualizing insights from a substantial volume of literature, providing objective references. Nonetheless, it is worth noting that the bibliometric approach, while highly valuable, cannot replace the manual systematic review undertaken by researchers, which extends the analysis with a critical perspective [16].

To complement the above quantitative approach, a secondary qualitative analysis has been performed. This qualitative review aims to identify existing related studies, meticulously selecting contributions and critically evaluating their relevance [17]. It is key to emphasize that this systematic review diverges from the conventional literature review in terms of its heightened objectivity, meticulous systematization, transparency, and replicability. This rigor is made possible by following a standardized and well-defined protocol [18]. The analysis conducted in this study adhered to the methodology outlined in the PRISMA review protocol (Preferred Reporting Items for Systematic Reviews and Meta-Analysis) [19]. This systematic approach encompasses six distinct stages: (1) formulation of the research question(s), selection of relevant databases, and identification of key search terms (keywords); (2) specification of inclusion and exclusion criteria for articles; (3) preliminary search and initial selection of relevant materials; (4) scrutiny of search results against predefined selection criteria; (5) comprehensive critical assessment of the literature; and (6) synthesis of the obtained results. Figure 1 summarizes the main steps involving the systematic, bibliometric, and thematic research.

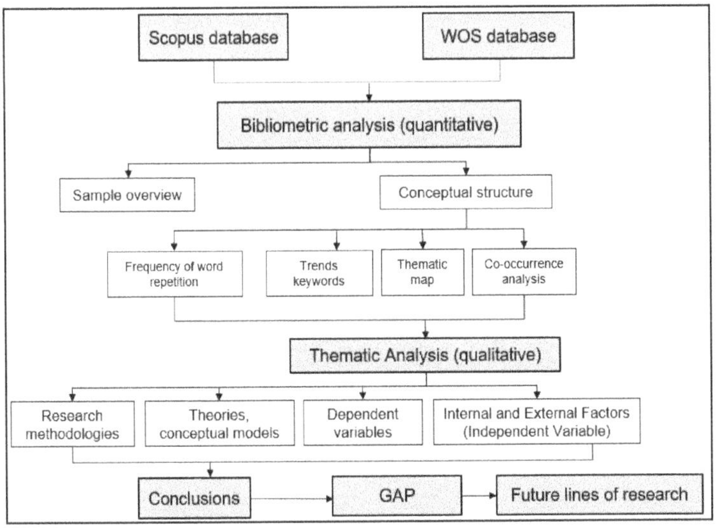

Figure 1. Stages in this bibliometric and systematic review. Source: Own elaboration, adapted from [16].

Step 1: Formulation of Research Questions, Database Selection, and Keyword Establishment

The primary focus of this research is to understand both internal factors (encompassing psychosocial and socio-demographic dimensions) and external (contextual) variables influencing household water-conservation behavior. Additionally, we aim to identify barriers hindering behavior change or adoption, along with its motivators. In light of this objective, the following research questions are stated:

1. What specific behavior is examined in the studies? (e.g., intention, behavior-reported or observed-, past behaviors, current behaviors).
2. Which theories or conceptual frameworks are used in these studies?
3. What are the main factors employed to explain the behavior, and what is their importance?
4. Which environmental psychology theories or factors have not been thoroughly explored in this context?
5. What are the main findings yielded by previous research?
6. What future research directions have been identified by scholars in this field?

To systematically search for research studies, two globally renowned databases, Web of Science (WOS) and Scopus, were selected for their respected peer review process, coverage of major international scientific publishers, and comprehensive inclusion of relevant works [16,17]. The substantial overlap between these databases ensures the inclusion of virtually all relevant articles, with Scopus, especially, offering comprehensive coverage across various research domains, crucial for the interdisciplinary nature of this study encompassing psychology, environmental psychology, marketing, economics, and communication [15,20].

The selection of search terms involved a comparative analysis of 23 literature review articles on water consumption and conservation from high-impact journals (see the list in Appendix A, Table A1), leading to the identification of keywords and thematic categories related to determinants of water behavior (Table A2). The search terms underwent refinement stages for precision, culminating in the compilation of terms in Table A3. Scopus and Web of Science (WOS) databases were used, employing Boolean operators "AND" and "OR". Keywords were entered hierarchically and grouped into blocks (context, behavior, water, motivators, barriers, behavioral determinants, theories), enhancing search efficiency. The search structure is detailed in Table A3.

Step 2: Defining the inclusion and exclusion criteria.

This literature review focuses on peer-reviewed journal articles aligned with the research goals of understanding motivating factors and barriers in household water consumption/conservation [12,18]. Inclusion criteria follow recommendations, considering only empirical research articles in English, excluding theoretical works, literature reviews, and non-journal sources [16,21,22]. The scope emphasizes studies investigating water-consumption or saving behavior in households and urban environments [11], excluding those in other domains such as water management, supply-related perspectives, or aggregate water demand [23].

Step 3: Search and preliminary selection of articles

The final article search in the WOS and Scopus databases was on 8 March 2023, encompassing all relevant research up to that date without setting any publication date restrictions. Out of the initial 9707 articles retrieved, 3018 duplicates were automatically detected and removed using the Mendeley management platform. A manual review, considering titles, authors, publication years, and DOIs, eliminated an additional 156 potential duplicates. The remaining 6533 articles underwent a detailed scrutiny of titles and abstracts, resulting in the exclusion of 5875 articles that did not meet inclusion criteria. [24]. Further refinement involved a meticulous examination of the methodology and conclusion sections, leading to the exclusion of an additional 503 records. The systematic process, detailed in Figure 2, culminated in a final sample of 155 articles.

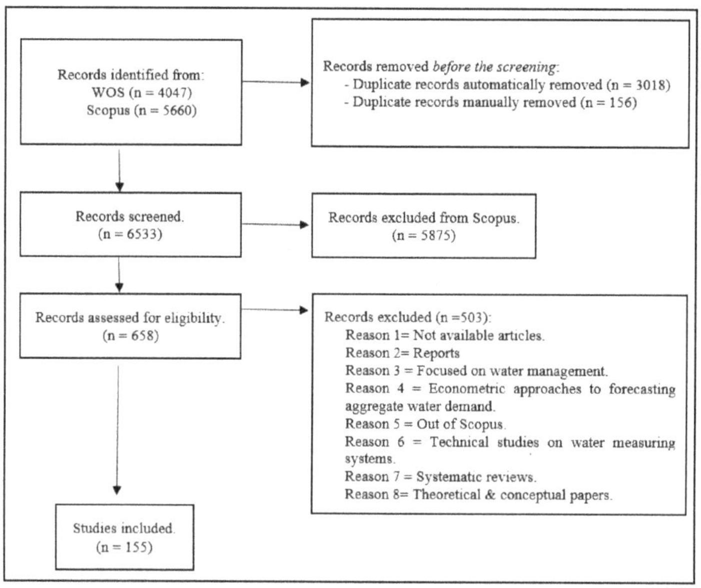

Figure 2. PRISMA diagram of the publication search and selection process. Source: own elaboration following PRISMA recommendations [19].

Step 4: Evaluation of the results related to the selection criteria.

To systematically organize and condense pertinent information, a working table was constructed. This table facilitated the thorough examination of key sections in each article, including the introduction, conceptual framework, methodology, results, discussions, and conclusions.

Step 5: Critical evaluation of the literature.

The article assessment involved a two-stage analysis [25]. The first stage included a bibliometric analysis of the 155 selected articles, following the model by Ricart et al. [23]. This initial stage focused on sample descriptive statistics. The second stage aimed to identify current and emerging research themes, patterns, and future directions. This involved keyword frequency analysis, thematic mapping, and co-occurrence networks. Similar methodologies have been applied in pro-environmental behavior studies, covering areas such as climate change [26], environmental communication [27], and general pro-environmental behaviors, along with specific domains such as recycling behaviors [15] and solar panel adoption [28]. Several tools are available for conducting bibliometric analyses. For this research, R version 4.2.2 was used. The analysis was performed using the Bibliometrix library, accessed through the Biblioshiny package, which simplifies data usage and analysis. Moreover, it can import data from a wide range of databases such as WOS, Scopus, and PubMed [29]. It has been extensively employed for conducting bibliometric studies in fields such as marketing and sustainability [30,31], pro-environmental behaviors [32], and, specifically, water-conservation behavior [23,33].

The second stage entailed a qualitative examination of article content through thematic analysis, a flexible and accessible method that identifies recurring patterns within data [34]. Adopting a theoretical thematic analysis approach, closely aligned with the researcher's theoretical or analytical interest [25,34], facilitated a comprehensive exploration of data facets [35,36]. This analysis focused on barriers and determinants influencing household water-consumption/conservation behavior, with data coded according to initial research objectives. Data were compiled in Microsoft Excel and included relevant variables such as, e.g., authorship, research objectives, models or theories employed, and research methodology. Subsequently, a content analysis was conducted, employing inductive reasoning to process the information while also considering insights derived from the bibliometric analysis [25,37]. Section 3 (Results) provides comprehensive insights into this critical evaluation and synthesis process.

Step 6: Synthesis of results.

The section labeled "Discussion and Conclusions" offers a condensed summary of the findings derived from the literature review.

3. Results

3.1. Bibliometric Analysis

3.1.1. Main Characteristics of Contributions

A summary of the studies included in the sample is depicted in Figure 3. These 155 articles were published spanning the years 1982 to 2023 and appeared in 80 different academic journals. On average, each article garnered approximately 36 citations. The research in this field is published across a broad spectrum of academic journals, encompassing both Social Sciences and Science disciplines. As indicated in Table A4 (Appendix A), some of the most prominent academic journals in this domain include the *Journal of Environmental Management* (11 times, 7.1%), *Water* (9, 5.8%), *Journal of Environmental Psychology* (8, 5.2%), *Sustainability* (7, 4.5%), *Journal of Applied Social Psychology* (5, 3.2%), and *Water Policy* (5, 3.2%), among others. This extensive array of publication outlets reflects the interdisciplinary nature of the field, with journals spanning disciplines such as Management, Environmental Psychology, Social Psychology, Economics, Sustainability, Public Policy, and the Natural Sciences.

Timespan 1982–2023	**Sources** 80	**Documents** 155	**Authors** 406
Authors of single-authored 13	**Co-authors/doc** 3.08	**International co-authorship** 20%	**Author's keywords** 469
Annual growth rate 2.72%	**References** 7534	**Document Avg. age** 7.31	**Average citations/doc** 35.87

Figure 3. Overview of the analyzed articles. Source: Result from Biblioshiny.

One interesting aspect to evaluate is the significance and contemporary relevance of the topic under study. As illustrated in Figure 4, it becomes readily apparent that the scientific community's interest in investigating behaviors related to water consumption, saving, or conservation has witnessed exponential growth since 2010, ultimately reaching a peak of 21 annual publications in 2021. When examining relative figures, a substantial 132% increase is observed between the periods of 1982–2010 and 2011–2023.

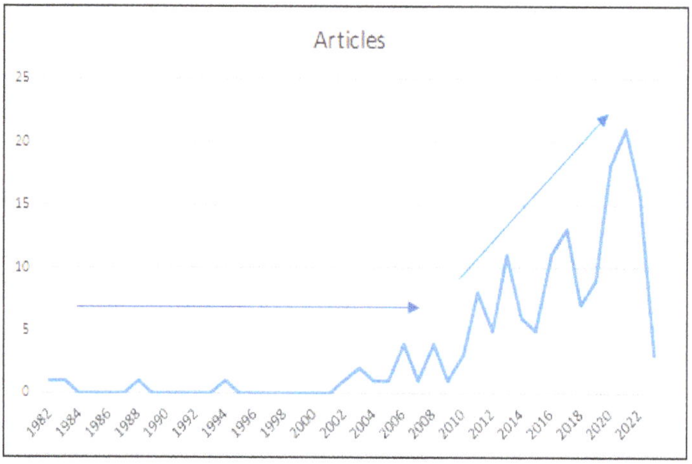

Figure 4. Annual scientific production. Source: Result from Biblioshiny. Note: By not fully including all months of 2023 in the analysis (see Step 3), the graph shows a very steep drop in the number of articles registered after 2022.

When assessing the global contributions to a particular area of knowledge, it is essential to consider their geographical distribution (Figure 5). In alignment with trends in sustainability research, the predominant regions were North America (USA, 93 articles, 60%, and Mexico, 13 articles, 8.3%). Additionally, Oceania, represented primarily by Australia (57 articles, 37%), has made significant contributions. Europe has also been a notable contributor, with Spain (34 articles, 22%), the United Kingdom (14 articles, 9%), and the Netherlands (11 articles, 7%) actively participating. Furthermore, though to a lesser extent, Asia has shown involvement, with China (17 articles, 11%) and Iran (7 articles, 4.5%) making contributions. Finally, Africa, primarily represented by South Africa (8 articles, 5.1%), and South America, where Chile (5 articles, 3.2%) is prominent, have also played roles in this research domain.

Examining the dispersion of research among authors and groups, Table A5 (Appendix A) outlines the frequency of author appearances in the sample. Prominent figures include Warner (5 articles, 1%), Corral-Verdugo (4 articles, 0.8%), Fielding (4 articles, 0.8%), and others, with 352 authors appearing only once. Assessing the impact of these publications, Table A6 presents citations and annual averages. Works by Willis et al. [38] (JEP, 22.9 citations/year), Schultz et al. [39] (E&B, 17.4 citations/year), and Fielding et al. [40] (JEM, 17.1 citations/year) stand out. Collaboration analysis in research is key to understanding the underlying structure of a particular knowledge domain. Results show that 9.03% of articles were single-authored, averaging 3.8 authors per study. International co-authorship is around 20% (Figure 6). Notably, the United States of America and Australia emerged as leaders in international research collaborations, closely followed by China, Spain, the Netherlands, and the United Kingdom. In contrast, research collaborations involving countries from Latin Northern Asia, South America, or Africa appear to be relatively scarce.

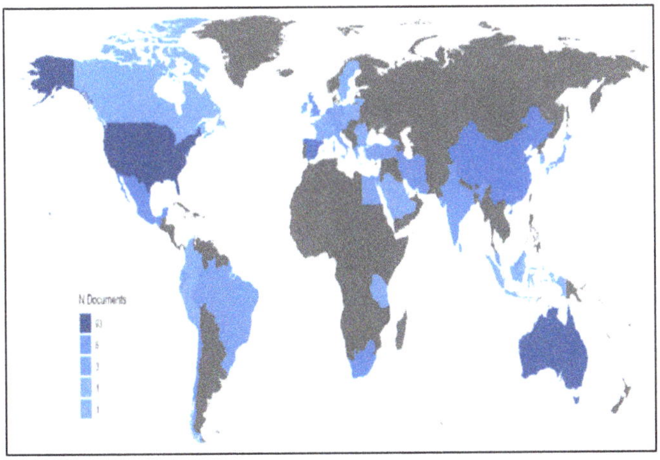

Figure 5. Scientific production by country researcher home institution. Source: Result from Biblioshiny.

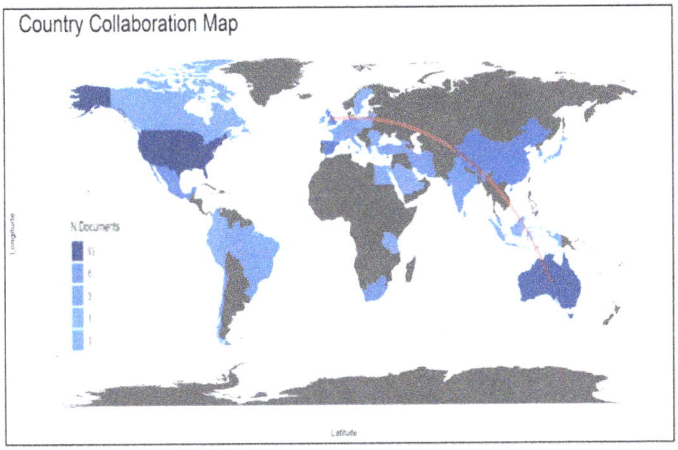

Figure 6. Author's collaboration network by country researcher home institution. Source: Result from Biblioshiny. Note: The strength of the blue means the intensity of publication by country, grey areas are countries without contributions in the sample. Pink lines indicate international collaborations.

To enhance the understanding of research dynamics, a collaborative network among authors was generated and is illustrated in Figure 7. This network visualizes the interactions among authors within the specified field of study, providing insights into the formation of author groups, influential figures, or author communities, as suggested by Aria and Cuccurullo [29]. Upon close examination of the figure, it becomes evident that research groups tend to be relatively small, with most consisting of two to three collaborators. Notably, there are a few cases with up to four collaborations. Judging by the size of the node and the number of collaborations, it can be inferred that Professor Kelly Fielding holds a prominent role as an influential author and a reference within the subject of study.

The joint analysis of the collaborating countries and the working groups of researchers reveals some interesting patterns. In comparison to other fields of knowledge, research teams tend to be relatively small, and international networks exhibit limited scope. Generally, authors tend to publish alongside co-authors from their own country or individuals with whom they have had prior academic interactions, such as sharing the same educational institution or originating from the same country. Moreover, it seems that cross-country collaborations are typically concentrated. For instance, the United States displays 16 international collaborations, followed by Australia with 6, Spain with 4, and both the Netherlands, China, and the United Kingdom with 3 each (The full Table A7 is available in Appendix A).

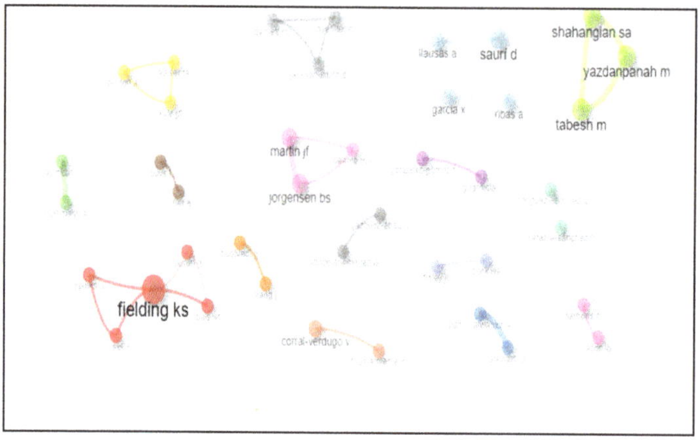

Figure 7. Collaboration networks between authors. Source: Result from Biblioshiny.

3.1.2. Conceptual Structure of Contributions

To conduct the conceptual analysis, several bibliometric instruments were used, including keyword frequency assessments, thematic mapping, and co-occurrence networks. These tools are instrumental in identifying present and emerging research themes and forecasting future areas of exploration [41]. The outcomes of this analysis provide insights into the conceptual frameworks and attributes associated with the topic under study [25,42].

This study involved a preliminary data cleansing aimed at removing synonyms and terms found in articles that are unrelated to the research objective [43]. Specifically, highly frequent words that were initially part of the article search criteria were excluded. For instance, following previous literature reviews (e.g., [43–45]) terms such as "water" or words related to research methodologies such as "survey" were removed (List of words deleted for these analyses in Biblioshiny: household survey, questionnaire, questionnaire survey, housing, surveys, surveys, water, water management, water supply, water conservation, water demand, water demand management, demand-side management, human, female, man, middle-aged, adult, controlled study, article, water, water resource, water use, water consumption, humans, aged, male, water resources, household, household water, priority journal, rural area, urban area, environmental issues, sampling, human behavior, local participation, conceptual framework, conservation of water resources, internal consistency, policymakers, resident population, environmental issue, theory).

A word cloud, shown in Figure 8, generated from "Authors' keywords" (The word cloud generated using the "keywords plus" approach was also examined, and its findings closely resembled those of the previous word cloud. Therefore, comparing both word clouds was deemed unnecessary), after data filtering, visually emphasizes prevalent terms [44,46]. "Social norms" stands out as an extensively studied variable in household water-conservation behavior, along with related terms such as "descriptive norms" and "injunctive norms". Other frequently mentioned words include "attitude", "habits", "feedback", "intention", "communication", "environmental knowledge", "credibility", and "environmental concern", identifying potential factors influencing water use/conservation. Terms such as "conservation behavior", "behavioral intention", "domestic water consumption", and "water saving" likely denote outcome variables in the studies. Notably, "theory of planned behavior" suggests Ajzen's theory [47] as a predominant conceptual framework.

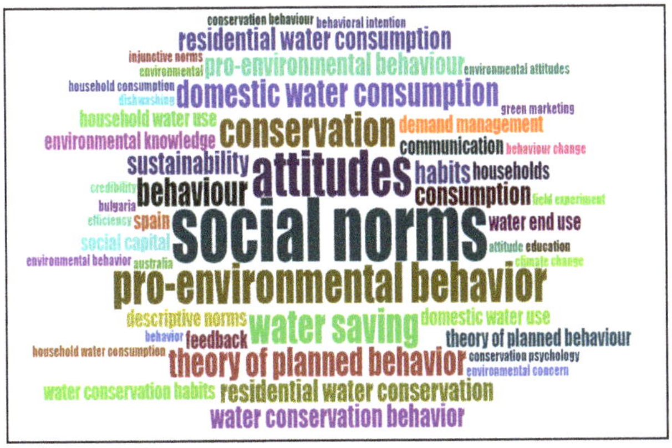

Figure 8. Word cloud based on "authors' keywords". Source: Result from Biblioshiny.

An analysis of the past decade's trends, with a focus on frequently occurring words, was performed using the "keyword plus" criterion generated by the Biblioshiny algorithm. These keywords, extracted from article titles in bibliographic references, may differ from the authors' original keywords or the article title (Refs. [48,49] used a similar approach). Notable trends since 2020 encompass terms such as "water insecurity", "perception", "motivation", "efficient water use", and "behaviors and psychology". Figure 9 underscores that key internal factors affecting water consumption/conservation are "perception", "attitude", and "motivation", while external factors beyond individual control encompass "water quality" and climatic variables such as "drought".

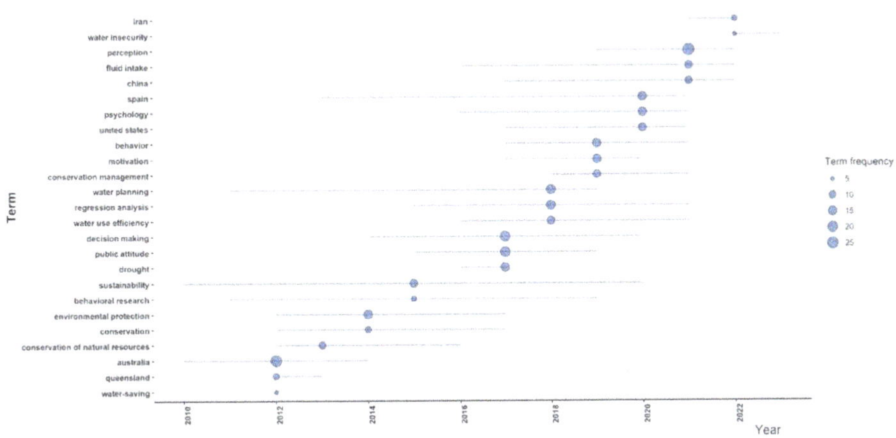

Figure 9. Trends "Keywords Plus", 2010–2023. Source: Result from Biblioshiny.

A thematic map, employing density (theme development) on the vertical axis and centrality (topic relevance) on the horizontal axis, defines key themes in four quadrants: (1) niche themes, highly developed or isolated; (2) motor themes, the most relevant and central; (3) emerging or declining themes; and (4) basic themes. This approach aligns with prior bibliometric studies [31,44]. Figure 10 displays the thematic map in this study using author keywords. In the "niche topics" quadrant, notable proximity is observed between "water tariffs" and "behavior change", reflecting interest in the relationship between water pricing and consumption. Keywords such as "attitude", "efficient water-saving behavior", and "attitude towards the environment" are present, suggesting a connection to efficient behavior, possibly involving devices such as "dishwashers" for conservation. Moving to the "motor themes" quadrant, terms such as "social norms", "habits", "environmental knowledge", "communication", and "feedback" are prominent. While "smart water meters" remains relevant, its development seems to decline. In the lower quadrants, the significance of studying the "theory of planned behavior" and "water use in the home" is evident, with a diminishing relevance.

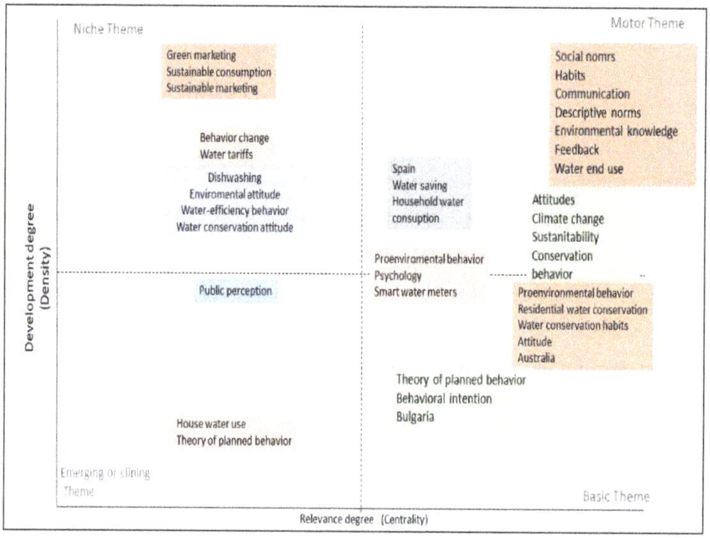

Figure 10. Thematic map based on *authors' keywords*. Source: Result from Biblioshiny.

Expanding on insights from the thematic map, the determinants impacting water use/conservation behavior fall into two groups: internal (individual factors) and external (outside the individual). Internal factors encompass "attitude", "intention", "perception", "habits", "social norms", and "knowledge", while external factors include "water tariffs", "water-saving devices", "water-consumption measurement systems", and the "feedback effect of that information". Using the same thematic mapping tool, temporal evolution was examined across two periods: (i) 1982 to 2017 and (ii) 2018 to 2023. Figure A1 in Appendix A provides a comparative analysis of these thematic maps.

The comparison between both periods reveals interesting results. First, it is clear that certain fundamental themes such as "perception", "motivation", "behavior change", and "attitude" remain relevant. Second, during 2017–2023, there was an emergence of pivotal themes, including "communication", "irrigation and landscaping systems", "social behavior", "intention", "environmental psychology", and "efficient water utilization". Third, interestingly the concept of "water efficiency" transitions from being an emerging theme to consolidating its place among the core themes. Fourth, the 2017–2023 period introduces new basic themes such as "environmental values and household structure" (encompassing factors such as household size and age), "household income", and the interrelation between "social norms and environmental determinants". Finally, the scrutiny of "feedback" (related to water consumption on an individual or household basis) is gradually becoming a focal research area, whereas the prominence of "incentives" seems to be diminishing.

This temporal review delves into the progression of water use and conservation behavior research. Rooted in environmental psychology, elements such as "attitude", "motivation", and "perception" engage scholars consistently. Intrinsic factors such as "values", "knowledge", "intention", and "social norms" remain significant. External determinants, including socio-demographics, household attributes, climate change, and economic incentives, are explored. Research methods exhibit shifts, with "regression" studies initially in the core themes but descending in later periods. "Structural equations", absent initially, emerge as a core theme, while "experimental studies" transition from niche to declining.

The co-occurrence network is the primary tool for understanding the conceptual structure of contributions, offering a comprehensive view of potential subjects in papers' content [25]. Graphical representations in the co-occurrence map capture synergies within bibliographic metadata [29]. By linking pivotal terms provided by authors, a matrix reveals how often term pairs co-appear, resulting in labeled circles (graphs) of varying sizes and colors, smoothly connected [43]. Graph size indicates occurrence frequency, reflecting a term's prevalence in articles [29]. Color signifies the assigned group or cluster. This analysis implicitly explores authors' established relationships between keywords [50], exemplified by "motivation" and "water saving".

In Figure 11, the co-occurrence network from 155 contributions reveals three distinct clusters with varying nodes. Prominent nodes include "perception" (blue cluster), "environmental protection" (red cluster), and "Australia" (green cluster). The blue cluster centers on perception, attitude, social behavior, water insecurity, knowledge, and water consumption, intertwining with terms such as marketing, conservation programs, water efficiency, and strategic planning. The red cluster, emphasizing environmental protection, includes themes such as motivation, attitude, education, public opinion, and conservation. The green cluster, labeled "Australia", predominantly addresses climate change, drought, Australian context, and demographic variables.

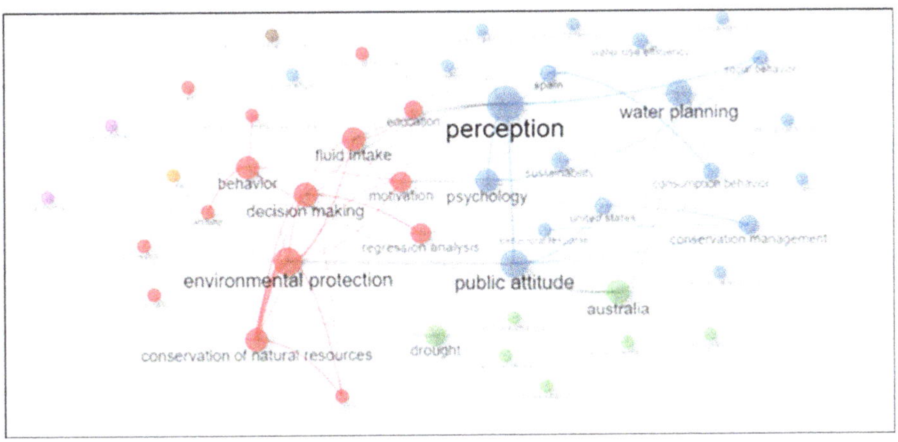

Figure 11. Co-occurrence of key terms. Source: Result from Biblioshiny.

3.2. *Thematic Analysis (Qualitative–Exploratory)*

In this section, a qualitative analysis of the 155 publications was conducted following the previous bibliometric analysis. In essence, this section summarizes the constructs, methodologies, theories, and variables applied in the examination of water-conservation/consumption behavior at home.

3.2.1. Research Methodologies Used in the Literature

The first aspect to be analyzed is the methodological characteristics of the empirical studies comprised by this literature review. More precisely, we focus on delineating the study type and the estimation procedure employed in each instance. Within this framework, studies can be categorized into four research domains: (i) qualitative and exploratory studies, (ii) quantitative and correlational studies, (iii) experimental and longitudinal studies, and (iv) simulation studies. See Table 1 for a comprehensive overview.

Table 1. Analysis of contributions by research approach and methodologies.

Research Approach	Data Analysis Method	Frequency	%
(i) Qualitative–exploratory	Qualitative research	6	3.6%
	Case studies	1	0.6%
	Mixed methods (quali–quanti)	9	5.5%
SUB-TOTAL QUALITATIVE EXPLORATORY		**16**	**9.7%**
(ii) Quantitative correlational	Structural Modeling: CB-SEM	31	18.8%
	Structural Modeling: PLS-SEM	2	1.2%
	Latent-growth curve modeling (SEM-based)	1	0.6%
	Factor analysis: EFA	3	1.8%
	Multiple regression model	25	15.2%
	Discrete data analysis (Probit, Logit, and Poisson)	20	12.1%
	Spatial autoregressive models (SARs)	1	0.6%
	Regression tree	2	1.2%
	Cluster analysis + Latent profile analysis (LPA)	5	3.0%
	Jackknife grouping approach	1	0.6%
	ANOVA	4	2.4%
	ANCOVA	1	0.6%
	MANOVA	3	1.8%
	Mixed methods (quali–quanti)	9	5.5%
	Descriptive statistics	8	4.8%
	Correlation analysis	2	1.2%
	Multivariate methods	1	0.6%
SUB-TOTAL QUANTITATIVE CORRELATIONAL		**119**	**72.1%**
(iii) Longitudinal and experimental quantitative	Experiments	25	15.2%
	Longitudinal studies	3	1.8%
SUB-TOTAL LONGITUDINAL AND EXPERIMENTAL		**28**	**17.0%**
(iv) Simulation models	Simulation models	1	0.6%
	Agent-based modeling (ABM)	1	0.6%
SUB-TOTAL SIMULATION		**2**	**1.2%**
TOTAL ANALYSIS TECHNIQUES		**165 ***	

Note: CB-SEM = Structural models of covariances; PLS-SEM = Structural models of variances. * n = 155. Some of the 155 papers use more than one analysis technique. Source: Own elaboration.

Firstly, it is important to note that several studies employed multiple research methods. Consequently, the sample size comprises 155 articles, with a total of 165 research methods utilized. Globally, the majority of studies (72.1%) rely on cross-sectional data with a quantitative and correlational approach. Common methodologies within this category include structural equation models (CB 18.8%, PLS 1.2%), multiple regression models (15.2%), and discrete choice models (12.1%). The next category involves studies based on experimental or longitudinal data (17%), followed by more qualitative or exploratory studies (9.7%), with fewer focusing on data simulation applications (1.2%). Quantitative studies dominate, with only 5.5% using a mixed methodology [51]. Notably, a limited 1.8% adopt a time series and longitudinal approach, despite calls for long-term monitoring [52–56]. Moreover, these studies are scarce, even considering high water-consumption seasonality [57,58].

3.2.2. Theoretical and Conceptual Approaches

In examining studies, a critical aspect requiring in-depth analysis is the conceptual framework and theoretical underpinnings. Notably, 54% of the analyzed studies lack explicit reference to the theoretical framework used for studying the barriers or motivators of the behavior (see Table A8 in the Appendix A). The majority present concepts and theoretical precedents without a direct linkage to a specific theory. Among the 46% that do reference theoretical foundations, the Theory of Planned Behavior (TPB, [58] (10%), (NAM, [59] (3%), and New Environmental Paradigm [60] (3%) are noted. However, this list is non-exhaustive, reflecting the interdisciplinary nature of research in psychology, behavioral economics, health, communication, persuasion, and environmental psychology. Furthermore, 8.4% explicitly draw on more than one theory or model, such as Construal Level Theory and TPB [61], TRA and NEP [62], TPB and Social Cognitive Theory [63], or TRA and ELM [64]. Combining theories is justified for enhancing predictive capacity and deepening understanding of the intention–behavior gap in water conservation.

3.2.3. Behaviors Analyzed: Dependent Variable

Another key consideration when comparing studies focused on pro-environmental behavior change is the specific dependent variables being examined. In our particular case, the primary dependent variables under investigation include (1) water-conservation or saving behavior and (2) water use or consumption (for specific measurements, see Appendix A Table A9), both at the household level. Thus, within the types of environmentally significant behavior most frequently used in the literature, we focus on private-sphere environmentalism [65]. Water consumption can be classified into two categories: efficiency and curtailment behaviors. Efficiency behavior requires the purchase of water-efficiency equipment to be able to save water, while water curtailment behaviors are highly dependent on consumers' awareness and understanding of how to save water [66]. However, in this review, only five articles (3%) explicitly categorized behaviors as efficient or curtailment (e.g., [63,67,68]).

The predominant method of measuring the dependent variable in the analyzed studies is self-reported measures (57%) (e.g., [68,69]), followed by behavioral intention to conserve or save water (27%) (e.g., [70,71]). To a lesser degree, actual water consumption has been used as a metric, encompassing variations such as "per-capita consumption" or "consumption per household" (7%). These data often come from water supply companies and/or smart water metering systems (e.g., [53,72]). It is noteworthy that only 3% of the studies employ a combination of different methods to measure water consumption or saving. For instance, Haeffner et al. [73] investigate water-conservation behavior by scrutinizing consumption bills (reflecting actual target consumption) and assessing behavioral intentions.

3.2.4. Determinants of Behavior: Independent Variables

In exploring the determinants of household water-conservation behavior, this review categorizes the factors based on the criteria established by Stern [65]. Initially, our analysis focuses on personal-sphere variables, which include both psychosocial and socio-demographic aspects. This is followed by an examination of contextual factors as outlined by Stern [65]. Personal-sphere variables reflect the internal attributes of an individual, whereas contextual factors denote external elements beyond an individual's control that affect behavior [74]. This review reveals that prior research has analyzed personal-sphere variables such as attitudes, knowledge, environmental awareness, moral obligation, social norms (descriptive and injunctive norms), perceived effectiveness and perceived response efficacy, adscription of responsibility, time distance or future orientation, emotions, and habits. The main socio-demographic variables analyzed are age, gender, income level, education, and homeownership status. In contrast, the contextual variable exploration has highlighted external factors, including household features (number of people), physical characteristics (size, age, presence of gardens and pools), financial costs, and incentives, along with broader economic, political, and social factors. Facilitating elements, including the availability of water-saving devices and climatic conditions, must also be considered as external factors.

Personal-Sphere (Internal) Factors Related to Water-Conservation Behavior

These antecedents are systematically detailed in Table A10 (included in Appendix A). An in-depth examination of the most salient ones follows below.

Attitudes

A substantial body of research has centered on analyzing attitudes. Although there is widespread agreement on evaluating attitudes toward water conservation and use, research has delved into other types of attitudes as well. These include attitudes toward "responsible consumption" [75], "water pricing and water restrictions" [76], "routine (curtailment) and non-routine (efficiency) behaviors" [67], "water-saving devices" [77], and so forth. While attitudes significantly influence intentions for water-saving behaviors, a persistent gap exists between positive attitudes and actual choices. Individuals predisposed to saving water (positive attitude) may not always translate this attitude into specific conservation efforts [53,78]. This incongruence underscores the complex relationships influencing water-related decisions. Attitudinal variables, while crucial, account for only a modest portion of behavioral variance [79]. Understanding water conservation requires considering contextual and structural household factors, highlighting the need for a comprehensive understanding of multifaceted influences on water-related behaviors [77,79–81].

Knowledge

Numerous studies, such as [33,82], emphasize the role of knowledge in water conservation. Madias et al. [83] argue that water-related knowledge directly influences the intention to adopt water-saving devices and indirectly impacts overall water-conservation intention. Lack of knowledge hinders understanding the environmental impact and may lead to a lack of responsibility and intent to save water. High environmental knowledge correlates with the positive attitudes, behaviors, and habits supporting efficient water use [82]. Addo et al. [84] emphasize the significance of water-saving knowledge, environmental education gaps, and inadequate information about personal water consumption as substantial psychological barriers to adopting water-saving behaviors. Studies such as [85,86] explore the impact of information provision on water consumption, revealing positive effects and behavioral changes in water use, especially under conditions of scarcity.

Environmental awareness

Environmental awareness is defined as individuals' understanding of the impact of human activities on the environment [87]. Several studies in the field of water-conservation behavior have examined this construct (e.g., [52,88]). Overall, this literature indicates that while awareness does play a role in shaping behavioral intentions, it alone is insufficient to drive behavioral changes [89,90]. Environmental awareness is frequently investigated together with environmental concerns. Environmental concern relates to individuals' awareness of environmental issues and their disposition to address those issues [91]. Within the scope of this thematic review, studies have documented a positive correlation between participants' degree of environmental concern and their self-reported behaviors [92]. Nevertheless, certain studies suggest that this correlation is relatively weak (e.g., [93,94]) or that they are unrelated constructs (e.g., [95,96]).

Moral obligation

Individuals, motivated by a sense of moral obligation, engage in influencing water-conservation attitudes and intentions [97–99]. However, conflicting findings arise as some express a moral duty to conserve water without aligning actual consumption with beliefs [100]. While Marzouk et al. [101] argue that moral obligation, combined with other factors, explains water conservation, Lowe et al. [102] find no association. The lack of consensus highlights the need for additional research to unravel the complexities surrounding moral obligation and water-conservation behavior.

Social norms

Social norms have received extensive attention in the domain of water-conservation research. They are usually defined as the informal guidelines that govern and shape social behaviors, determining whether a specific behavior is deemed acceptable within a given society or group [103]. They reflect whether significant others endorse or discourage a certain behavior [64]. Despite their positive impact on water conservation [73], Landon et al. [79] suggest social norms explain only a small portion of variance in water use. Some studies explore the combined impacts of social norms and water-consumption feedback, revealing contributions to reducing consumption, though this effect diminishes over time [40,104]. Furthermore, social norms are often categorized into two distinct types: descriptive norms, referring to the perceptions of how most people commonly behave, and injunctive norms, which pertain to the societal perceptions of behaviors that are generally deemed acceptable or unacceptable. Seventy-one percent of studies make no norm distinction, 24% distinguish both descriptive and injunctive norms, and 5% analyze only descriptive norms. While descriptive norms influence conservation (e.g., [67,105]), injunctive norms, especially considering neighbors' behaviors, often exert a more profound impact on water-saving actions. Messages with explicit social judgments amplify this effect, with individuals seeking approval from neighbors more than other significant figures [106]. Studies linked to descriptive norms and consumption information suggest a bias in self-consumption perception, where individuals tend to either underestimate or overestimate their consumption compared to others [73,107]. Associating social norms with social identity enhances normative messages' efficacy, emphasizing the norm's association with the referent group [108].

Perceived efficacy

This variable has been denoted by different terms within the literature, even when not always referencing the same concept. This can generate confusion and misinterpretation. Specifically, perceived efficacy is also referred to as (1) perceived effectiveness, (2) outcome expectations, or (3) personal response efficacy. These three terms share a common definition, including the extent to which individuals believe their actions can contribute to solving an environmental problem. Notably, it is crucial to distinguish between the concept of perceived efficacy and self-efficacy. Self-efficacy relates to individuals' beliefs regarding their capability to perform specific actions or whether they perceive proposed behaviors as easy or challenging to execute [68]. This construct bears similarity to perceived behavioral control, as proposed in Ajzen's TPB [47].

Adscription of responsibility

Adscription of responsibility involves the sense of accountability for adverse consequences resulting from environmentally unfriendly consumption behaviors [109]. This sense also includes opinions on who should be held responsible for such conduct [65]. Limited research within this thematic review explores the connection between adscription of responsibility and water-conservation behavior [110–112]. Antecedents of responsibility adscription include knowledge of environmental problems, awareness of consequences, and awareness of water care [83,113]. For responsibility to be triggered, individuals must possess knowledge about environmental problems and/or the impacts of their consumption behaviors. Studies diverge on the role of adscription of responsibility, with some linking it to social norms and intention to save water [83,113], while others find no connection to pro-environmental behavior intention and actual behavior [112]. The literature also explores attributions of responsibility to different actors, such as local or national governments, companies, individuals, social groups, or society as a whole [114].

Emotions

A scarce number of studies explore emotional variables in water consumption/conservation. Andrade et al. [70] examine moral emotions related to irresponsible water use, finding a modest relationship with water objective knowledge. Díaz et al. [69] show that perceived happiness predicts current behavior, while stress predicts both present and future behavior. "Subjective wellness or well-being" is tied to positive emotions; however, there is a lack of consensus regarding its relationship with water consumption [115]. Some authors argue that well-being consistently predicts conservation behavior (e.g., [69]), while others find limited evidence (e.g., [95]). Finally, Manríquez-Betanzos et al. [116] explore gratitude and eudaimonia's effects on water-saving practices, revealing that eudaimonia promotes water saving and is negatively affected by water scarcity, suggesting a need for further research on eudaimonia due to limited evidence [116].

Habits

A habit is an automatic, unconscious behavior, resistant to change [64,117]. While some studies aim to explore habits, most of them operationalize the concept as past behavior (e.g., [40,56,81,82,118]). Past water-conservation behavior predicts intentions [40,56,81,118,119], indicating a link between self-efficacy and adopting new conservation behaviors. Individuals who reported performing simple (easy) water-conservation behaviors had greater intentions to adopt new, more complex water-conservation behaviors. However, Jorgensen et al. [120] find evidence of a negative association between past and future saving behavior. Participants who reported more savings in the past were likely to show less water-saving behavior in the future [120].

Socio-demographic variables

Researchers have scrutinized socio-demographic variables such as age, gender, education, income, and homeownership to understand their impact on water-saving behavior. Despite some consensus, differences in findings persist. Gender's role remains mixed; while some studies suggest that females tend to exhibit higher levels of water-saving behavior (e.g., [52,121]), others support the opposite [122]. Older individuals tend to consume more water than younger counterparts (e.g., [53,123]). Education's impact on water-saving behavior varies, with some studies finding no significant link (e.g., [52,90]), while others observe differences based on educational attainment (e.g., [124]). Higher-income households with advanced education tend to have lower water consumption [125], attributed to greater resources for water-saving devices [121].

Contextual (External) Factors Related to Water-Conservation Behavior

An additional aim of this review is to identify the external factors that impact water-conservation/saving behaviors. These antecedents are thoroughly presented in Table A11 (Appendix A) and are further elaborated upon in this.

Climatic and seasonal factors

The literature strongly supports the impact of external factors such as climate and season on household water consumption. Geographical location [78], exposure to drought or restrictions [125], seasonal variations [72], and temperature and rainfall patterns [126] significantly influence both intention and behavior in conserving water. Regions facing water stress exhibit lower consumption [49]. Water scarcity affects individual variables such as environmental concern and trust in conservation information [127]. Seasonality also influences perception, with individuals underestimating water consumption in summer and aligning more closely with actual use in winter [72].

Household composition

Previous research explores factors such as family size (e.g., [126,128]) and the presence of children or adolescents in relation to water consumption [129] but yields inconclusive results. Some studies suggest larger households exhibit lower per-capita water consumption (e.g., [121]), while others report a positive relationship [130]. The presence of children and adolescents consistently correlates with increased water consumption, with the number of adolescents having a substantial impact, especially in shower water usage [129,131].

Characteristics of the property

Property attributes affecting water consumption include house size and building age, correlating with indoor water use. Conversely, factors such as swimming pools, gardens, park presence, landscaping irrigation systems, and vegetation type impact outdoor water use. Larger homes, gardens, and pools drive higher water consumption, influencing consumption variations [52,132]. The literature indicates larger homes consume more water for cleaning, irrigation, and appliances, while mortgaged or rented households show water-consumption mitigation. The existing literature states that (i) larger homes tend to consume more water for activities such as cleaning, irrigation, and various water-consuming appliances [133]; (ii) households with mortgages or rentals tend to exhibit water-consumption mitigation [131]; and (iii) garden irrigation accounts for the highest proportion of external water consumption, primarily in outdoor settings [134].

4. Discussion and Conclusions

Bibliometric Analysis (Quantitative)

Analyzing household water-conservation/consumption behavior is a complex task due to the multifaceted relationship of diverse social, individual, and contextual factors influencing consumer decisions [12]. Consequently, our findings show that this is a highly multidisciplinary research field, drawing contributions from disciplines such as environmental psychology, social psychology, economics, management, marketing, engineering, and ecology, among others. Notably, since 2010, there has been a significant increase in interest within the scientific community regarding this topic. This heightened attention likely reflects the growing global concerns surrounding water scarcity in numerous regions and the imperative of addressing the United Nations' Sustainable Development Goals. A closer examination of the scientific production by country reveals that an extensive number of studies originate in regions struggling with water crises, including Australia, certain areas in the United States, Spain, South Africa, and Chile, among others. However, it might also be of interest to conduct water-conservation studies in regions where water scarcity issues are not present to determine if the results can be extrapolated to other hydrological contexts. Likewise, it would be worthwhile to carry out studies comparing both hydrological situations (e.g., [135]). Additionally, it is necessary to conduct studies in countries where this topic has not been previously investigated (e.g., in Russia and countries in Northern Africa). Conceptual analysis has also been used to identify key variables, current study trends, and important insights to design future lines of research. This valuable information, in turn, has facilitated a comprehensive response to the research inquiries articulated in the subsequent phase of the systematic literature review (qualitative thematic analysis). During this subsequent stage, a more profound examination of the observed statistical outcomes has been feasible, enabling the formulation of recommendations for future research directions. The main findings will be discussed further below.

Thematic analysis (qualitative)

Despite the growing number of studies regarding the determinants of household water conservation/consumption, it is surprising that the vast majority do not integrate guiding theories or frameworks into their investigations. This finding diverges from the foundational principles of CBSM programs. As emphasized by the CBSM, the formulation and execution of effective social marketing strategies require a foundational understanding of the perceived benefits and barriers (whether internal or external) that individuals associate with that specific activity [3]. This prior knowledge is key because it will be used to design a social marketing strategy that overcomes the barriers and increases the perceived benefits of the behavior targeted to generate long-term voluntary behavioral changes [136]. Nevertheless, it is notable that a substantial number of environmental CBSM-based interventions do not incorporate theories or models into their environmental social marketing strategies. For instance, Anibaldi et al. [137] found in their literature review on environmentally sustainable farming practices that most studies do not explicitly detail how theories were selected and how they were applied in the design of the intervention.

Among those studies that do explicitly mention their grounding in particular theories, three predominant frameworks stand out: The Theory of Planned Behavior (TPB, [59]), the Norm Activation model (NAM, [60]), and the New Environmental Paradigm [61]. A subset of studies has opted for a combination of theories and models that, while not entirely novel, increase their explanatory capacity. For example, Shahangian et al. [63] combine TPB and Social Cognitive Theory, Maduku [64] extend TRA with ELM and habits, and Deng et al. [61] study Construal level theory and TPB. However, other theories can also play an essential role in bridging the gap between intention and behavior, but they have been underexplored in the domain of household water behavior [91]. One of them is the Construal Level Theory [138]. This framework suggests that individuals perceive people, objects, or events as psychologically proximate or distant. This perceived distance—whether social, spatial, or temporal—subsequently shapes attitudes, emotions, and actions [139]. For example, water-saving actions are typically perceived as tangible and near, resulting in a low structural level [62]. In contrast, concepts such as climate change assume a more abstract form, rendering them psychologically distant with a high construal level. Future research into the role of perceived psychological distances in water conservation is essential [62]. Thus, Zhuang et al. [140] suggest a better understanding of the role of culture (social distance) as a moderating variable that influences attitude and behavior. Likewise, this review shows that the Value-Belief-Norm model (VBN, [65]) has received scant attention in examining household water-conservation behaviors. Furthermore, Rodriguez-Sanchez et al. [4] have recently suggested the Goal Framing Theory [60] as a potential avenue. This theory supplements existing models such as the NAM, the TPB, and the VBN by focusing on goal attainment spanning hedonic, gain-based, and normative objectives. Owing to its comprehensive approach to addressing goal conflicts, situational variables, and both conscious and unconscious processes, the Goal Framing Theory presents a promising foundation for instigating pro-environmental behaviors such as water-conservation behavior [141].

Regarding the dependent variables used in previous research, most studies rely on self-reported measures to assess household water conservation or consumption. However, self-reported measures often exhibit perceptual biases, suggesting that individuals may either underestimate or overestimate their actual water consumption [73]. This cognitive distortion acts as a barrier to water conservation [142]. The need to observe real water-consumption behaviors is highlighted. Furthermore, there is a tangible interest in understanding the duration for which a behavior change persists over time; however, longitudinal measurements have been infrequently conducted [52,53,143]. Moreover, given the influence of climatic and seasonal elements on water consumption, it becomes imperative to perform measurements at different times of the year [57,58]. In addition, Rusell and Knoeri [56] call for a longitudinal approach to understand why the installation of water-efficiency technology does not result in a reduction in water use. Lastly, the academic landscape shows a scarce amount (15%) of causal research, especially experimental designs that could shed light on the impact of specific factors on individuals' real-time behaviors [73]. Furthermore, only five studies have explicitly distinguished between curtailment behavior and efficiency behavior, while in the rest of the sample the behavior (water saving or water use) is analyzed generically without specifying the type of behavior, and to a lesser extent both behaviors are mixed. Previous studies have shown that the determinants of curtailment and efficiency behavior are different [143] and call to explore the differences between these two types of behaviors [144]. For example, Pérez Urdiales and García Valiñas [145] demonstrate that the type of water device (e.g., electric or non-electric) influences the water-conservation habit and intention, which shows that a future line of research could understand the barriers or motivators to water-efficiency intention or behavior depending on the type of device.

Focusing on the determinants of water-conservation/consumption behavior, several key factors emerge in this review. Regarding personal-sphere (internal) factors, attitude is the most frequently examined variable. However, while attitude undeniably serves as an antecedent to intention, it offers a limited explanation for actual behavior, suggesting a myriad of other variables at play. Thus, it is essential for studies to look beyond attitudinal variables, and if they employ them, to do so in conjunction with other more explanatory variables. Likewise, social norms have also been examined by a significant number of studies. This is further corroborated by the bibliometric analysis (word cloud). Regarding descriptive and injunctive norms, this review shows that the majority of studies use the concept of social norms, without distinguishing between descriptive and injunctive norms, even though both constructs are different [146]. In addition, however, researchers usually analyzed both constructs together. Warner [106] proposes an independent exploration of each to reveal their individual impacts on behavior. The revised literature exhibits gaps concerning how descriptive and injunctive social norms affect actual water-use behaviors [101,147]. For instance, descriptive norms may not be effective for individuals with a high level of involvement in water conservation [40]. Future research could analyze the influence of descriptive and injunctive norms moderated by personal involvement, considering that involvement influences conservation behavior [148]. Still, the implications of injunctive norms, when contrasted in different populations or within varied contexts, remain ambiguous [106]. For example, for some individuals, it is more significant to obtain approval for conservation practices from their neighbors (closer) rather than from those whom they consider important (more distant) [106]. In this context, the notion of spatial psychological distance [139], together with social comparison theory, offers a promising avenue for forthcoming investigations.

On the contrary, the factors that have been less examined in household water-conservation studies, and which should be analyzed in greater depth due to their potential explanatory value, are perceived efficacy, emotions, and habits. The evidence indicated that perceived efficacy is directly and positively linked to intention, and indirectly to actual behavior [144,149]. It is quite an important construct because it helps people to recognize the tangible consequences of their behavior [148]. On the contrary, it is becoming a barrier to behavior if individuals perceive their actions will not be effective in resolving water problems [148]. Additionally, future research should analyze personal and collective response efficacy. In the domain of communication and social marketing, Rodriguez-Sanchez et al. [4] state that personal response efficacy can offer a suitable framework for fostering changes in individual pro-environmental behaviors. This approach centers on the individual, avoiding the diffusion of responsibility within society or to "others". This phenomenon is based on the idea that "when people perceive that their actions contribute to solving a specific environmental problem, they are more likely to perform such behaviors" ([148], p. 195).

Concerning emotions, while there is a general agreement that they influence behavioral intentions, a more in-depth examination is essential to identify the specific emotions triggered by water-consumption patterns [69,150]. In past research, the primary focus has been on positive emotions, such as happiness, eudaimonia, gratitude, mood, and well-being. Positive emotions are positively linked to engagement with climate change, but positive emotions do not always motivate more pro-environmental engagement [150], so it could be interesting to analyze future research on the relationship between positive emotions and engagement in water-conservation behavior. However, only two negative emotions have been extensively studied: stress and emotions linked to irresponsible water use. In addition, further research is needed to understand the moderation effect that positive and negative emotions cause in cognitive determinants of water-conservation behavior [69]. Past research states that including emotion in cognitive models enhances their model explanatory capacity regarding pro-environmental behavior [70]. Finally, concerning habits, our findings show that most research predominantly focuses on the link between past behavior and water consumption. A very limited number of studies have thoroughly analyzed and operationalized the habit construct (habit strength). Consequently, future research should delve deeper into the correlation between habit construct and water consumption. This emphasis is critical, given that habits are an important barrier to water behavior change [151]. The challenge of promoting changes in these habits remains largely unaddressed [64]. Some scholars propose the application of communication or persuasion frameworks to encourage habit change [64], for instance, by appealing to self-efficacy by showing an audience that habit change is easy to achieve or by simply describing water-saving tips [119].

The predictability of socio-demographic variables for water conservation actions remains inconsistent [152]. Demographics might be examined as potential moderators that might be found to influence the relationship between conservation behaviors and other internal variables such as attitudes, values, and moral norms [153]. For example,

Kang et al. [92] suggest the need to explore the differences in water beliefs and perceptions according to gender and age.

Regarding the external determinants of household water use, scholars advocate for deeper inquiries into contemporary urban lifestyles and more understanding of how shifts in family structures might affect water-consumption levels [132]. It is crucial to integrate family characteristics and seasonal variations into research models since both factors are key in shaping water-consumption habits [154]. Prior experiences in water-scarce environments shape attitudes toward water conservation and seasonal consumption patterns [15,40,72]. Households with children, especially adolescents, tend to consume more water [129,131], while single-occupancy households show higher per-capita consumption compared to larger households [128]. Future research should analyze how external factors influence individual-level variables, for example, by exploring the influences of water-conservation messages in different climatic regions [155], or how water scarcity affects the credibility of water-conservation information [127] or the influence of seasonality on bias perception of consumption [72].

In conclusion, our review underscores the need for future research in the domain of household water conservation, presenting three overarching areas worthy of exploration. Firstly, expanding the geographical scope beyond regions with known water scarcity issues would allow us to assess the generalizability of findings to diverse hydrological contexts. Additionally, comparative studies involving regions with different hydrological situations could offer valuable insights. Secondly, despite the increasing number of studies on household water behavior, a noteworthy gap persists as most fail to integrate guiding theories or frameworks. Aligning with the principles of Community-Based Social Marketing (CBSM), effective social marketing strategies require a foundational understanding of perceived benefits and barriers. Incorporating relevant theories and underexplored theories such as Construal Level Theory and Goal Framing Theory could bridge existing gaps. Importantly, relying on self-reported measures to assess water behavior introduces perceptual biases, emphasizing the imperative for real-time observations. Longitudinal measurements, especially considering climatic and seasonal influences, are warranted to deepen our understanding of behavior persistence. Furthermore, distinguishing between curtailment and efficiency behaviors, examining the influence of psychological distances, and exploring the moderating effects of emotions on cognitive determinants are areas requiring more comprehensive exploration. Thirdly, future research should prioritize less-explored internal factors such as perceived efficacy, emotions, and habits, along with key external factors. Finally, investigating the inconsistent predictability of socio-demographic variables and their potential moderation effects on conservation behaviors is crucial for a comprehensive understanding of the factors influencing water-saving actions.

4.1. Managerial Implications

Our research provides insights into how to develop effective interventions following a social marketing approach. Firstly, household water-conservation programs must clearly define the behavior they aim to promote, distinguishing between curtailment and efficiency behaviors due to their distinct internal and external determinants. Even further specification is recommended, such as differentiating curtailment behaviors (e.g., indoor vs. outdoor) or efficiency types (e.g., electric vs. non-electric water devices). Secondly, audience segmentation is crucial, encompassing socio-demographic factors, family composition (e.g., households with children, teenagers, or singles), and homeownership status. Additionally, climatic and seasonal variables, as well as neighborhood housing features (e.g., the presence of swimming pools, gardens, or the age of the residences), should be considered. Once the target audience has been segmented, the next step is to research and understand the determinants that act as barriers or motivators associated with the behavior, and finally design an intervention that targets these key determinants [146].

According to our findings, there are several determinants that should be triggered by interventions (The recommendations outlined below are primarily based on the work conducted by van Valkengoed et al. [147], recently published in the journal *Nature Human Behavior*) either because they play a significant role in explaining water-conservation intention or behavior, or because they have been underutilized in the past. Further research is needed on the subjects of attitudes, social norms, outcome efficacy, emotions, and habits.

Attitudes towards water conservation could be influenced by the following three strategies. First, providing information about the environmental consequences associated with specific water-related actions, such as excessive lawn watering or extended shower durations. In this sense, individuals are anticipated to view these behaviors less favorably, thus encouraging more sustainable water use. Second, providing information about the (non-environmental) co-benefits and costs associated with behavior. Highlighting, for instance, the financial savings from reduced water bills or the long-term property benefits of maintaining a drought-resistant garden can further motivate households to embrace water conservation. Third, introducing direct incentives, such as rebates for installing rainwater harvesting systems or discounts for using water-efficient appliances. By highlighting these additional benefits, people may be more likely to perceive a behavior positively and engage in it.

Furthermore, the following managerial strategies leveraging social norms can also be performed. First, providing people with descriptive norm information. This intervention reveals what the majority of people are doing concerning water-saving behaviors. For instance, if individuals learn that most households in their neighborhood are collecting rainwater for gardening, they might be more inclined to adopt the same. Second, provide dynamic norm information. This intervention involves providing people with information that indicates that an increasing number of people are changing their behavior. Such information may signal to people what behavior may be normative in the near future, to which people may already want to conform. Finally, providing information about injunctive norms. This intervention involves providing people with information about whether a behavior is commonly approved or disapproved of by people or groups that are important to them. For example, knowing that the local community values households that have drought-resistant gardens can spur others to consider such practices.

One possible intervention that could enhance outcome efficacy is providing households with detailed instructions on how to execute water-conservation measures, such as rainwater harvesting or fixing leaky faucets. This can bolster individuals' confidence in their capability to implement the behavior appropriately and realize the anticipated benefits. Furthermore, offering feedback on the outcomes of their actions, such as quantifying the amount of water saved by shortening shower durations, can allow individuals to recognize the positive impact of their endeavors and amplify their assurance in achieving the intended water-saving results.

Regarding emotions, several interventions can be effective by eliciting specific emotions. Firstly, providing feedback on behavioral outcomes can heighten a sense of achievement. For instance, informing households of the liters of water saved by fixing leaks or using efficient fixtures can foster a sense of pride in their proactive choices. Secondly, employing prompts and reminders can serve as continual nudges toward sustainable actions. A sticker near the sink reminding occupants to turn off the tap when brushing their teeth, for example, can stimulate a sense of responsibility and motivation to conserve. Lastly, the strategy of social comparison capitalizes on the power of peer influence. When households receive data illustrating their water usage in comparison to their neighbors, emotions such as pride, for those excelling, or guilt, for those lagging behind, can be triggered. Such emotional responses can be strong catalysts driving households toward more judicious water use.

Finally, the following interventions can be effective for triggering automatic decision-making (habits). Predominantly, choice architecture interventions or "nudges" have been employed to subtly direct individuals toward pro-environmental behaviors without constricting their choices or altering perceived costs and benefits. For instance, setting water-saving behaviors as default options, such as a washing machine automatically starting on an eco-friendly setting, simplifies pro-environmental choices, making them more instinctual. Additionally, integrating visual cues, such as installing water meters in visible areas, makes water consumption more apparent, nudging individuals towards conservation. Lastly, placing reminders, such as stickers near showers prompting shorter water usage, serves as cues, seamlessly guiding individuals towards water-saving behaviors without overtly dictating their actions.

4.2. Limitations of the Study

This study presents a series of limitations that it is important to highlight. First, the exhaustive review process spanned several months. As a result, there is potential that the most recent publications from the latter stages of this period may not have been incorporated into this analysis. Second, the keyword selection plays a crucial role in a systematic review. Despite meticulous efforts to curate a comprehensive set of keywords and Boolean operators to include all relevant literature (see Tables A1–A3), there remains a possibility that some significant publications could have been missed. Third, this systematic research is based on bibliographic databases such as Scopus and Web of Science (WoS), which predominantly includes studies published in English. As a result, potentially significant research from non-traditional sources or those embedded within grey literature might have been overlooked. This could also introduce a geographical bias, potentially constraining the applicability of findings to regions that are underrepresented. Fourth, the bibliometric review carries its own set of limitations. Outcomes rely on citations and bibliometric metrics (e.g., h-index, impact factor, etc.) that might not necessarily reflect the quality or influence of a given publication. Inherent biases in this approach include issues such as self-citations and the temporal gap between the publication date and the bibliometric review. To mitigate this latter limitation, the average annual citation count is computed to gauge the significance and relevance of the research articles.

Author Contributions: Conceptualization, C.S., C.R.-S. and F.S.-E.; methodology, C.S. and F.S.-E.; software, C.S.; validation, C.S., C.R.-S. and F.S.-E.; formal analysis, C.S. and F.S.-E.; investigation, C.S., C.R.-S. and F.S.-E. data curation, C.S.; writing—original draft preparation, C.S., C.R.-S. and F.S.-E.; writing—review and editing, C.S., C.R.-S. and F.S.-E.; visualization, C.S., C.R.-S. and F.S.-E.; supervision, C.R.-S. and F.S.-E.; project administration, C.R.-S. and F.S.-E.; funding acquisition, C.S., C.R.-S. and F.S.-E. All authors have read and agreed to the published version of the manuscript.

Funding: This research was funded by Generalitat Valenciana (Emerging Project GV2022 number: CIGE/2022/051), Consejo Nacional de Investigaciones Científicas y Técnicas (CONICET) doctoral research scholarship, and Universidad Católica de Córdoba (Argentina).

Data Availability Statement: Data are available upon request.

Conflicts of Interest: The authors declare no conflict of interest.

Appendix A

Table A1. Literature reviews used to select the keywords for this review.

Author	Article Title	Journal
Abu-Bakar et al. (2021) [156]	A review of household water demand management and consumption measurement	Journal of Cleaner Production
Asprilla Echeverria, (2020) [157]	Cross-country evidence for social dimensions of urban water consumption during droughts	Journal of Cleaner Production
Benzoni & Telenko (2016) [158]	A Review of Intervention Studies Aimed at Domestic Water Conservation	Springer International Pub.
Carvalho et al. (2013) [159]	Sustainable airport environments: A review of water conservation practices in airports	Resources, Conservation, & Recycling

Table A1. *Cont.*

Author	Article Title	Journal
Ehret et al. (2021) [11]	Systematic Review of Household Water-Conservation Interventions Using the Information–Motivation– Behavioral Skills Model	Environment and Behavior
Grilli & Curtis (2021) [160]	Encouraging pro-environmental behaviors: A review of methods and approaches	Renewable and Sustainable Energy Reviews
Hall et al. (2016) [161]	Accommodation Consumers and Providers' Attitudes, Behaviors and Practices for Sustainability: A Systematic Review	Sustainability
Hurlimann et al. (2009) [162]	Understanding behavior to inform water supply management in developed nations—A review of literature, conceptual model and research agenda	Journal of Environmental Management
Inman & Jeffrey (2007) [163]	A review of residential water conservation tool performance and influences on implementation effectiveness	Urban Water Journal
Jorgensen et al. (2009) [164]	Household water use behavior: An integrated model	Journal of Environmental Management
Koop et al. (2019) [165]	Enhancing domestic water conservation behavior: A review of empirical studies on influencing tactics	Journal of Environmental Management
Liu & Mukheibir (2018) [166]	Digital metering feedback and changes in water consumption—A review	Resources, Conservation & Recycling
Moglia et al. (2018) [13]	Promoting Water Conservation: Where to from here?	Water
Moore & Boldero (2017) [167]	Designing Interventions that Last: A Classification of Environmental Behaviors in Relation to the Activities, Costs, and Effort Involved for Adoption and Maintenance	Frontiers in Psychology
Ricart et al. (2021) [168]	Extending Natural Limits to Address Water Scarcity? The Role of Non-Conventional Water Fluxes in Climate Change Adaptation Capacity: A Review	Sustainability
Russell & Fielding (2010) [74]	Water demand management research: A psychological perspective	Water Resources Research
Sanguinetti et al. (2018) [169]	Information, timing, and display: A design-behavior framework for improving the effectiveness of eco-feedback	Energy Research & Social Science
Stankuniene et al. (2020) [170]	Systematic Literature Review on Behavioral Barriers of Climate Change Mitigation in Households	Sustainability
Syme et al. (2000) [171]	The evaluation of information campaigns to promote voluntary household water conservation	Evaluation Review
Warren & Becken (2017) [172]	Saving energy and water in tourist accommodation: A systematic literature review (1987–2015)	International Journal of Tourism Research
Weis (2019) [173]	Systematic literature review on impacts and indicators for measuring costs and benefits of water sector-related interventions	SSRN
Voskamp et al. (2020) [174]	A systematic review of factors influencing spatiotemporal variability in urban water and energy consumption	Journal of Cleaner Production

Note: Source: Own elaboration.

Table A2. Thematic categories and keywords initially identified.

Thematic Category	Search Terms Used in the Search Engines
General	Factors, determinants, antecedents, influences, psychological-social drivers, economics drivers.
Contextual	Household/domestic /residential water.
	Indoor/outdoor uses. Internal/external consumption. Urban/local. Droughts. Climate/seasonal factors. Physical environmental variables.
	Property characteristics: lot size, pool, garden, house size, house age.
	Household characteristics or situational influences: household composition, household income, home ownership, water-saving technology, water supply technology.
	Household culture of water conservation.
Behavioral	Behavior, behavioral change, community-based behavior change. Social change. Curtailment/efficiency behavior.
Water	Water use. Actual water use. Water save/saving, water conservation, water consumption, Water scarcity, waste/wasting water.
Motivators	Drivers, motivation, conservation motives.
	Non-rational behavioral drivers. Incentives.
Barriers	Barrier. Resistance.
Factors determinants of behavior	Attitude/attitudinal factors. Intentions. Perceived self-efficacy. Social and personal Norms. Subjective norm.
	Cognitive behavior. Habits behavior. Past water-use behavior. Routines.
	Personal capabilities: Awareness, knowledge, education, environmental conscious/concerns.
	Beliefs. Normative beliefs. Cultural/environmental beliefs. Trust.
	Personal involvement. Perceived behavioral control. Locus of control. Perceptions of other behavior.
	Values. Moral obligation. Perceived responsibility. Hedonic values.
	Negative/positive emotions.
	Cost: time cost, cognitive cost. Lifestyle.
Theories	Theory of Reasoned action (TRA).
	Value-Belief-Norms (VBN).
	The goal norm.
	Behavioral economics.

Note: Source: Own elaboration.

Table A3. Final key search terms and Boolean operators used in Scopus and WoS.

Database	Search Terms
Scopus	(TITLE-ABS-KEY ((“water us*” OR “us* water” OR “actual water” OR “water sav*” OR “sav* water” OR “water conserv*” OR “conserv* water” OR “water consumpt*” OR “consum* water” OR “water scarc*” OR “water demand”)) AND TITLE-ABS-KEY ((“individual*” OR “household” OR “behavi*” OR “action”) AND TITLE-ABS-KEY ((“factor*” OR “determinant*” OR “force*” OR “antecedent*” OR “influenc*” OR “driver*” OR “motiv*” OR “conserv*” OR “incentive*” OR “barrier” OR “resistance” OR “inhibit*”)) AND TITLE-ABS-KEY ((“domestic” OR “residential” OR “indoor” OR “outdoor” OR “internal” OR “external” OR “urban” OR “local” OR “drought*” OR “climate” OR “season*” OR “property*” OR “house*” OR “ownership”)) AND TITLE-ABS-KEY ((“inform*” OR “attitu*” OR “intention” OR “self-efficacy” OR (“social” OR “personal *” OR “subjective” AND “norm”) OR “cogniti*” OR “habit*” OR “routine*” OR “capabilit*” OR “awareness” OR “knowledge” OR “educat*” OR “environment*” OR “concern*” OR “belie*” OR “cultur*” OR “trust” OR “involve*” OR “control” OR “locus” OR “values” OR “moral” OR “responsib*” OR (“hedonic” AND “values”) OR “emot*” OR “cost” OR “lifestyle” OR “demographic”) AND (LIMIT-TO (LANGUAGE, “English”) AND (LIMIT-TO (DOCTYPE, “ar”) OR LIMIT-TO (DOCTYPE, “re”))

Table A3. *Cont.*

Database	Search Terms
Web of Science	(TS = (("water us*" OR "us* water" OR "actual water" OR "water sav*" OR "sav* water" OR "water conserv*" OR "conserv* water" OR "water consumpt*" OR "consum* water" OR "water scarc*" OR "water demand")) AND TS = (("individual*" OR "household" OR "behavi*" OR "action"))) AND TS = (("factor*" OR "determinant*" OR "force*" OR "antecedent*" OR "influenc*" OR "driver*" OR "motiv*" OR "conserv*" OR "incentive*" OR "barrier" OR "resistance" OR "inhibit*")) AND TS = (("domestic" OR "residential" OR "indoor" OR "outdoor" OR "internal" OR "external" OR "urban" OR "local" OR "drought*" OR "climate" OR "season*" OR "property*" OR "house*" OR "ownership")) AND TS = (("inform*" OR "attitu*" OR "intention" OR "self-efficacy" OR ("social" OR "personal *" OR "subjective" AND "norm") OR "cogniti*" OR "habit*" OR "routine*" OR "capabilit*" OR "awareness" OR "knowledge" OR "educat*" OR "environment*" OR "concern*" OR "belie*" OR "cultur*" OR "trust" OR "involve*" OR "control" OR "locus" OR "values" OR "moral" OR "responsib*" OR ("hedonic" AND "values") OR "emot*" OR "cost" OR "lifestyle" OR "demographic")))) AND (DT == ("ARTICLE" OR "REVIEW") AND LA == ("ENGLISH"))

Note: Source: Own elaboration. * = truncation sign in Boolean search. For instance, "sav*" indicates that the search is done for all terms beginning by "sav" and with any ending letters.

Table A4. Academic journals where included contributions were published.

Source (Journal Name)	Publisher	Articles	%
Journal of Environmental Management	Academic Press Inc.	11	7.1%
Water	MDPI	9	5.8%
Journal of Environmental Psychology	Academic Press Inc.	8	5.2%
Sustainability	Springer Nature Switz.	7	4.5%
Journal of Applied Social Psychology	Wiley-Blackwell	5	3.2%
Water Policy	IWA	5	3.2%
Ecological Economics	Elsevier	4	2.6%
Environment & Behavior	SAGE Pub. Ltd.	4	2.6%
Resources, Conservation & Recycling	Elsevier	4	2.6%
Science of The Total Environment	Elsevier	4	2.6%
Society & Natural Resources	Taylor and Francis Ltd.	4	2.6%
International Journal of Consumer Studies	Wiley-Blackwell Pub. Ltd.	3	1.9%
Journal of Cleaner Production	Elsevier Ltd.	3	1.9%
Urban Water Journal	Taylor and Francis Ltd.	3	1.9%
Water International	Taylor and Francis Ltd.	3	1.9%
Water Resources Research	Wiley-Blackwell Pub. Ltd.	3	1.9%
Australasian Journal of Environmental Management	Taylor and Francis Ltd.	2	1.3%
Frontiers In Water	Frontiers Media S.A.	2	1.3%
International Journal of Water Resources Development	Routledge	2	1.3%
Journal of Environmental Economics & Management	Academic Press Inc.	2	1.3%
Landscape And Urban Planning	Elsevier	2	1.3%
Proceedings of The National Academy of Sciences of the USA	National Academy of Sciences	2	1.3%
Psyecology	Taylor and Francis Ltd.	2	1.3%
Sustainable Cities & Society	Elsevier BV	2	1.3%
Sustainable Water Resources Management	Springer Nature Switz.	2	1.3%
Urban Forestry & Urban Greening	Urban und Fischer Verlag GmbH und Co. KG	2	1.3%
Water Resources Management	Springer Netherlands	2	1.3%

Table A4. *Cont.*

Source (Journal Name)	Publisher	Articles	%
Ahuri Final Report	Australian Housing and Urban Research Institute (AHURI)	1	0.6%
Applied Environmental Education & Communication	Routledge	1	0.6%
Applied Geography	Elsevier BV	1	0.6%
Applied Research in Quality & Life	Springer Netherlands	1	0.6%
Applied Water Science	Springer Science and Business Media Deutschland GmbH	1	0.6%
Australian Journal & Water Resources	Taylor and Francis Ltd.	1	0.6%
Behavior & Information Technology	Taylor and Francis Ltd.	1	0.6%
Design Journal	Taylor and Francis Ltd.	1	0.6%
Ecopsychology	Mary Ann Liebert Inc.	1	0.6%
Environment & Ecology Research	Horizon Research Publishing	1	0.6%
Environmental Engineering & Management Journal	Gh. Asachi Technical University of Iasi	1	0.6%
Environmental Management	Academic Press Inc.	1	0.6%
Environmental Science & Policy	Elsevier BV	1	0.6%
Environmental Science & Pollution Research	Springer Science + Business Media	1	0.6%
Frontiers In Environmental Science	Frontiers Media S.A.	1	0.6%
Geoforum	Elsevier BV	1	0.6%
Global Business Review	Sage Publications India Pvt. Ltd.	1	0.6%
Great Plains Research	Center for Great Plains Studies	1	0.6%
H2open Journal	IWA	1	0.6%
Health Communication	Routledge	1	0.6%
International Journal of Advertising	Taylor and Francis Ltd.	1	0.6%
International Journal of Environmental Research	Springer International Publishing AG	1	0.6%
International Journal of Environmental Research & Public Health	MDPI	1	0.6%
International Journal of Sustainable Energy	Taylor and Francis Ltd.	1	0.6%
Irish Geography	Routledge	1	0.6%
Khawra Journal of The American Water Resources Association	Wiley-Blackwell Pub. Ltd.	1	0.6%
Journal of Agricultural Education & Extension	Association for International Agricultural and Extension Education	1	0.6%
Journal of Consumer Behavior	Wiley-Blackwell	1	0.6%
Journal of Economic Psychology	Elsevier	1	0.6%
Journal of Environmental Planning & Management	Routledge	1	0.6%
Journal of Extension	Extension Journal, Inc.	1	0.6%
Journal of Global Marketing	Routledge	1	0.6%
Journal of Health Communication	Taylor and Francis Ltd.	1	0.6%
Journal of Hydrology	Elsevier	1	0.6%
Journal of Marketing Management	Taylor and Francis Ltd.	1	0.6%
Journal of Policy Analysis & Management	Wiley-Liss Inc.	1	0.6%
Journal of Water Resources Planning & Management	American Society of Civil Engineers (ASCE)	1	0.6%

Table A4. *Cont.*

Source (Journal Name)	Publisher	Articles	%
Journal of Water Sanitation & Hygiene for Development	IWA	1	0.6%
Journal of Water Supply: Research & Technology—Aqua	IWA	1	0.6%
Methodsx	Elsevier BV	1	0.6%
Organizational Behavior & Human Decision Processes	Academic Press Inc.	1	0.6%
PLOS One	Public Library of Science	1	0.6%
Population And Environment	Springer Netherlands	1	0.6%
Social Influence	Taylor and Francis Ltd.	1	0.6%
Social Science Journal	Taylor and Francis Ltd.	1	0.6%
Sociological Perspectives	SAGE Publications Inc.	1	0.6%
South East European Journal & Economics & Business	School of Economics and Business in Sarajevo	1	0.6%
Urban Climate	Elsevier BV	1	0.6%
Urban Studies	SAGE Publications Inc.	1	0.6%
Water And Environment Journal	Wiley-Blackwell	1	0.6%
Water Conservation & Management	Zibeline International Publishing Sdn. Bhd.	1	0.6%
Water Science & Technology: Water Supply	IWA	1	0.6%
World Development Perspectives	Elsevier Ltd.	1	0.6%
Total		155	100.0%

Note: Source: Own elaboration.

Table A5. Number of articles by author in the sample.

Author	Number Articles	%
Warner	5	1.0%
Corral-Verdugo V	4	0.8%
Fielding KS	4	0.8%
Dolnicar S	3	0.6%
Hurlimann A	3	0.6%
Jorgensen BS	3	0.6%
Martin JF	3	0.6%
Panuwatwanich K	3	0.6%
Sauri D	3	0.6%
Shahangian SA	3	0.6%
Stewart RA	3	0.6%
Tabesh M	3	0.6%
Yazdanpanah M	3	0.6%
Addo IB	2	0.4%
Al-Maadid A	2	0.4%
Barnett MJ	2	0.4%
Bhanot SP	2	0.4%
Buys L	2	0.4%
Clark WA	2	0.4%

Table A5. *Cont.*

Author	Number Articles	%
Demetriades SZ	2	0.4%
Finley JC	2	0.4%
Frías-Armenta M	2	0.4%
Garcia X	2	0.4%
Gonzalez-Gomez F	2	0.4%
Guardiola J	2	0.4%
Gázquez-Abad JC	2	0.4%
Haeffner M	2	0.4%
Hustvedt G	2	0.4%
Jackson-Smith D	2	0.4%
Kaiser RA	2	0.4%
Kang J	2	0.4%
Katz D	2	0.4%
Kyle GT	2	0.4%
LandonAC	2	0.4%
Lauren N	2	0.4%
Llausàs A	2	0.4%
Louis WR	2	0.4%
Miller E	2	0.4%
Mondéjar-Jiménez JA	2	0.4%
Otaki AND	2	0.4%
Parsons M	2	0.4%
Pearce MW	2	0.4%
Ribas A	2	0.4%
Ritcher CP	2	0.4%
Rodriguez-Sanchez C	2	0.4%
Russell S	2	0.4%
Sarabia-Sanchez FJ	2	0.4%
Schultz PW	2	0.4%
Spinks A	2	0.4%
Syme GJ	2	0.4%
Thoms MC	2	0.4%
Walter N	2	0.4%
Willis EM	2	0.4%
Willis RM	2	0.4%
Authors with only one article	352	73.8%
Total	477	100%

Source: Own elaboration.

Table A6. Contributions included in the review by number of citations.

Author	Year	Contribution	Total Cites	Cites/Year
Willis et al. [38]	2011	Willis, R. M., Stewart, R. A., Panuwatwanich, K., Williams, P. R., & Hollingsworth, A. L. (2011). Quantifying the influence of environmental and water conservation attitudes on household end use water consumption. Journal of Environmental Management, 92(8), 1996–2009.	275	22.9
Domene et al. [132]	2006	Domene, E., & Saurí, D. (2006). Urbanisation and water consumption: Influencing factors in the metropolitan region of Barcelona. Urban Studies, 43(9), 1605–1623.	264	15.5
Gilg & Barr [175]	2006	Gilg, A., & Barr, S. (2006). Behavioral attitudes towards water saving? Evidence from a study of environmental actions. Ecological Economics, 57(3), 400–414.	249	14.6
Gregoy & Di Leo [81]	2003	Gregory, G. D., & Di Leo, M. (2003). Repeated Behavior and Environmental Psychology: The Role of Personal Involvement and Habit Formation in Explaining Water Consumption. Journal of Applied Social Psychology, 33(6), 1261–1296.	229	11.5
Fielding et al. [40]	2012	Fielding, K. S., Russell, S., Spinks, A., & Mankad, A. (2012). Determinants of household water conservation: The role of demographic, infrastructure, behavior, and psychosocial variables. Water Resources Research, 48(10).	183	16.6
Lam [176]	2006	Lam, S. P. (2006). Predicting intention to save water: Theory of planned behavior, response efficacy, vulnerability, and perceived efficiency of alternative solutions. Journal of Applied Social Psychology, 36(11), 2803–2824.	177	10.4
Corral-Verdugo et al. [122]	2003	Corral-Verdugo, V., Bechtel, R. B., & Fraijo-Sing, B. (2003). Environmental beliefs and water conservation: An empirical study. Journal of Environmental Psychology, 23(3), 247–257.	172	8.6
Fielding et al. [40]	2013	Fielding, K. S., Spinks, A., Russell, S., McCrea, R., Stewart, R., & Gardner, J. (2013). An experimental test of voluntary strategies to promote urban water demand management. Journal of Environmental Management, 114, 343–351.	171	17.1
Grafton et al. [96]	2011	Grafton, R. Q., Ward, M. B., To, H., & Kompas, T. (2011). Determinants of residential water consumption: Evidence and analysis from a 10-country household survey. Water Resources Research, 47(8).	162	13.5
Randolph & Troy [177]	2008	Randolph, B., & Troy, P. (2008). Attitudes to conservation and water consumption. Environmental Science and Policy, 11(5), 441–455.	159	10.6
Syme et al. [134]	2004	Syme, G. J., Shao, Q., Po, M., & Campbell, E. (2004). Predicting and understanding home garden water use. Landscape and Urban Planning, 68(1), 121–128.	151	7.9
Harlan et al. [178]	2009	Harlan, S. L., Yabiku, S. T., Larsen, L., & Brazel, A. J. (2009). Household water consumption in an arid city: Affluence, affordance, and attitudes. Society and Natural Resources, 22(8), 691–709.	138	9.9
Clark & Finley [93]	2007	Clark, W. A., & Finley, J. C. (2008). Household water conservation challenges in Blagoevgrad, Bulgaria: A descriptive study. Water International, 33(2), 175–188.	134	8.4

Table A6. *Cont.*

Author	Year	Contribution	Total Cites	Cites/Year
Attari [179]	2014	Attari, S. Z. (2014). Perceptions of water use. Proceedings of the National Academy of Sciences of the United States of America, 111(14), 5129–5134.	131	14.6
Schultz et al. [39]	2016	Schultz, P. W., Messina, A., Tronu, G., Limas, E. F., Gupta, R., & Estrada, M. (2016). Personalized Normative Feedback and the Moderating Role of Personal Norms: A Field Experiment to Reduce Residential Water Consumption. Environment and Behavior, 48(5), 686–710.	122	17.4
Kurz et al. [180]	2005	Kurz, T., Donaghue, N., & Walker, I. (2005). Utilizing a social-ecological framework to promote water and energy conservation: A field experiment. Journal of Applied Social Psychology, 35(6), 1281–1300.	110	6.1
Lauren et al. [119]	2016	Lauren, N., Fielding, K. S., Smith, L., & Louis, W. R. (2016). You did, so you can and you will: Self-efficacy as a mediator of spillover from easy to more difficult pro-environmental behavior. JOURNAL OF ENVIRONMENTAL PSYCHOLOGY, 48, 191–199.	102	14.6
Corral-Verdugo et al. [123]	2002	Corral-Verdugo, V., Frías-Armenta, M., Pérez-Urias, F., Orduña-Cabrera, V., & Espinoza-Gallego, N. (2002). Residential water consumption, motivation for conserving water and the continuing tragedy of the commons. Environmental Management, 30(4), 527–535.	97	4.6
Dolnicar et al. [97]	2012	Dolnicar, S., Hurlimann, A., & Grun, B. (2012). Water conservation behavior in Australia. Journal of Environmental Management, 105, 44–52.	95	8.6
Makki et al. [129]	2013	Makki, A. A., Stewart, R. A., Panuwatwanich, K., & Beal, C. (2013). Revealing the determinants of shower water end use consumption: Enabling better targeted urban water conservation strategies. Journal of Cleaner Production, 60, 129–146.	92	9.2
Bronfman et al. [111]	2015	Bronfman, N. C., Cisternas, P. C., López-Vázquez, E., la Maza, C., & Oyanedel, J. C. (2015). Understanding attitudes and pro-environmental behaviors in a Chilean community. Sustainability (Switzerland), 7(10), 14133–14152.	86	10.8
Corral-Verdugo & Frías-Armenta [123]	2006	Corral-Verdugo, V., & Frías-Armenta, M. (2006). Personal normative beliefs, antisocial behavior, and residential water conservation. Environment and Behavior, 38(3), 406–421.	80	4.7
Gilbertson et al. [181]	2011	Gilbertson, M., Hurlimann, A., & Dolnicar, S. (2011). Does water context influence behavior and attitudes to water conservation? Australasian Journal of Environmental Management, 18(1), 47–60.	76	6.3
Miller & Buys [112]	2008	Miller, E., & Buys, L. (2008a). The impact of social capital on residential water-affecting behaviors in a drought-prone Australian community. Society and Natural Resources, 21(3), 244–257.	73	4.9
Seyranian et al. [57]	2015	Seyranian, V., Sinatra, G. M., & Polikoff, M. S. (2015). Comparing communication strategies for reducing residential water consumption. Journal of Environmental Psychology, 41, 81–90.	70	8,8
Aprile & Fiorillo [182]	2017	Aprile, M. C., & Fiorillo, D. (2017). Water conservation behavior and environmental concerns: Evidence from a representative sample of Italian individuals. Journal of Cleaner Production, 159, 119–129.	62	10.3

Table A6. *Cont.*

Author	Year	Contribution	Total Cites	Cites/Year
Dolnicar & Hurlimann [77]	2010	Dolnicar, S., & Hurlimann, A. (2010). Australians' water conservation behaviors and attitudes. Australian Journal of Water Resources, 14(1), 43–53.	60	4.6
Kantola et al. [183]	1982	Kantola, S. J., Syme, G. J., & Campbell, N. A. (1982). The Role of Individual Differences and External Variables in a Test of the Sufficiency of Fishbein's Model to Explain Behavioral Intentions to Conserve Water. Journal of Applied Social Psychology, 12(1), 70–83.	60	1.5
Wolters [62]	2014	Wolters, E. A. (2014). Attitude-behavior consistency in household water consumption. Social Science Journal, 51(3), 455–463.	59	6.6
Lowe et al. [102]	2015	Lowe, B., Lynch, D., & Lowe, J. (2015). Reducing household water consumption: a social marketing approach. Journal of Marketing Management, 31(3–4), 378–408.	55	6.9
Stewart et al. [184]	2013	Stewart, R. A., Willis, R. M., Panuwatwanich, K., & Sahin, O. (2013). Showering behavioral response to alarming visual display monitors: Longitudinal mixed method study. Behavior and Information Technology, 32(7), 695–711.	53	5.3
Deng et al. [61]	2017	Deng, Y., Wang, M., & Yousefpour, R. (2017). How do people's perceptions and climatic disaster experiences influence their daily behaviors regarding adaptation to climate change?—A case study among young generations. Science of the Total Environment, 581–582, 840–847.	45	7.5
Jaeger & Schultz [148]	2017	Jaeger, C. M., & Schultz, P. W. (2017). Coupling social norms and commitments: Testing the underdetected nature of social influence. Journal of Environmental Psychology, 51, 199–208.	44	7.3
Suárez Varela et al. [185]	2016	Suárez Varela, M., Guardiola, J., & González Gómez, F. (2016). Do Pro-environmental Behaviors and Awareness Contribute to Improve Subjective Well-being? Applied Research in Quality of Life, 11(2), 429–444.	42	6.0
Mondéjar Jiménez et al. [186]	2011	Mondéjar Jiménez, J. A., Cordente Rodríguez, M., Meseguer Santamaría, M. L., & Gázquez Abad, J. C. (2011). Environmental Behavior and Water Saving in Spanish Housing. International Journal of Environmental Research, 5(1), 1–10.	41	3.4
Lede et al. [108]	2019	Lede, E., Meleady, R., & Seger, C. R. (2019). Optimizing the influence of social norms interventions: Applying social identity insights to motivate residential water conservation. JOURNAL OF ENVIRONMENTAL PSYCHOLOGY, 62, 105–114.	40	10.0
Russell & Knoeri [56]	2020	Russell, S. V, & Knoeri, C. (2020). Exploring the psychosocial and behavioral determinants of household water conservation and intention. International Journal of Water Resources Development, 36(6), 940–955.	39	13.0
Hamilton [187]	1983	Hamilton, L. C. (1983). Saving water: A Causal Model of Household Conservation. Sociological Perspectives, 26(4), 355–374.	39	1.0

Table A6. *Cont.*

Author	Year	Contribution	Total Cites	Cites/Year
Moore et al. [188]	1994	Moore, S., Murphy, M., & Watson, R. (1994). A longitudinal study of domestic water conservation behavior. Population and Environment, 16(2), 175–189.	37	1.3
Torres & Carlsson [189]	2018	Torres, M. M. J., & Carlsson, F. (2018). Direct and spillover effects of a social information campaign on residential water-savings. Journal of Environmental Economics and Management, 92, 222–243.	35	7.0
Richter [190]	2011	Richter, C. P. (2011). Usage of dishwashers: Observation of consumer habits in the domestic environment. International Journal of Consumer Studies, 35(2), 180–186.	35	2,9
Rajapaksa et al. [191]	2019	Rajapaksa, D., Gifford, R., Torgler, B., Garcia-Valiñas, M., Athukorala, W., Managi, S., & Wilson, C. (2019). Do monetary and non-monetary incentives influence environmental attitudes and behavior? Evidence from an experimental analysis. Resources, Conservation and Recycling, 149, 168–176.	34	8.5
Jorgensen et al. [76]	2014	Jorgensen, B. S., Martin, J. F., Pearce, M. W., & Willis, E. M. (2014). Predicting Household Water Consumption With Individual-Level Variables. Environment and Behavior, 46(7), 872–897.	34	3.8
Martínez Espiñeira & García Valiñas [192]	2013	Martínez Espiñeira, R., & García Valiñas, M. Á. (2013). Adopting versus adapting: Adoption of water-saving technology versus water conservation habits in Spain. International Journal of Water Resources Development, 29(3), 400–414.	33	3.3
Otaki et al. [86]	2017	Otaki, Y., Ueda, K., & Sakura, O. (2017). Effects of feedback about community water consumption on residential water conservation. Journal of Cleaner Production, 143, 719–730.	32	5,3
Fan et al. [133]	2013	Fan, L., Liu, G., Wang, F., Geissen, V., Ritsema, C. J., & Tong, Y. (2013). Water use patterns and conservation in households of Wei River Basin, China. Resources, Conservation and Recycling, 74, 45–53.	32	3.2
Segev [193]	2015	Segev, S. (2015). Modelling household conservation behavior among ethnic consumers: The path from values to behaviors. International Journal of Consumer Studies, 39(3), 193–202.	30	3.8
Sarabia Sánchez et al. [149]	2014	Sarabia Sánchez, F. J., Rodríguez Sánchez, C., & Hyder, A. (2014). The role of personal involvement, credibility and efficacy of conduct in reported water conservation behavior. Journal of Environmental Psychology, 38, 206–216.	29	3.2
Ramsey et al. [90]	2017	Ramsey, E., Berglund, E. Z., & Goyal, R. (2017). The impact of demographic factors, beliefs, and social influences on residential water consumption and implications for non-price policies in urban India. Water (Switzerland), 9(11).	27	4.5
Landon et al. [79]	2017	Landon, A. C., Kyle, G. T., & Kaiser, R. A. (2017). An Augmented Norm Activation Model: The Case of Residential Outdoor Water Use. Society and Natural Resources, 30(8), 903–918.	27	4.5
Pérez Urdiales & García Valiñas [145]	2016	Pérez Urdiales, M., & García Valiñas, M. T. (2016). Efficient water-using technologies and habits: A disaggregated analysis in the water sector. Ecological Economics, 128, 117–129.	27	3.9

Table A6. *Cont.*

Author	Year	Contribution	Total Cites	Cites/Year
Dascher et al. [150]	2014	Dascher, E. D., Kang, J., & Hustvedt, G. (2014). Water sustainability: Environmental attitude, drought attitude and motivation. International Journal of Consumer Studies, 38(5), 467–474.	27	3.0
Richter & Stamminger [194]	2012	Richter, C. P., & Stamminger, R. (2012). Water Consumption in the Kitchen—A Case Study in Four European Countries. Water Resources Management, 26(6), 1639–1649.	27	2.5
Gómez-Llanos et al. [54]	2020	Gómez-Llanos, E., Durán-Barroso, P., & Robina-Ramírez, R. (2020). Analysis of consumer awareness of sustainable water consumption by the water footprint concept. Science of the Total Environment, 721.	26	8.7
Garcia et al. [195]	2013	Garcia, X., Ribas, A., Llausàs, A., & Saurí, D. (2013a). Socio-demographic profiles in suburban developments: Implications for water-related attitudes and behaviors along the Mediterranean coast. Applied Geography, 41, 46–54.	26	2.6
Shahangian et al. [153]	2021	Shahangian, S. A., Tabesh, M., & Yazdanpanah, M. (2021b). How can socio-psychological factors be related to water-efficiency intention and behaviors among Iranian residential water consumers? Journal of Environmental Management, 288.	25	12.5
Straus et al. [118]	2016	Straus, J., Chang, H., & Hong, C.-Y. (2016). An exploratory path analysis of attitudes, behaviors and summer water consumption in the Portland Metropolitan Area. Sustainable Cities and Society, 23, 68–77.	25	3,6
Maas et al. [130]	2017	Maas, A., Goemans, C., Manning, D., Kroll, S., Arabi, M., & Rodriguez-McGoffina, M. (2017). Evaluating the effect of conservation motivations on residential water demand. Journal of Environmental Management, 196, 394–401.	23	3.8
Chang [196]	2013	Chang, G. (2013). Factors influencing water conservation behavior among urban residents in China's arid areas. Water Policy, 15(5), 691–704.	22	2.2
Bhanot [197]	2021	Bhanot, S. P. (2021). Isolating the effect of injunctive norms on conservation behavior: New evidence from a field experiment in California. Organizational Behavior and Human Decision Processes, 163, 30–42.	21	10.5
Addo et al. [84]	2018	Addo, I. B., Thoms, M. C., & Parsons, M. (2018). Barriers and Drivers of Household Water-Conservation Behavior: A Profiling Approach. Water, 10(12).	21	4.2
Landon et al. [79]	2016	Landon, A. C., Kyle, G. T., & Kaiser, R. A. (2016). Predicting compliance with an information-based residential outdoor water conservation program. Journal of Hydrology, 536, 26–36.	21	3.0
Marzouk & Mahrous [101]	2020	Marzouk, O. A., & Mahrous, A. A. (2020). Sustainable Consumption Behavior of Energy and Water-Efficient Products in a Resource-Constrained Environment. Journal of Global Marketing, 33(5), 335–353.	20	6.7
Jorgensen et al. [120]	2013	Jorgensen, B. S., Martin, J. F., Pearce, M., & Willis, E. (2013). Some difficulties and inconsistencies when using habit strength and reasoned action variables in models of metered household water conservation. Journal of Environmental Management, 115, 124–135.	20	2.0

Table A6. *Cont.*

Author	Year	Contribution	Total Cites	Cites/Year
Liobikiene & Minelgaite [198]	2021	Liobikiene, G., & Minelgaite, A. (2021). Energy and resource-saving behaviors in European Union countries: The Campbell paradigm and goal framing theory approaches. Science of the Total Environment, 750.	19	9.5
Gu et al. [199]	2020	Gu, D., Jiang, J., Zhang, Y., Sun, Y., Jiang, W., & Du, X. P. (2020). Concern for the future and saving the earth: When does ecological resource scarcity promote pro-environmental behavior? Journal of Environmental Psychology, 72.	19	6.3
Bhanot et al. [200]	2017	Bhanot, S. P. (2017). Rank and response: A field experiment on peer information and water use behavior. Journal of Economic Psychology, 62, 155–172.	19	3.2
Schultz et al. [201]	2019	Schultz, W., Javey, S., & Sorokina, A. (2019). Social Comparison as a Tool to Promote Residential Water Conservation. Frontiers in Water, 1.	18	4.5
Matikinca et al. [202]	2020	Matikinca, P., Ziervogel, G., & Enqvist, J. P. (2020). Drought response impacts on household water use practices in Cape Town, South Africa. Water Policy, 22(3), 483–500.	17	5,7
Goette et al. [203]	2019	Goette, L., Leong, C., & Qian, N. (2019). Motivating household water conservation: A field experiment in Singapore. PLOS ONE, 14(3).	17	4,3
Chenoweth et al. [95]	2016	Chenoweth, J., López-Avilés, A., Morse, S., & Druckman, A. (2016). Water consumption and subjective wellbeing: An analysis of British households. Ecological Economics, 130, 186–194.	17	2,4
Addo et al. [84]	2019	Addo, I. B., Thoms, M. C., & Parsons, M. (2019). The influence of water-conservation messages on reducing household water use. Applied Water Science, 9(5).	16	4.0
Arbués et al. [78]	2016	Arbués, F., Bolsa, M. Á., & Villanúa, I. (2016). Which factors determine water saving behavior? evidence from Spanish households. Urban Water Journal, 13(5), 511–520.	16	2.3
Keramitsoglou & Tsagarakis [89]	2011	Keramitsoglou, K. M., & Tsagarakis, K. P. (2011). Raising effective awareness for domestic water saving: evidence from an environmental educational programme in Greece. Water Policy, 13(6), 828–844.	15	1.3
Clark & Finley [93]	2008	Clark, W. A., & Finley, J. C. (2007). Determinants of water conservation intention in Blagoevgrad, Bulgaria. Society and Natural Resources, 20(7), 613–627.	15	1,0
Lindsay & Supski [204]	2017	Lindsay, J., & Supski, S. (2017). Changing household water consumption practices after drought in three Australian cities. Geoforum, 84, 51–58. https://doi.org/10.1016/j.geoforum.2017.06.001	14	2,3
Kang et al. [92]	2017	Kang, J., Grable, K., Hustvedt, G., & Ahn, M. (2017). Sustainable water consumption: The perspective of Hispanic consumers. Journal of Environmental Psychology, 50, 94–103.	14	2,3
Bruvold & Smith [126]	1988	Bruvold, W. H., & Smith, B. R. (1988). Developing and assessing a model of residential water conservation. JAWRA Journal of the American Water Resources Association, 24(3), 661–669.	14	0.4

Table A6. *Cont.*

Author	Year	Contribution	Total Cites	Cites/Year
Dean et al. [105]	2021	Dean, A. J., Kneebone, S., Tull, F., Lauren, N., & Smith, L. D. G. (2021). 'Stickiness' of water-saving behaviors: What factors influence whether behaviors are maintained or given up? Resources, Conservation and Recycling, 169.	13	6.5
Rogers & Bragg [205]	2012	Rogers, Z., & Bragg, E. (2012). The power of connection: Sustainable lifestyles and sense of place. Ecopsychology, 4(4), 307–318.	13	1.2
Tom et al. [206]	2011	Tom, G., Tauchus, G., Williams, J., & Tong, S. (2011). The role of communicative feedback in successful water conservation programs. Applied Environmental Education and Communication, 10(2), 80–90.	13	1.1
Wang & Dong [207]	2017	Wang, C. H., & Dong, H. (2017). Responding to the drought: A spatial statistical approach to investigating residential water consumption in Fresno, California. Sustainability (Switzerland), 9(2).	12	2.0
Garcia et al. [208]	2013	Garcia, X., Muro, M., Ribas, A., Llausàs, A., Jeffrey, P., & Saurí, D. (2013b). Attitudes and behaviors towards water conservation on the Mediterranean coast: the role of socio-demographic and place-attachment factors. Water International, 38(3), 283–296.	12	1.2
Céspedes Restrepo & Morales-Pinzón [85]	2020	Céspedes Restrepo, J. D., & Morales-Pinzón, T. (2020). Effects of feedback information on the household consumption of water and electricity: A case study in Colombia. Journal of Environmental Management, 262.	11	3.7
Zhuang et al. [140]	2018	Zhuang, J., Lapinski, M. K., & Peng, W. (2018). Crafting messages to promote water conservation: Using time-framed messages to boost conservation actions in the United States and China. Journal of Applied Social Psychology, 48(5), 248–256.	11	2.2
Tijs et al. [209]	2017	Tijs, M. S., Karremans, J. C., Veling, H., de Lange, M. A., van Meegeren, P., & Lion, R. (2017). Saving water to save the environment: contrasting the effectiveness of environmental and monetary appeals in a residential water saving intervention. Social Influence, 12(2–3), 69–79.	11	1.8
Sadalla et al. [210]	2014	Sadalla, E., Berlin, A., Neel, R., & Ledlow, S. (2014). Priorities in Residential Water Use: A Trade-Off Analysis. Environment and Behavior, 46(3), 303–328.	11	1,2
Jorgensen et al. [120]	2015	Jorgensen, B. S., Martin, J. F., Pearce, M. W., & Willis, E. M. (2015). Aligning theory and measurement in behavioral models of water conservation. Water Policy, 17(4), 762–776.	10	1,3
Shahangian et al. [153]	2021	Shahangian, S. A., Tabesh, M., & Yazdanpanah, M. (2021b). Psychosocial determinants of household adoption of water-efficiency behaviors in Tehran capital, Iran: Application of the social cognitive theory. Urban Climate, 39.	9	4.5
Warner [106]	2021	Warner, L. A. (2021). Who conserves and who approves? Predicting water conservation intentions in urban landscapes with referent groups beyond the traditional 'important others.' Urban Forestry and Urban Greening, 60.	9	4.5

Table A6. *Cont.*

Author	Year	Contribution	Total Cites	Cites/Year
Díaz et al. [69]	2020	Díaz, J., Odera, E., & Warner, L. (2020). Delving deeper: Exploring the influence of psycho-social wellness on water conservation behavior. Journal of Environmental Management, 264.	9	3.0
Rondinel Oviedo & Sarmiento Pastor [121]	2020	Rondinel Oviedo, D. R., & Sarmiento Pastor, J. M. (2020). Water: consumption, usage patterns, and residential infrastructure. A comparative analysis of three regions in the Lima metropolitan area. Water International, 45(7–8), 824–846.	9	3.0
Wang et al. [211]	2019	Wang, Y. H., Chang, M. C., & Liou, J. R. (2019). Effects of water-saving education in Taiwan on public water knowledge, attitude, and behavior intention change. Water Policy, 21(5), 964–979.	9	2,3
Katz et al. [212]	2018	Katz, D., Kronrod, A., Grinstein, A., & Nisan, U. (2018). Still Waters Run Deep: Comparing Assertive and Suggestive Language in Water Conservation Campaigns. WATER, 10(3).	9	1.8
Walter et al. [154]	2017	Walter, N., Demetriades, S. Z., & Murphy, S. T. (2017). Involved, United, and Efficacious: Could Self-Affirmation Be the Solution to California's Drought? Health Communication, 32(9), 1161–1170.	9	1.5
Manríquez Betanzos et al. [116]	2016	Manríquez Betanzos, J. C., Corral Verdugo, V., Vanegas Rico, M. C., Fraijo Sing, B. S., & Tapia Fonllem, C. O. (2016). Positive (Gratitude, eudaimonia) and negative (scarcity, costs) determinants of water conservation behavior [Determinantes positivos (Gratitud, eudaimonia) y negativos (escasez, costos) del ahorro de agua]. Psyecology, 7(2), 178–200.	9	1.3
Rodríguez Sánchez et al. [135]	2020	Rodríguez Sánchez, C., & Sarabia Sanchez, F. J. (2020). Does Water Context Matter in Water Conservation Decision Behavior? Sustainability, 12(7).	8	2.7
Chaudhary et al. [213]	2019	Chaudhary, A. K., Warner, L. A., & Ali, A. D. (2019). Using perceived benefits to segment residential landscape irrigation users. Urban Forestry & Urban Greening, 38, 318–329.	8	2.0
Holland et al. [127]	2019	Holland, D., Janet, K., & Landrum, A. (2019). Experience is Key: Examining the Relative Importance of Factors Influencing Individuals' Water Conservation. Water, 11(9).	8	2.0
Demetriades & Walter [154]	2016	Demetriades, S. Z., & Walter, N. (2016). You Should Know Better: Can Self-Affirmation Facilitate Information-Seeking Behavior and Interpersonal Discussion? Journal of Health Communication, 21(11), 1131–1140.	8	1.1
Fielding et al. [67]	2010	Fielding, K. S., Thompson, A., Louis, W. R., & Warren, C. (2010). Environmental sustainability: Understanding the attitudes and behavior of Australian households. AHURI Final Report, 152, 1–132.	8	0,6
Miller & Buys [112]	2008	Miller, E., & Buys, L. (2008). The role of social capital in predicting and promoting 'feelings of responsibility' for local environmental issues in an Australian community. Australasian Journal of Environmental Management, 15(4), 231–240.	8	0.5
Hasan et al. [214]	2021	Hasan, H. H., Razali, S. F. M., & Razali, N. H. M. (2021). Does the household save water? Evidence from behavioral analysis. Sustainability (Switzerland), 13(2), 1–20.	7	3.5

Table A6. *Cont.*

Author	Year	Contribution	Total Cites	Cites/Year
Maduku [64]	2021	Maduku, D. K. (2021). Water conservation campaigns in an emerging economy: how effective are they? International Journal of Advertising, 40(3), 452–472.	7	3.5
Araya et al. [72]	2020	Araya, F., Osman, K., & Faust, K. M. (2020). Perceptions versus reality: Assessing residential water conservation efforts in the household. Resources, Conservation and Recycling, 162.	7	2.3
Timm & Deal [80]	2018	Timm, S. N., & Deal, B. M. (2018). Understanding the behavioral influences behind Singapore's water management strategies. Journal of Environmental Planning and Management, 61(10), 1654–1673.	7	1.4
Aisa & Larramona [215]	2012	Aisa, R., & Larramona, G. (2012). Household water saving: Evidence from Spain. Water Resources Research, 48(12).	7	0.6
Shahangian et al. [153]	2022	Shahangian, S. A., Tabesh, M., Yazdanpanah, M., Zobeidi, T., & Raoof, M. A. (2022). Promoting the adoption of residential water conservation behaviors as a preventive policy to sustainable urban water management. Journal of Environmental Management, 313.	6	6,0
Barnett et al. [53]	2020	Barnett, M. J., Jackson-Smith, D., Endter-Wada, J., & Haeffner, M. (2020). A multilevel analysis of the drivers of household water consumption in a semi-arid region. Science of the Total Environment, 712.	6	2.0
Lamm et al. [216]	2018	Lamm, A. J., Warner, L. A., Lundy, L. K., Bommidi, J. S., & Beattie, P. N. (2018). Informing water-saving communication in the United States using the situational theory of problem solving. Landscape and Urban Planning, 180, 217–222.	6	1.2
Untaru et al. [99]	2020	Untaru, E.-N., Ispas, A., & Han, H. (2020). Exploring the synergy between customer home-based and hotel-based water consumption and conservation behaviors: An empirical approach. Journal of Consumer Behavior, 19(6), 542–555.	5	1.7
Cahn et al. [217]	2020	Cahn, A., Katz, D., & Ghermandi, A. (2020). Analyzing Water Customer Preferences for Online Feedback Technologies in Israel: A Prototype Study. Journal of Water Resources Planning and Management, 146(4).	5	1.7
Ananga et al. [110]	2019	Ananga, E. O., Becerra, T. A., Peaden, C., & Pappas, C. (2019). Examining water conservation behaviors and attitudes: evidence from the city of Ada, Oklahoma, USA. Sustainable Water Resources Management, 5(4), 1651–1663.	5	1.3
Lavelle & Fahy [94]	2016	Lavelle, M. J., & Fahy, F. (2016). What's consuming Ireland? Exploring expressed attitudes and reported behaviors towards the environment and consumption across three case study locations on the island of Ireland. Irish Geography, 49(2), 29–54.	5	0.7
Balnave & Adeyeye [143]	2013	Balnave, J., & Adeyeye, K. (2013). A comparative study of attitudes and preferences for water efficiency in homes. Journal of Water Supply: Research and Technology—AQUA, 62(8), 515–524.	5	0.5
Daniel et al. [218]	2022	Daniel, D., Pande, S., & Rietveld, L. (2022). Endogeneity in water use behavior across case studies of household water treatment adoption in developing countries. World Development Perspectives, 25.	4	4,0

Table A6. *Cont.*

Author	Year	Contribution	Total Cites	Cites/Year
Alvarado Espejo et al. [52]	2021	Alvarado Espejo, J. M., Ontaneda, W. I. T., Padilla, N. I. A., Ochoa-Moreno, W. S., Alvarado Espejo, J. M., Torres Ontaneda, W. I., Aguirre Padilla, N. I., & Ochoa-Moreno, W. S. (2021). Water saving practices conditioned by socioeconomic factors: A case study of Ecuadorian households. Journal of Environmental Management, 293.	4	2,0
Koop et al. [12]	2021	Koop, S. H. A., Clevers, S. H. P., Blokker, E. J. M., & Brouwer, S. (2021). Public attitudes towards digital water meters for households. Sustainability (Switzerland), 13(11).	4	2,0
Wang & Chermak [139]	2021	Wang, J., & Chermak, J. M. (2021). Is less always more? Conservation, efficiency and water education programs. Ecological Economics, 184.	4	2.0
Warner et al. [219]	2021	Warner, L. A., Diaz, J. M., Díaz, J. M., & Diaz, J. M. (2021). Amplifying the Theory of Planned behavior with connectedness to water to inform impactful water conservation program planning and evaluation. Journal of Agricultural Education and Extension, 27(2), 229–253.	4	2.0
Sarabia Sánchez & Rodríguez Sánchez [51]	2013	Sarabia Sánchez, F. J., & Rodríguez Sánchez, C. (2013). Attitudes towards saving water, household structural characteristics and water consumption [Actitudes hacia el ahorro de agua, características estructurales del hogar y consumo de agua]. Psyecology, 4(2), 115–137.	4	0.4
Graymore et al. [220]	2010	Graymore, M. L. M., Wallis, A., & O'Toole, K. (2010). Understanding drivers and barriers: The key to water use behavior change. Water Science and Technology: Water Supply, 10(5), 679–688.	4	0.3
Ibáñez-Rueda et al. [221]	2022	Ibáñez-Rueda, N., Guardiola, J., & González-Gómez, F. (2022). The role of nature contact and connectedness to nature as determinants of household water use: A case study from Spain. Water and Environment Journal, 36(2), 282-291.	3	3.0
Martinez et al. [222]	2021	Martinez, D. M., Maia, A. G., Martínez, D. M., & Maia, A. G. (2021). The Effect of Social Behavior on Residential Water Consumption. Water (Switzerland), 13(9).	3	1.5
Hodges et al. [223]	2020	Hodges, H., Kuehl, C., Anderson, S. E., Ehret, P. J., & Brick, C. (2020). How Managers Can Reduce Household Water Use Through Communication: A Field Experiment. Journal of Policy Analysis and Management, 39(4), 1076–1099.	3	1.0
Caspers [75]	2020	Caspers, C. G. W. (2020). Role of Trust in Adopting Consumer Social Responsible Behavior in the Context of Water Use in Domestic Households. South East European Journal of Economics and Business, 15(1), 1–13.	3	1.0
Liu et al. [155]	2020	Liu, H., Zhao, Y., Li, H., Wang, L., & Wang, Q. (2020). Individual water-saving response based on complex adaptive system theory: Case study of Beijing City, China. Water (Switzerland), 12(5).	3	1.0
Barberán et al. [224]	2022	Barberán, R., López-Laborda, J., Rodrigo, F., Barberan, R., Lopez-Laborda, J., & Rodrigo, F. (2022). The Perception of Residential Water Tariff, Consumption, and Cost: Evidence of its Determinants Using Survey Data. Water Resources Management, 36(9), 2933–2952.	2	2.0

Table A6. *Cont.*

Author	Year	Contribution	Total Cites	Cites/Year
Jessoe et al. [225]	2021	Jessoe, K., Lade, G. E., Loge, F., & Spang, E. (2021). Residential water conservation during drought: Experimental evidence from three behavioral interventions. Journal of Environmental Economics and Management, 110.	2	1.0
Delistavrou [146]	2021	Delistavrou, A. (2021). Water and energy conservation in Greece: the impact of values and attitudes. International Journal of Sustainable Energy, 40(6), 602–615.	2	1.0
Akpinar et al. [88]	2018	Akpinar, M. G., Gul, M., Ceylan, R. F., & Gulcan, S. (2018). Evaluation of the factors affecting water-saving attitudes of urban life on the verge of the next century: a case study of the Mediterranean region of Turkey. Journal of Water Sanitation and Hygiene for Development, 8(2), 340–348.	2	0.4
Gázquez-Abad et al. [226]	2011	Gázquez-Abad, J. C., Mondéjar-Jiménez, J.-A., & Vargas-Vargas, M. (2011). Factors influencing water saving behavior for Spanish households. Environmental Engineering and Management Journal, 10(12), 1873–1881.	2	0.2
Haeffner et al. [73]	2023	Haeffner, M., Jackson-Smith, D., & Barnett, M. J. (2023). Categorizing relative water use perception bias using household surveys and monthly water bills. Journal of Environmental Management, 334.	1	1.0
Long et al. [128]	2022	Long, H., Shi, S., Tang, Z., & Zhang, S. (2022). Does living alone increase the consumption of social resources? Environmental Science and Pollution Research, 29(47), 71911–71922.	1	1.0
Li et al. [91]	2022	Li, Y., Wang, B., & Cui, M. (2022). Environmental Concern, Environmental Knowledge, and Residents' Water Conservation Behavior: Evidence from China. Water (Switzerland), 14(13).	1	1.0
Wahid et al. [113]	2022	Wahid, N. A., Fadzil, S. F. S., & Ariffin, S. K. (2022). Influences of Problem Awareness, Awareness of Consequences and Ascription of Responsibility on Consumer's Personal Norm to Prevent Water Wastage Behavior. Environment and Ecology Research, 10(2), 275–283.	1	1.0
Vivek et al. [227]	2021	Vivek, Malghan, D., & Mukherjee, K. (2021). Toward achieving persistent behavior change in household water conservation. Proceedings of the National Academy of Sciences of the United States of America, 118(24).	1	0,5
Andrade et al. [70]	2021	Andrade, E., Seoane, G., Vila-Tojo, S., Gómez-Román, C., & Sabucedo, J.-M. (2021). Psychological and situational variables associated with objective knowledge on water-related issues in a northern Spanish city. International Journal of Environmental Research and Public Health, 18(6), 1–16.	1	0.5
Bermejo-Martín et al. [228]	2021	Bermejo-Martín, G., Rodríguez-Monroy, C., & Núñez-Guerrero, Y. M. (2021). Water consumption range prediction in Huelva's households using classification and regression trees. Water (Switzerland), 13(4).	1	0.5
Kalifa et al. [100]	2021	Kalifa, A., Al-Maadid, A., Koutiva, I., & Makropoulos, C. (2021). Individual water consumption behavior in relation to urban residential dynamics: The Case of Qatar. Urban Water Journal, 18(10), 806–816.	1	0.5

Table A6. *Cont.*

Author	Year	Contribution	Total Cites	Cites/Year
Warner et al. [229]	2020	Warner, L. A., Turner, S., & Lundy, L. (2020). Comparing Linkages Between Descriptive Norms and Current and Intended Outdoor Water Conservation. Journal of Extension, 58(6), 1–9.	1	0.3
Lyach & Remr [230]	2023	Lyach, R., & Remr, J. (2023). Motivations of Households towards Conserving Water and Using Purified Water in Czechia. Sustainability (Switzerland), 15(3).	0	0.0
Thakur et al. [231]	2022	Thakur, R., Onwubu, S. C., Harris, G., & Thakur, S. (2022). Examining the factors influencing water conservation intentions amongst peri urban communities of Ethekwini Municipality, South Africa. Water Conservation and Management, 6(2), 81–88.	0	0.0
Reddy et al. [98]	2023	Reddy, R. A., Sengupta, R., Jackson, B. M., & Lewis, C. (2023). Development of a new measure to check attitude towards water conservation☆. MethodsX, 10.	0	0.0
Grespan et al. [131]	2022	Grespan, A., Garcia, J., Brikalski, M. P., Henning, E., & Kalbusch, A. (2022). Assessment of water consumption in households using statistical analysis and regression trees. Sustainable Cities and Society, 87.	0	0.0
Madias et al. [33]	2022	Madias, K., Borusiak, B., & Szymkowiak, A. (2022). The role of knowledge about water consumption in the context of intentions to use IoT water metrics. Frontiers in Environmental Science, 10.	0	0.0
Sarpong & Amankwaa [82]	2022	Sarpong, K. A., & Amankwaa, G. (2022). Household behavioral intention, environmental habit and attitude related to efficient water management: an empirical analysis on pro-environmental behavior among urban residents. H2Open Journal, 5(3), 438–455.	0	0.0
Otaki & Maeda [86]	2022	Otaki, Y., & Maeda, A. (2022). Water-Saving Tips With a Visualized Indicator Related to the Environment. Frontiers in Water, 4.	0	0.0
Khodadad et al. [124]	2022	Khodadad, M., Sanei, M., Narvaez-Montoya, C., & Aguilar-Barajas, I. (2022). Climatic Hazards and the Associated Impacts on Households' Willingness to Adopt Water-Saving Measures: Evidence from Mexico. Sustainability (Switzerland), 14(10).	0	0.0
Oğur Aydın & Doğan [232]	2022	Oğur Aydın, D., & Doğan, Ç. (2022). Exploring water-consuming personal care and hygiene practices in the bathroom environment and user intentions for improving effective water consumption. Design Journal, 25(5), 828–848.	0	0.0
Al-Maadid et al. [107]	2022	Al-Maadid, A., Akesson, J., Bernstein, D. H., Chakravarti, J., & Khalifa, A. (2022). Understanding Water Consumption in Qatar: Evidence From a Nationally Representative Survey. Urban Water Journal.	0	0.0
Njoku et al. [125]	2022	Njoku, P. O., Durowoju, O. S., Uhunamure, S. E., & Makungo, R. (2022). Investigating the Attitude of Domestic Water Use in Urban and Rural Households in South Africa. Water (Switzerland), 14(2).	0	0.0

Table A6. *Cont.*

Author	Year	Contribution	Total Cites	Cites/Year
Lameck et al. [233]	2021	Lameck, E., Sesabo, J., & Mkuna, E. (2021). Household behavior towards water conservation activities in Mvomero District in Tanzania: a convergent parallel mixed approach. Sustainable Water Resources Management, 7(3).	0	0.0
Buday et al. [71]	2021	Buday, A., Zollinger, B., Hammersmith, A., & Heine, K. (2021). Thirsting for sustainability: Water conservation in a great plains city. Great Plains Research, 31(1), 1–16.	0	0.0
Sengupta [234]	2020	Sengupta, J. (2020). The Effect of Non-pecuniary-based Incentive Mechanisms to Reduce Water Usage at the Household Level and to Achieve Positive Environmental Outcomes. Global Business Review, 21(5), 1232–1248.	0	0.0

Note: Source: Own elaboration.

Table A7. International collaboration between countries.

Country 1	Country 2	Frequency
USA	Australia	2
USA	Bulgaria	1
USA	Chile	2
USA	China	1
USA	India	1
USA	Israel	1
USA	Italy	1
USA	Mexico	2
USA	Netherlands	2
USA	Qatar	1
USA	UK	2
Australia	c	1
Australia	Saudi Arabia	1
Australia	Spain	1
Australia	UK	3
Spain	Canada	1
Spain	France	2
Spain	UK	1
Netherlands	Belgium	1
Netherlands	Indonesia	1
Netherlands	Israel	1
UK	Netherlands	1
UK	Qatar	1
UK	Switzerland	1
China	Germany	1
China	Hong Kong	1
China	Netherlands	1
France	Canada	1
Greece	Qatar	1
Iran	Canada	1
Chile	Sweden	1
Mexico	Chile	1
South Korea	Romania	1

Note: Source: Own elaboration.

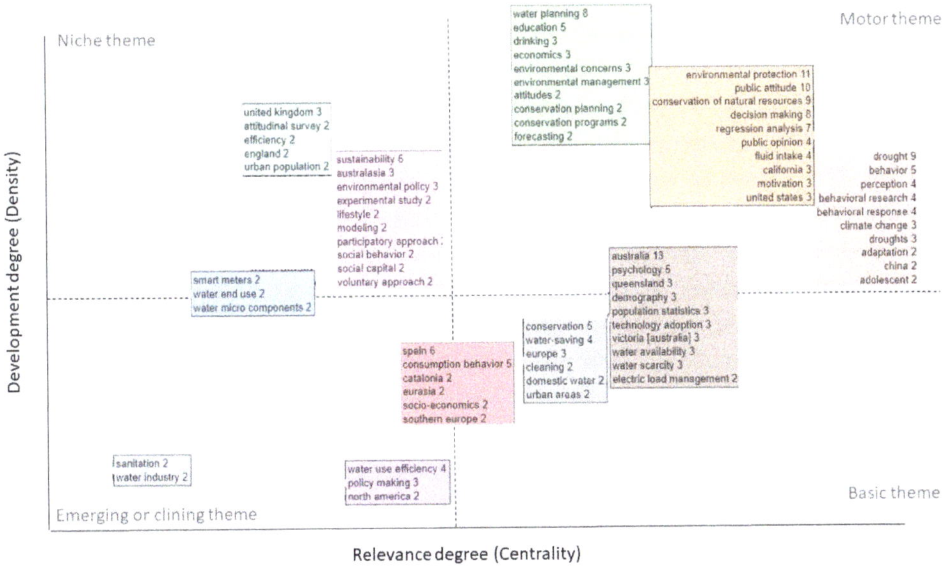

(**a**)

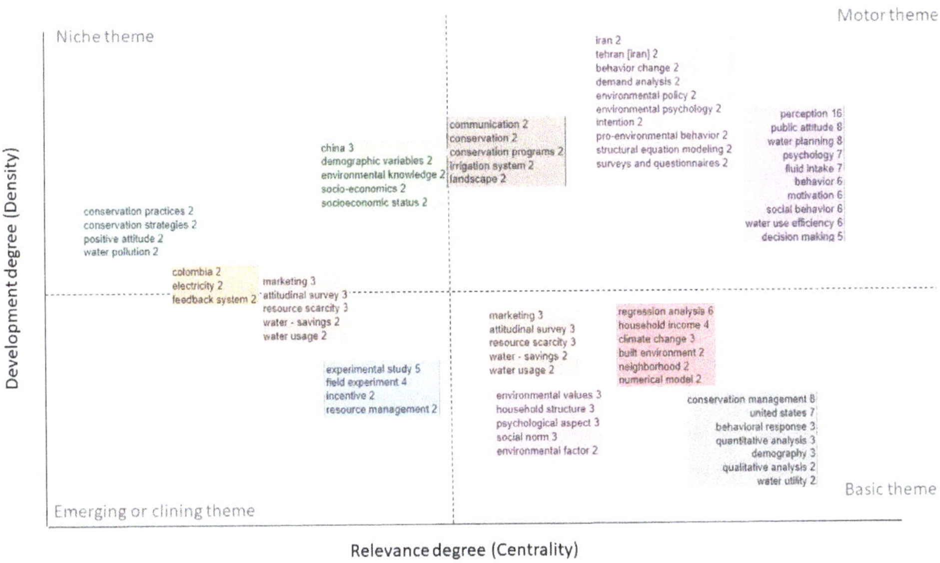

(**b**)

Figure A1. Thematic maps: temporal comparisons 1982–2017 and 2018–2023. (**a**) Thematic map based on authors' keywords: 1982–2017. (**b**) Thematic map based on authors' keywords: 2018–2023. Source: Result from Biblioshiny.

Table A8. Main theories and theoretical frameworks.

Theories and/or Theoretical Frameworks	Frequency	%
Studies that applied a single theory or model		
Theory of Planned Behavior (TPB)	16	10%
New Environmental Paradigm (NEP)	4	3%
Standards Activation Method (NAM)	4	3%
Behavior Change Wheel (BCW) Model	3	2%
Social Influence Approach	2	1%
Theory of Reasoning Action (TRA)	2	1%
Values–Attitudes–Behavior	2	1%
Value-Belief Norms (VBN)	2	1%
Consumer Behavior Model	1	1%
Behavioral Economics	1	1%
Theory of Commitment	1	1%
Theory of Complex Adaptive Systems	1	1%
Construal Level Theory (CLT)	1	1%
Demarketing	1	1%
Ecological Economics	1	1%
Grounded Theory	1	1%
Theory of Habits	1	1%
Health Belief Model (HBM)	1	1%
Information Motivation Behavior Model (IMB)	1	1%
Knowledge Deficit Model	1	1%
Situational Problem-Solving Theory (STOPS)	1	1%
Randomized Controlled Trials (RCTs)	1	1%
Self-affirmation Theory	1	1%
Trade-off Paradigm	1	1%
Socio-ecological Framework	1	1%
Social Identity Framework	1	1%
Social Impact Theory	1	1%
Theory of Social Norms	1	1%
Theory of Social Practice	1	1%
Theory of the Tragedy of the Commons	1	1%
Theory of Ecological Attitude	1	1%
Studies that combined theories and/or models		
Level of Interpretation Theory (CLT) + Theory of Planned Behavior (TPB)	1	1%
Self-Affirmation Theory + Planned Behavior Theory (BPT)	1	1%
Propagation Theory (Spillover theory) + Self-affirmation theory	1	1%
The Campbell Paradigm + The Goal Framework Theory	1	1%
Social Norms Theory + Social Comparison Theory	1	1%
Theory of Normative Conduct	1	1%
Theory of Planned Behavior (TPB) + Connection with Nature (CTN)	1	1%
Theory of Planned Behavior (TPB) + Extended TPB	1	1%

Table A8. *Cont.*

Theories and/or Theoretical Frameworks	Frequency	%
Theory of Planned Behavior (TPB) + Social Marketing	1	1%
Theory of Planned Behavior (TPB) + Utilitarian Belief of Water	1	1%
Theory of Reasoned Action (ART) + Elaboration Probability Model (ELM) + Habits	1	1%
Reasoned Action Theory (ART) + New Environmental Paradigm (NEP)	1	1%
Prospect Theory + Communication Frameworks + Political Ideology	1	1%
Values + Intention Model + Social Cognitive Theory	1	1%
Does not explicitly present a theory or framework	83	54%
TOTAL	155	100%

Note: Source: Own elaboration.

Table A9. Dependent variables used in the contributions.

Dependent Variable	Frequency	%
Water Conservation	40	26%
Water Consumption	30	19%
Water Use	19	12%
Water Saving	16	10%
Behavioral Intention	11	7%
Water Conservation Intention	8	5%
Water Consumption (Water meter)	5	3%
Water Saving Attitude	4	3%
Current Water Consumption	3	2%
Showering Behavior	2	1%
Current Water Conservation	2	1%
Actual Behavior	2	1%
Spillover Effect	2	1%
Pro-environmental Behavior	2	1%
Water Objective Knowledge	1	1%
Subjective Well-being	1	1%
Personal Norms	1	1%
Past Water Conservation	1	1%
Intention to Adopt a Smart Water Meter	1	1%
Household Responses	1	1%
Engagement in Sustainability Actions	1	1%
Communicative Action	1	1%
Difficult Behavior	1	1%
Total	155	100%

Note: Source: Own elaboration.

Table A10. Internal factors to the individual related to water-conservation behavior and/or consumption.

PERSONAL-SPHERE VARIABLES		
Variable/Factor	**Specific Example**	**Contributions**
1.1. Habits related to water user	Habit. Past water consumption/saving behavior.	Aisa and Larramona (2012) [215]; García et al. (2013) [195]; Gregory and Di Leo (2003) [81]; Jorgensen et al. (2013) [76]; Jorgensen et al. (2015) [120]; Maduku (2021) [64]; Lauren et al. (2016) [119]; Martínez Espiñeira and García Valiñas (2013) [192]; Pérez Uridales and García Valiñas (2016) [145]; Russell and Knoeri (2020) [56]; Sarabia Sánchez et al. (2014) [149]; Sarpong and Amankwaa (2022) [82]; Straus et al. (2016) [118].
1.2. Familiarity with the behavior	Familiarity with water-related behavior	Shahangian et al. (2021) [153].
1.3. Perception regarding water consumption/saving.	Perception regarding water consumption/saving.	Al-Maadid et al. (2022) [107]; Andrade et al. (2021) [70]; Araya et al. (2020) [72]; Attari (2014) [179]; Deng et al. (2017) [61]; Domene and Sauri (2006) [132]; Hasan et al. (2021) [214].
1.4. Commitment to water conservation	Commitment to water conservation	Jorgensen et al. (2014) [76].
1.5. Antisocial behavior	Antisocial behavior linked to water	Corral Verdugo and Frias Armenta (2006) [123].
1.6. Information on water consumption	Information on water consumption. Councils. Feedback (smart meter data).	Addo et al. (2019) [84]; Al-Maadid et al. (2022) [107]; Bhanot (2017) [200]; Cahn et al. (2020) [217]; Céspedes Restrepo and Morales Pinzon (2020) [85]; Dascher et al. (2014) [150]; Dolnicar et al. (2012) [97]; Goette et al. (2019) [203]; Gu et al. (2020) [199]; Hodges et al. (2020) [223]; Holland et al. (2019) [127]; Jaeger and Schultz (2017) [148]; Katz et al. (2018) [212]; Kurz et al. (2005) [180]; Lede et al. (2019) [108]; Liu et al. (2020) [155]; Otaki and Maeda (2022) [55]; Otaki et al. (2017) [86]; Ramli (2021) [104]; Schultz et al. (2016) [39]; Schultz et al. (2019) [201]; Tijs et al. (2017) [209]; Tom et al. (2011) [206]; Torres and Carlsson (2018) [189].
1.7. Participation in water-related practices/behaviors	Participation in water-related practices/behaviors	Chaudhary et al. (2019) [213].
1.8. Descriptive and injunctive norms	Social norms. Subjective norms. Injunctive norms. Precautionary and descriptive rules. Social comparison, relating to water.	Barnett et al. (2020) [53]; Bhanot (2021) [197]; Cahn et al. (2020) [217]; Daniel et al. (2018) [220]; Dean et al. (2021) [105]; Fielding et al. (2012) [40]; Fielding et al. (2010) [67]; Harlan et al. (2009) [178]; Kantola et al. (1982) [183]. Goette et al. (2019) [203]; Gómez Llanos et al. (2020) [54]; Haeffner et al. (2023) [73]; Hodges et al. (2020) [223]; Jaeger and Schultz (2017) [148]; Jorgensen et al. (2014) [76]; Kang et al. (2017) [92]. Landon et al. (2016) [79]; Lavelle and Fahy (2016) [94]; Lede et al. (2019) [108]; Lowe et al. (2015) [102]; Maduku (2021) [64]; Martínez and Maia (2021) [222]; Ramli (2021) [104]; Ramsey et al. (2017) [90]; Russell and Knoeri (2020) [56]; Sengupta (2020) [234]; Seyranian et al. (2015) [57]; Schultz et al. (2019) [201]; Schultz et al. (2016) [39]; Thakur et al. (2022) [231]; Timm and Deal (2017) [80]; Torres and Carlsson (2018) [189]; Wahid et al. (2022) [113]; Warner et al. (2020) [229]; Warner (2021) [106]; Warner and Diaz (2021) [219].
1.9. Perception of the behavior of other people	Perception of other people's water consumption behavior	Shahangian et al. (2021) [63].
1.10. Social awareness	Social awareness. Awareness of consequences/actions. Environmental knowledge. Understanding of the actions, regarding water.	Addo et al. (2018) [84]; Akpinar et al. (2018) [88]; Al-Maadid et al. (2022) [107]; Alvarado Espejo et al. (2021) [52]; Andrade et al. (2021) [70]; Aprile and Fiorillo (2017) [182]; Bronfman et al. (2015) [111]; Dean et al. (2021) [105]; Gazquez-Abad et al. (2011) [226]; Gregory and Di Leo (2003) [81]; Hasan et al. (2021) [214]; Hodges et al. (2020) [223]; Landon et al. (2017) [79]; Li et al. (2022) [91]; Madias et al. (2022) [33]; Matikinca et al. (2020) [202]; Moore et al. (1994) [188]; Ramsey et al. (2017) [90]; Rajapaksa et al. (2019) [191]; Sarpong and Amankwaa (2022) [82]; Segev (2015) [193]; Suarez Varela et al. (2016) [185]; Wang and Chermak (2021) [139]; Wahid et al. (2022) [113]; Wang et al. (2019) [211]; Willis et al. (2011) [38].
1.11. Identity	Environmental identity. Social identity. Personal identity.	Dean et al. (2021) [105]; Seyranian et al. (2015) [57].
1.12. Community attachment	Community attachment.	Landon et al. (2017) [79]; Miller and Buys (2008) [112].
1.13. Collectivism	Collectivism	Segev (2015) [193].

Table A10. *Cont.*

PERSONAL-SPHERE VARIABLES		
Variable/Factor	**Specific Example**	**Contributions**
1.14. Political ideology. Political affiliation.	Political ideology. Political affiliation.	Andrade et al. (2021) [70]; Buday et al. (2021) [71]; Holland et al. (2019) [127]; Wolters (2014) [62].
1.15. Support for the policy	Policy support	Walter et al. (2017) [154].
1.16. Moral norms	Moral obligation. Moral norm concerning water. Personal norm.	Addo et al. (2018) [84]; Bronfman et al. (2015) [111]; Dolnicar et al. (2012) [97]; Kang et al. (2017) [92]; Landon et al. (2017) [79]; Lowe et al. (2015) [102]; Madias et al. (2022) [33]; Rajapaksa et al. (2019) [191]; Reddy et al. (2023) [98]; Shahangian et al. (2021) [153]; Torres and Carlsson (2018) [189]; Untaru et al. (2020) [99].
1.17. Emotions	Emotions (guilt, shame) related to saving water.	Andrade et al. (2021) [70]; Chenoweth et al. (2016) [95]; Martínez Betanzos et al. (2016) [116]; Walter et al. (2017) [154].
1.18. Perceived risk	Perception of risk of water scarcity.	Daniel et al. (2022) [218]; Rodríguez Sánchez and Sarabia Sánchez (2017) [135]; Shahangian et al. (2021) [153]; Walter et al. (2017) [154].
1.19. Impact of individual actions	Perceived importance of actions	Buday et al. (2021) [71]; Matikinca et al. (2020) [202]; Sarabia Sánchez et al. (2014) [149].
1.20. Attitude	Attitude towards saving water. Attitude towards water consumption. Attitude towards the price of water. Attitude towards efficient water devices. Attitude towards routine behaviors (curtailment). Attitude towards water restrictions.	Addo et al. (2018) [84]; Al-Maadid et al. (2022) [117]; Ananga et al. (2019) [110]; Andrade et al. (2021) [70]; Barnett et al. (2020) [53]; Bermejo et al. (2021) [228]; Casper (2020) [75]; Chenoweth et al. (2016) [95]; Daniel et al. (2022) [218]; Fielding et al. (2010) [67]; Fielding et al. (2012) [40]; Gazquez Abad et al. (2011) [226]; Gilbertson et al. (2011) [181]; Gregory and Di Leo (2003) [81]; Haeffner et al. (2023) [73]; Harlan et al. (2009) [178]; Hasan et al. (2021) [214]; Jorgensen et al. (2014) [76]; Kalifa et al. (2021) [100]; Kantola et al. (1982) [183]; Kang et al. (2017) [92]; Kurz et al. (2005) [180]; Landon et al. (2016) [79]; Lowe et al. (2015) [102]; Moore et al. (1994) [188]; Reddy et al. (2023) [98]; Russell and Knoeri (2020) [56]; Sarpong and Amankwaa (2022) [82]; Shahangian et al. (2021) [153]; Syme et al. (2004) [134]; Timm and Deal (2017) [80]; Untaru et al. (2020) [99]; Wang et al. (2019) [211]; Wang and Dong (2017) [207]; Warner et al. (2020) [229]; Warner (2021) [106]; Warner and Diaz (2021) [219]; Willis et al. (2011) [38]; Zhuang et al. (2018) [140].
1.21. Control	Perceived control of water-related behavior.	Addo et al. (2018) [84]; Fielding et al. (2012) [40]; Jorgensen et al. (2013) [73]; Kang et al. (2017) [92]; Landon et al. (2016) [79]; Lowe et al. (2015) [102]; Russell and Knoeri (2020) [56]; Shahangian et al. (2021) [153]; Timm and Deal (2017) [80]; Warner (2021) [106]; Warner and Diaz (2021) [221]. Warner et al. (2020) [230].
1.22. Perceived effectiveness	Perceived self-efficacy and perceived collective efficacy. Effectiveness of results related to water.	Dascher et al. (2014) [150]; Fielding et al. (2010) [67]; Lauren et al. (2016) [119]; Ramsey et al. (2017) [90]; Sarabia Sánchez et al. (2014) [149]; Segev (2015) [193]; Shahangian et al. (2022) [68]; Shahangian et al. (2021) [63]; Walter et al. (2017) [154].
1.23. Impact of individual actions	Importance of saving water. Perceived importance of actions	Buday et al. (2021) [71]; Matikinca et al. (2020) [202]; Sarabia Sánchez et al. (2014) [149].
1.24. Responsibility	Environmental responsibility. Assignment of liability.	Alvarado Espejo et al. (2021) [52]; Ananga et al. (2019) [110]; Bronfman et al.](2015) [111]; Madias et al. (2022) [33]; Wahid et al. (2022) [113].
1.25. Beliefs	Beliefs. Personal normative beliefs. Belief in utilitarian water and ecological water.	Bermejo et al. (2021) [228]; Corral Verdugo and Frias (2006) [123]; Kalifa et al. (2021) [10]; Kang et al. (2017) [92]; Russell and Knoeri (2020) [56].
1.26. Motivation	Motivation to save water. Motivation to reduce water according to different climatic contexts. Motivation to use devices to save water. Motivation to adopt sustainable behaviors.	Ananga et al. (2019) [110]; Fan et al. (2013 [133]); Hodges et al. (2020) [223]; Lamm et al. (2016) [218]; Lyach and Remr (2023) [230]; Maas et al. (2017) [130].
1.27. Psychological distance	Psychological distance from the consequences of water use, psychological distance from the effects of climate change. Psychological distance with future water scarcity.	Gu et al. (2020) [199]; Zhuang et al. (2018) [140].
1.28. Environmental awareness	Environmental awareness	Akpinar et al. (2018) [88]; Kalifa et al. (2021) [100]; Lindsay and Supski (2017) [204]; Sadalla et al. (2014) [211].

Table A10. *Cont.*

PERSONAL-SPHERE VARIABLES		
Variable/Factor	**Specific Example**	**Contributions**
1.29. Environmental concern	Selfish/altruistic/biospheric environmental concern.	Addo et al. (2018) [84]; Akpinar et al. (2018) [88]; Alvarado Espejo et al. (2021) [52]; Aprile and Fiorillo (2017) [182]; Barnett et al. (2020) [53]; Bronfman et al. (2015) [111]; Chenoweth et al. (2016) [95]; Dascher et al. (2014) [150]; Delistavrou (2021) [146]; Gilbertson et al. (2011) [181]; Kang et al. (2017) [92]; Lavelle and Fahy (2016) [94]; Li et al. (2022) [91]; Segev (2015) [193]; Suarez Varela et al. (2016) [185]; Untaru et al. (2020) [99]; Wang et al. (2019) [211]; Willis et al. (2011) [38]; Wolters (2014) [62]; Zhuang et al. (2018) [140].
1.30. Perception regarding climate change	Perception of climate change	Deng et al. (2017) [61].
1.31. Perception regarding the right to water	Perception regarding the right to water	Lowe et al. (2015) [102].
1.32. Environmental values	Environmental values.	Bermejo et al. (2021) [228]; Bronfman et al. (2015) [111]; Sarpong and Amankwaa (2022) [82]; Sengupta (2020) [234]; Segev (2015) [193]; Wang et al. (2019) [211].
1.33. Trust and credibility	Confidence. Credibility (source of information, government). Credibility in the face of scarcity/problem	Addo et al. (2018) [84]; Caspers (2020) [75]; Maduku (2021) [64]; Miller and Buys (2008) [112]; Rodríguez Sánchez and Sarabia Sánchez (2020) [135]. Sarabia Sánchez et al. (2014) [149].
1.34. Personal involvement	Personal involvement	Gazquez Abad et al. (2011) [226]; Gregory and Di Leo (2003) [81]; Rodríguez Sánchez and Sarabia Sánchez (2020) [135]; Sarabia Sánchez et al. (2014) [149].
1.35. Connection and contact with nature.	Connection and contact with nature.	Ibañez Rueda et al. (2022) [221]; Warner and Diaz (2021) [219].
1.36. Life satisfaction	Life satisfaction	Dean et al. (2021) [105]; Syme et al. (2004) [134].
1.37. Self-transcendence	Self-transcendence (universalism vs. benevolence)	Delistavrou (2021) [146].

Note: Source: Own elaboration.

Table A11. External factors to the individual related to water-conservation behavior and/or consumption].

Variable/Factor	Specific Example	Contributions
2.1. Climatic/seasonal.	Drought, water stress (experience of drought), water scarcity, rainfall. Temperature.	Addo at al. (2019) [84]; Akpinar et al. (2018) [88]; Ananga et al. (2019) [110]; Araya et al. (2020) [72]; Arbues et al. (2016) [78]; Bermejo et al. (2021) [228]; Dascher et al. (2014) [150]; Dean et al. (2021) [105]; Deng et al. (2017) [62]; Dolnicar et al. (2012) [97]; Gilbertson et al. (2011) [181]; Gu et al. (2020) [199]; Holland et al. (2019) [127]; Kang et al. (2017) [92]; Khodadad et al. (2022) [124]; Martinez and Maia (2022) [224]; Njoku et al. (2022) [125]; Reddy et al. (2023) [98]; Shahangian et al. (2022) [68]; Wang and Chermak (2021) [139].
2.2. Household composition	Members, age of members, income, religion, culture, education, water-saving devices, smart meters	Addo et al. (2018) [84]; Aisa and Larramona (2012) [215]; Al-Maadid et al. (2022) [107]; Alvarado Espejo et al. (2021) [52]; Andrade et al. (2021) [70]; Aprile and Fiorillo (2017) [182]; Araya et al. (2020) [72]; Arbues et al. (2016) [78]; Barnett et al. (2020) [53]; Bermejo et al. (2021) [228]; Bhanot (2021) [197]; Buday et al. (2021) [71]; Chaudhary et al. (2019) [213]; Daniel et al. (2022) [218]; Fielding et al. (2010) [67]; Fielding et al. (2012) [40]; Gazquez Abad et al. (2011) [226]; Gomez Llanos et al. (2020) [54]; Grespan et al. (2022) [131]; Haeffner et al. (2023) [73]; Harlan et al. (2009) [178]; Hasan et al. (2021) [214]; Jorgensen et al. (2014) [76]; Kalifa et al. (2021) [100]; Kantola et al. (1982) [183]; Khodadad et al. (2022) [124]; Landon et al. (2017) [79]; Landon et al. (2016) [79]; Lavelle and Fahy (2016) [94]; Liu et al. (2020) [155]; Li et al. (2022) [91]; Long et al. (2022) [128]; Martinez Espiñeira and Garcia Valiñas (2013) [192]; Martinez and Maia (2021) [222]; Mass et al. (2017) [130]; Miller and Buys (2008) [112]; Njoku et al. (2022) [125]; Ramsey et al. (2017) [90]; Russell & Knoeri (2020) [56]; Sadalla et al. (2014) [210]; Sarpong and Amankwaa (2022) [82]; Schultz et al. (2019) [39]; Otaki and Maeda (2021) [55]; Pérez Uridales and Garcia Valiñas (2016) [145]; Untaru et al. (2020) [99]; Wang and Dong (2017) [207]; Wolters (2014) [62].

Table A11. *Cont.*

Variable/Factor	Specific Example	Contributions
2.3. Characteristics of the property	Age of the house, size, type of housing, garden, pool, owner/tenant.	Grespan et al. (2022) [131]. Wang and Chermak (2021) [139]. Dean et al. (2021) [105]. Martínez and Maia (2021) [222]. Buday et al. (2021) [71]. Bermejo et al. (2021) [228]. Russell & Knoeri (2020) [56]. Sengupta (2020) [234]. Barnett et al. (2020) [53]. Wang et al. (2019) [211]. Chaudhary et al. (2019) [213]. Landon et al. (2017) [79]. Aprile and Fiorillo (2017) [182]. Mass et al. (2017) [130]. Wang and Dong (2017) [207]. Arbues et al. (2016) [78]. Lavelle and Fahy (2016) [94]. Landon et al. (2016) [79]. Sadalla et al. (2014) [210]. Xavier Garcia et al. (2013) [195]. Fan et al. (2013) [133]. Fielding et al. (2010) [67]. Harlan et al. (2009) [178]. Domene and Sauri (2006) [132]. Syme et al. (2004) [134].
2.4. Incentives/policies to discourage consumption.	Economic incentives. Water tariff. Economic measures. Water consumption/cost information. Water restrictions.	Addo et al. (2018) [84]; Akpinar et al. (2018) [88]; Alvarado Espejo et al. (2021) [52]; Barnett et al. (2020) [53]; Cahn et al. (2020) [217]; Corral Verdugo and Frias Armenta (2006) [123]; Dascher et al. (2014) [150], Dean et al. (2021) [105]; Goette et al. (2019) [203]; Hasan et al. (2021) [214]; Lindsay and Supski (2017) [204]; Liu et al. (2020) [155]; Martinez and Maia (2021) [222]; Mass et al. (2017) [130]; Matikinca et al. (2020) [202]; Rajapaksa et al. (2019) [191]; Tijs et al. (2017) [209]; Wang et al. (2019) [211]; Wang and Chermak (2021) [139].
2.5. Social behavior of the home	Membership in social organizations and/or social activities. Share capital.	Aprile and Fiorillo (2017) [182]; Bermejo et al. (2021) [228]; Syme et al. (2004) [134].
2.6. Contextual factors	Water pollution.	Alvarado Espejo et al. (2021) [52]

Note: Source: Own elaborations.

References

1. United Nations (Ed.) *Water and Climate Change*; United Nations: New York, NY, USA, 2023. Available online: https://www.unwater.org/water-facts/water-and-climate-change (accessed on 11 August 2023).
2. IPCC Water. Contribution of Working Group II to the Sixth Assessment Report of the Intergovernmental Panel on Climate. In *Climate Change 2022: Impacts, Adaptation and Vulnerability*; Cambridge University Press: Cambridge, UK; New York, NY, USA, 2022; pp. 551–712. Available online: https://www.ipcc.ch/report/ar6/wg2/ (accessed on 10 July 2023).
3. Mckenzie-Mohr, D. New ways to promote proenvironmental behavior: Promoting sustainable behavior: An introduction to community-based social marketing. *J. Soc. Issues* **2000**, *56*, 543–554. [CrossRef]
4. Rodriguez-Sanchez, C.; Sancho Esper, F.M.; Campayo-Sánchez, F. A Systematic Review of Social Marketing Interventions to Promote Pro-Environmental Behavior Using CBSM Benchmark Criteria. *Res. Innov. Sustain. Mark.* **2023**, *1*, 32–34. [CrossRef]
5. Buyucek, N.; Kubacki, K.; Rundle-Thiele, S.; Pang, B. A systematic review of stakeholder involvement in social marketing interventions. *Australas. Mark. J.* **2016**, *24*, 8–19. [CrossRef]
6. Pang, B.; Kubacki, K.; Rundle-Thiele, S. Promoting active travel to school: A systematic review (2010–2016). *BMC Public Health* **2017**, *17*, 1–15. [CrossRef]
7. Rundle-Thiele, S.; David, P.; Willmott, T.; Pang, B.; Eagle, L.; Hay, R. Social marketing theory development goals: An agenda to drive change. *J. Mark. Manag.* **2019**, *35*, 160–181. [CrossRef]
8. Carins, J.E.; Rundle-Thiele, S.R.; Fidock, J.J. Seeing through a glass onion: Broadening and deepening formative research in social marketing through a mixed methods approach. *J. Mark. Manag.* **2016**, *32*, 1083–1102. [CrossRef]
9. Rundle-Thiele, S.; Pang, B.; Knox, K.; David, P.; Parkinson, J.; Hussenoeder, F. Generating new directions for reducing dog and koala interactions: A social marketing formative research study. *Australas. J. Environ. Manag.* **2019**, *26*, 173–187. [CrossRef]
10. Spotswood, F.; French, J.; Tapp, A.; Stead, M. Some reasonable but uncomfortable questions about social marketing. *J. Soc. Mark.* **2012**, *2*, 163–175. [CrossRef]
11. Ehret, P.J.; Hodges, H.E.; Kuehl, C.; Brick, C.; Mueller, S.; Anderson, S.E. Systematic Review of Household Water Conservation Interventions Using the Information–Motivation–Behavioral Skills Model. *Environ. Behav.* **2021**, *53*, 485–519. [CrossRef]
12. Koop, S.H.A.; Clevers, S.H.P.; Blokker, E.J.M.; Brouwer, S. Public attitudes towards digital water meters for households. *Sustainability* **2021**, *13*, 6440. [CrossRef]
13. Moglia, M.; Cook, S.; Tapsuwan, S. Promoting water conservation: Where to from here? *Water* **2018**, *10*, 1510. [CrossRef]
14. Zhang, L.; Wang, M.H.; Hu, J.; Ho, Y.S. A review of published wetland research, 1991–2008: Ecological engineering and ecosystem restoration. *Ecol. Eng.* **2010**, *36*, 973–980. [CrossRef]
15. Phulwani, P.R.; Kumar, D.; Goyal, P. A Systematic Literature Review and Bibliometric Analysis of Recycling Behavior. *J. Glob. Mark.* **2020**, *33*, 354–376. [CrossRef]
16. Si, H.; Shi, J.G.; Tang, D.; Wen, S.; Miao, W.; Duan, K. Application of the theory of planned behavior in environmental science: A comprehensive bibliometric analysis. *Int. J. Environ. Res. Public Health* **2019**, *16*, 2788. [CrossRef]
17. Fleith de Medeiros, J.; Bisognin Garlet, T.; Duarte Ribeiro, J.L.; Nogueira Cortimiglia, M. Success factors for environmentally sustainable product innovation: An updated review. *J. Clean. Prod.* **2022**, *345*, 131039. [CrossRef]

18. Esfandiar, K.; Pearce, J.; Dowling, R.; Goh, E. Pro-environmental behaviors in protected areas: A systematic literature review and future research directions. *Tour. Manag. Perspect.* **2022**, *41*, 100943. [CrossRef]
19. Page, M.J.; McKenzie, J.E.; Bossuyt, P.M.; Boutron, I.; Hoffmann, T.C.; Mulrow, C.D.; Moher, D. The PRISMA 2020 statement: An updated guideline for reporting systematic reviews. *Int. J. Surg.* **2021**, *88*, 105906. [CrossRef]
20. Vieira, L.C.; Amaral, F.G. Barriers and strategies applying Cleaner Production: A systematic review. *J. Clean. Prod.* **2016**, *113*, 5–16. [CrossRef]
21. Butler, G.; Ross, K.; Beaman, J.; Hoepner, C.; Baring, R.; Burke da Silva, K. Utilising tourist-generated citizen science data in response to environmental challenges: A systematic literature review. *J. Environ. Manag.* **2023**, *339*, 117889. [CrossRef]
22. Mishra, A.N.; Raj, A.; Pani, A.K. Construal Level Research in Decision Making: Analysis and Pushing Forward the Debate Using Bibliometric Review and Thematic Analysis. *Am. Bus. Rev.* **2020**, *23*, 106–135. [CrossRef]
23. Ricart, S.; Villar-Navascués, R.; Reyes, M.; Rico-Amorós, A.M.; Hernández-Hernández, M.; Toth, E.; Bragalli, C.; Neri, M.; Amelung, B. Water–tourism nexus research in the Mediterranean in the past two decades: A systematic literature review. *Int. J. Water Resour. Dev.* **2023**. *In press*. [CrossRef]
24. Andor, M.A.; Fels, K.M. Behavioral Economics and Energy Conservation—A Systematic Review of Non-price Interventions and Their Causal Effects. *Ecol. Econ.* **2018**, *148*, 178–210. [CrossRef]
25. Souza-Neto, V.; Marques, O.; Mayer, V.F.; Lohmann, G. Lowering the harm of tourist activities: A systematic literature review on nudges. *J. Sustain. Tour.* **2022**, *31*, 2173–2194. [CrossRef]
26. Díaz Tautiva, J.A.; Huaman, J.; Ponce Oliva, R.D. Trends in research on climate change and organizations: A bibliometric analysis (1999–2021). *Manag. Rev. Q.* **2022**. [CrossRef]
27. Wu, M.; Long, R.; Bai, Y.; Chen, H. Knowledge mapping analysis of international research on environmental communication using bibliometrics. *J. Environ. Manag.* **2021**, *298*, 113475. [CrossRef]
28. Fauzi, M.A.; Abidin, N.H.Z.; Suki, N.M.; Budiea, A.M.A. Residential rooftop solar panel adoption behavior: Bibliometric analysis of the past and future trends. *Renew. Energy Focus* **2023**, *45*, 1–9. [CrossRef]
29. Aria, M.; Cuccurullo, C. Bibliometrix: An R-tool for comprehensive science mapping analysis. *J. Informetr.* **2017**, *11*, 959–975. [CrossRef]
30. Kar, S.K.; Harichandan, S. Green marketing innovation and sustainable consumption: A bibliometric analysis. *J. Clean. Prod.* **2022**, *361*, 132290. [CrossRef]
31. Rita, P.; Ramos, R.F. Global research trends in consumer behavior and sustainability in E-Commerce: A bibliometric analysis of the knowledge structure. *Sustainability* **2022**, *14*, 9455. [CrossRef]
32. Zaidi, H.; Azmi, F.T. Workplace pro-environmental behavior: A review and bibliometric analysis. *Int. J. Product. Perform. Manag.* **2022**. *In press*. [CrossRef]
33. Madias, K.; Szymkowiak, A. Residential Sustainable Water Usage and Water Management: Systematic Review and Future Research. *Water* **2022**, *14*, 1027. [CrossRef]
34. Braun, V.; Clarke, V. Using thematic analysis in psychology. *Qual. Res. Psychol.* **2006**, *3*, 77–101. [CrossRef]
35. Byrne, D. A worked example of Braun and Clarke's approach to reflexive thematic analysis. *Qual. Quant.* **2022**, *56*, 1391–1412. [CrossRef]
36. Willig, C. Interpretation and Analysis. In *The Oxford Handbook of Qualitative Research*; Leavy, P., Ed.; Oxford University Press: Oxford, UK, 2013; pp. 259–277.
37. Yang, E.C.L.; Khoo-Lattimore, C.; Arcodia, C. A systematic literature review of risk and gender research in tourism. *Tour. Manag.* **2017**, *58*, 89–100. [CrossRef]
38. Willis, R.M.; Stewart, R.A.; Panuwatwanich, K.; Williams, P.R.; Hollingsworth, A.L. Quantifying the influence of environmental and water conservation attitudes on household end use water consumption. *J. Environ. Manag.* **2011**, *92*, 1996–2009. [CrossRef]
39. Schultz, P.W.; Messina, A.; Tronu, G.; Limas, E.F.; Gupta, R.; Estrada, M. Personalized Normative Feedback and the Moderating Role of Personal Norms: A Field Experiment to Reduce Residential Water Consumption. *Environ. Behav.* **2016**, *48*, 686–710. [CrossRef]
40. Fielding, K.S.; Spinks, A.; Russell, S.; McCrea, R.; Stewart, R.; Gardner, J. An experimental test of voluntary strategies to promote urban water demand management. *J. Environ. Manag.* **2013**, *114*, 343–351. [CrossRef]
41. Aparicio, G.; Iturralde, T.; Maseda, A. Conceptual structure and perspectives on entrepreneurship education research: A bibliometric review. *Eur. Res. Manag. Bus. Econ.* **2019**, *25*, 105–113. [CrossRef]
42. Rejeb, A.; Rejeb, K.; Abdollahi, A.; Treiblmaier, H. The big picture on Instagram research: Insights from a bibliometric analysis. *Telemat. Inform.* **2022**, *73*, 101876. [CrossRef]
43. Siccardi, S.; Villa, V. Trends in Adopting BIM, IoT and DT for Facility Management: A Scientometric Analysis and Keyword Co-Occurrence Network Review. *Buildings* **2023**, *13*, 15. [CrossRef]
44. Casado-Aranda, L.A.; Sánchez-Fernández, J.; Bigne, E.; Smidts, A. The application of neuromarketing tools in communication research: A comprehensive review of trends. *Psychol. Mark.* **2023**, *40*, 1737–1756. [CrossRef]
45. Wang, M.H.; Yu, T.C.; Ho, Y.S. A bibliometric analysis of the performance of Water Research. *Scientometrics* **2010**, *84*, 813–820. [CrossRef]
46. Kalia, P.; Mladenović, D.; Acevedo-Duque, Á. Decoding the Trends and the Emerging Research Directions of Digital Tourism in the Last Three Decades: A Bibliometric Analysis. *SAGE Open* **2022**, 1–23. [CrossRef]

47. Ajzen, I. The theory of planned behavior. *Organ. Behav. Hum. Decis. Process.* **1991**, *50*, 179–211. [CrossRef]
48. Bhatnagar, S.; Sharma, D. Evolution of green finance and its enablers: A bibliometric analysis. Renewable and Sustainable. *Energy Rev.* **2022**, *162*, 112405. [CrossRef]
49. Della Corte, V.; Del Gaudio, G.; Sepe, F.; Sciarelli, F. Sustainable tourism in the open innovation realm: A bibliometric analysis. *Sustainability* **2019**, *11*, 6114. [CrossRef]
50. Mariani, M.M.; Perez-Vega, R.; Wirtz, J. AI in marketing, consumer research and psychology: A systematic literature review and research agenda. *Psychol. Mark.* **2022**, *39*, 755–776. [CrossRef]
51. Sarabia Sánchez, F.J.; Rodríguez Sánchez, C. Attitudes towards saving water, household structural characteristics and water consumption. *Psyecology* **2013**, *4*, 115–137. [CrossRef]
52. Alvarado Espejo, J.M.A.; Ontaneda, W.I.T.; Padilla, N.I.A.; Ochoa-Moreno, W.S. Water saving practices conditioned by socioeconomic factors: A case study of Ecuadorian households. *J. Environ. Manag.* **2021**, *293*, 112818. [CrossRef]
53. Barnett, M.J.; Jackson-Smith, D.; Endter-Wada, J.; Haeffner, M. A multilevel analysis of the drivers of household water consumption in a semi-arid region. *Sci. Total Environ.* **2020**, *712*, 136489. [CrossRef]
54. Gómez-Llanos, E.; Durán-Barroso, P.; Robina-Ramírez, R. Analysis of consumer awareness of sustainable water consumption by the water footprint concept. *Sci. Total Environ.* **2020**, *721*, 137743. [CrossRef] [PubMed]
55. Otaki, Y.; Maeda, A. Water-Saving Tips with a Visualized Indicator Related to the Environment. *Front. Water* **2022**, *4*, 914665. [CrossRef]
56. Russell, S.V.; Knoeri, C. Exploring the psychosocial and behavioral determinants of household water conservation and intention. *Int. J. Water Resour. Dev.* **2020**, *36*, 940–955. [CrossRef]
57. Seyranian, V.; Sinatra, G.M.; Polikoff, M.S. Comparing communication strategies for reducing residential water consumption. *J. Environ. Psychol.* **2015**, *41*, 81–90. [CrossRef]
58. Ajzen, I.; Fishbein, M. *Theory of Reasoned Action-Theory of Planned Behavior 1988*; University of South Florida: Tampa, FL, USA, 2007; pp. 67–98.
59. Schwartz, S.H.; Howard, J.A. Internalized values as motivators of altruism. In *Development and Maintenance of Prosocial Behavior*; Springer: Boston, MA, USA, 1984; pp. 229–255. [CrossRef]
60. Dunlap, R. The new environmental paradigm scale: From marginality to worldwide use. *J. Environ. Educ.* **2008**, *40*, 3–18. [CrossRef]
61. Deng, Y.; Wang, M.; Yousefpour, R. How do people's perceptions and climatic disaster experiences influence their daily behaviors regarding adaptation to climate change?—A case study among young generations. *Sci. Total Environ.* **2017**, *581–582*, 840–847. [CrossRef]
62. Wolters, E.A. Attitude-behavior consistency in household water consumption. *Soc. Sci. J.* **2014**, *51*, 455–463. [CrossRef]
63. Shahangian, S.A.; Tabesh, M.; Yazdanpanah, M. How can socio-psychological factors be related to water-efficiency intention and behaviors among Iranian residential water consumers? *J. Environ. Manag.* **2021**, *288*, 112466. [CrossRef]
64. Maduku, D.K. Water conservation campaigns in an emerging economy: How effective are they? *Int. J. Advert.* **2021**, *40*, 452–472. [CrossRef]
65. Stern, P.C. Toward a coherent theory of environmentally significant behavior. *J. Soc. Issues* **2000**, *56*, 407–424. [CrossRef]
66. Savari, M.; Mombeni, A.S.; Izadi, H. Socio-psychological determinants of Iranian rural households' adoption of water consumption curtailment behaviors. *Sci. Rep.* **2022**, *12*, 13077. [CrossRef] [PubMed]
67. Fielding, K.S.; Thompson, A.; Louis, W.R.; Warren, C. Environmental sustainability: Understanding the attitudes and behavior of Australian households. *AHURI Final Rep.* **2010**, *152*, 1–132.
68. Shahangian, S.A.; Tabesh, M.; Yazdanpanah, M.; Zobeidi, T.; Raoof, M.A. Promoting the adoption of residential water conservation behaviors as a preventive policy to sustainable urban water management. *J. Environ. Manag.* **2022**, *313*, 115005. [CrossRef]
69. Díaz, J.; Odera, E.; Warner, L. Delving deeper: Exploring the influence of psycho-social wellness on water conservation behavior. *J. Environ. Manag.* **2020**, *264*, 110404. [CrossRef] [PubMed]
70. Andrade, E.; Seoane, G.; Vila-Tojo, S.; Gómez-Román, C.; Sabucedo, J.-M. Psychological and situational variables associated with objective knowledge on water-related issues in a northern Spanish city. *Int. J. Environ. Res. Public Health* **2021**, *18*, 3213. [CrossRef] [PubMed]
71. Buday, A.; Zollinger, B.; Hammersmith, A.; Heine, K. Thirsting for Sustainability: Water Conservation in a Great Plains City. *Great Plains Res.* **2021**, *31*, 1–16. [CrossRef]
72. Araya, F.; Osman, K.; Faust, K.M. Perceptions versus reality: Assessing residential water conservation efforts in the household. *Resour. Conserv. Recycl.* **2020**, *162*, 105020. [CrossRef]
73. Haeffner, M.; Jackson-Smith, D.; Barnett, M.J. Categorizing relative water use perception bias using household surveys and monthly water bills. *J. Environ. Manag.* **2023**, *334*, 117443. [CrossRef]
74. Russell, S.; Fielding, K. Water demand management research: A psychological perspective. *Water Resour. Res.* **2010**, *46*, W05302. [CrossRef]
75. Caspers, C.G.W. Role of Trust in Adopting Consumer Social Responsible Behavior in the Context of Water Use in Domestic Households. *South East Eur. J. Econ. Bus.* **2020**, *15*, 1–13. [CrossRef]
76. Jorgensen, B.S.; Martin, J.F.; Pearce, M.W.; Willis, E.M. Predicting Household Water Consumption with Individual-Level Variables. *Environ. Behav.* **2014**, *46*, 872–897. [CrossRef]

77. Dolnicar, S.; Hurlimann, A. Australians' water conservation behaviors and attitudes. *Aust. J. Water Resour.* **2010**, *14*, 43–53. [CrossRef]
78. Arbués, F.; Bolsa, M.Á.; Villanúa, I. Which factors determine water saving behavior? evidence from Spanish households. *Urban Water J.* **2016**, *13*, 511–520. [CrossRef]
79. Landon, A.C.; Kyle, G.T.; Kaiser, R.A. Predicting compliance with an information-based residential outdoor water conservation program. *J. Hydrol.* **2016**, *536*, 26–36. [CrossRef]
80. Timm, S.N.; Deal, B.M. Understanding the behavioral influences behind Singapore's water management strategies. *J. Environ. Plan. Manag.* **2018**, *61*, 1654–1673. [CrossRef]
81. Gregory, G.D.; Di Leo, M. Repeated Behavior and Environmental Psychology: The Role of Personal Involvement and Habit Formation in Explaining Water Consumption. *J. Appl. Soc. Psychol.* **2003**, *33*, 1261–1296. [CrossRef]
82. Sarpong, K.A.; Amankwaa, G. Household behavioral intention, environmental habit and attitude related to efficient water management: An empirical analysis on pro-environmental behavior among urban residents. *H2Open J.* **2022**, *5*, 438–455. [CrossRef]
83. Madias, K.; Borusiak, B.; Szymkowiak, A. The role of knowledge about water consumption in the context of intentions to use IoT water metrics. *Front. Environ. Sci.* **2022**, *10*, 934965. [CrossRef]
84. Addo, I.B.; Thoms, M.C.; Parsons, M. The influence of water-conservation messages on reducing household water use. *Appl. Water Sci.* **2019**, *9*, 126. [CrossRef]
85. Céspedes Restrepo, J.D.; Morales-Pinzón, T. Effects of feedback information on the household consumption of water and electricity: A case study in Colombia. *J. Environ. Manag.* **2020**, *262*, 110315. [CrossRef] [PubMed]
86. Otaki, Y.; Ueda, K.; Sakura, O. Effects of feedback about community water consumption on residential water conservation. *J. Clean. Prod.* **2017**, *143*, 719–730. [CrossRef]
87. Kollmuss, A.; Agyeman, J. Mind the Gap: Why do people act environmentally and what are the barriers to pro-environmental behavior? *Environ. Educ. Res.* **2002**, *8*, 239–260. [CrossRef]
88. Akpinar, M.G.; Gul, M.; Ceylan, R.F.; Gulcan, S. Evaluation of the factors affecting water-saving attitudes of urban life on the verge of the next century: A case study of the Mediterranean region of Turkey. *J. Water Sanit. Hyg. Dev.* **2018**, *8*, 340–348. [CrossRef]
89. Keramitsoglou, K.M.; Tsagarakis, K.P. Raising effective awareness for domestic water saving: Evidence from an environmental educational programme in Greece. *Water Policy* **2011**, *13*, 828–844. [CrossRef]
90. Ramsey, E.; Berglund, E.Z.; Goyal, R. The impact of demographic factors, beliefs, and social influences on residential water consumption and implications for non-price policies in urban India. *Water* **2017**, *9*, 844. [CrossRef]
91. Li, Y.; Wang, B.; Cui, M. Environmental Concern, Environmental Knowledge, and Residents' Water Conservation Behavior: Evidence from China. *Water* **2022**, *14*, 2087. [CrossRef]
92. Kang, J.; Grable, K.; Hustvedt, G.; Ahn, M. Sustainable water consumption: The perspective of Hispanic consumers. *J. Environ. Psychol.* **2017**, *50*, 94–103. [CrossRef]
93. Clark, W.A.; Finley, J.C. Determinants of water conservation intention in Blagoevgrad, Bulgaria. *Soc. Nat. Resour.* **2007**, *20*, 613–627. [CrossRef]
94. Lavelle, M.J.; Fahy, F. What's consuming Ireland? Exploring expressed attitudes and reported behaviors towards the environment and consumption across three case study locations on the island of Ireland. *Ir. Geogr.* **2016**, *49*, 29–54. [CrossRef]
95. Chenoweth, J.; López-Avilés, A.; Morse, S.; Druckman, A. Water consumption and subjective wellbeing: An analysis of British households. *Ecol. Econ.* **2016**, *130*, 186–194. [CrossRef]
96. Grafton, R.Q.; Ward, M.B.; To, H.; Kompas, T. Determinants of residential water consumption: Evidence and analysis from a 10-country household survey. *Water Resour. Res.* **2011**, *47*, W08537. [CrossRef]
97. Dolnicar, S.; Hurlimann, A.; Grun, B. Water conservation behavior in Australia. *J. Environ. Manag.* **2012**, *105*, 44–52. [CrossRef] [PubMed]
98. Reddy, R.A.; Sengupta, R.; Jackson, B.M.; Lewis, C. Development of a new measure to check attitude towards water conservation. *MethodsX* **2023**, *10*, 101992. [CrossRef]
99. Untaru, E.-N.; Ispas, A.; Han, H. Exploring the synergy between customer home-based and hotel-based water consumption and conservation behaviors: An empirical approach. *J. Consum. Behav.* **2020**, *19*, 542–555. [CrossRef]
100. Kalifa, A.; Al-Maadid, A.; Koutiva, I.; Makropoulos, C. Individual water consumption behavior in relation to urban residential dynamics: The Case of Qatar. *Urban Water J.* **2021**, *18*, 806–816. [CrossRef]
101. Marzouk, O.A.; Mahrous, A.A. Sustainable Consumption Behavior of Energy and Water-Efficient Products in a Resource-Constrained Environment. *J. Glob. Mark.* **2020**, *33*, 335–353. [CrossRef]
102. Lowe, B.; Lynch, D.; Lowe, J. Reducing household water consumption: A social marketing approach. *J. Mark. Manag.* **2015**, *31*, 378–408. [CrossRef]
103. Graf, C.; Suanet, B.; Wiepking, P.; Merz, E.M. Social norms offer explanation for inconsistent effects of incentives on prosocial behavior. *J. Econ. Behav. Organ.* **2023**, *211*, 429–441. [CrossRef]
104. Ramli, U. Social Norms Based Eco-Feedback for Household Water Consumption. *Sustainability* **2021**, *13*, 2796. [CrossRef]
105. Dean, A.J.; Kneebone, S.; Tull, F.; Lauren, N.; Smith, L.D.G. 'Stickiness' of water-saving behaviors: What factors influence whether behaviors are maintained or given up? *Resour. Conserv. Recycl.* **2021**, *169*, 105531. [CrossRef]

106. Warner, L.A. Who conserves and who approves? Predicting water conservation intentions in urban landscapes with referent groups beyond the traditional 'important others'. *Urban For. Urban Green.* **2021**, *60*, 127070. [CrossRef]
107. Al-Maadid, A.; Akesson, J.; Bernstein, D.H.; Chakravarti, J.; Khalifa, A. Understanding Water Consumption in Qatar: Evidence from a Nationally Representative Survey. *Urban Water J.* **2022**. *In press*. [CrossRef]
108. Lede, E.; Meleady, R.; Seger, C.R. Optimizing the influence of social norms interventions: Applying social identity insights to motivate residential water conservation. *J. Environ. Psychol.* **2019**, *62*, 105–114. [CrossRef]
109. De Groot, J.I.; Steg, L. Mean or green? Values, morality and environmental significant behavior. *Conserv. Lett.* **2009**, *2*, 61–66. [CrossRef]
110. Ananga, E.O.; Becerra, T.A.; Peaden, C.; Pappas, C. Examining water conservation behaviors and attitudes: Evidence from the city of Ada, Oklahoma, USA. *Sustain. Water Resour. Manag.* **2019**, *5*, 1651–1663. [CrossRef]
111. Bronfman, N.C.; Cisternas, P.C.; López-Vázquez, E.; la Maza, C.; Oyanedel, J.C. Understanding attitudes and pro-environmental behaviors in a Chilean community. *Sustainability* **2015**, *7*, 14133–14152. [CrossRef]
112. Miller, E.; Buys, L. The impact of social capital on residential water-affecting behaviors in a drought-prone Australian community. *Soc. Nat. Resour.* **2008**, *21*, 244–257. [CrossRef]
113. Wahid, N.A.; Fadzil, S.F.S.; Ariffin, S.K. Influences of Problem Awareness, Awareness of Consequences and Ascription of Responsibility on Consumer's Personal Norm to Prevent Water Wastage Behavior. *Environ. Ecol. Res.* **2022**, *10*, 275–283. [CrossRef]
114. Chen, L.; Dong, C.; Zhang, Y. An Online Experiment Evaluating the Effects of Social Endorsement Cues, Message Source, and Responsibility Attribution on Young Adults' COVID-19 Vaccination Intentions. *SAGE Open* **2022**, *12*, 1–12. [CrossRef]
115. Diener, E. Subjective Well-Being. *Psychol. Bull.* **1984**, *95*, 542–575. [CrossRef]
116. Manríquez-Betanzos, J.C.; Corral-Verdugo, V.; Vanegas-Rico, M.C.; Fraijo-Sing, B.S.; Tapia-Fonllem, C.O. Positive (gratitude, eudaimonia) and negative (scarcity, costs) determinants of water conservation behaviour. *Psyecology* **2016**, *7*, 178–200. [CrossRef]
117. MacInnes, S.; Grün, B.; Dolnicar, S. Habit drives sustainable tourist behavior. *Ann. Tour. Res.* **2022**, *92*, 103329. [CrossRef]
118. Straus, J.; Chang, H.; Hong, C.Y. An exploratory path analysis of attitudes, behaviors and summer water consumption in the Portland Metropolitan Area. *Sustain. Cities Soc.* **2016**, *23*, 68–77. [CrossRef]
119. Lauren, N.; Fielding, K.S.; Smith, L.; Louis, W.R. You did, so you can and you will: Self-efficacy as a mediator of spillover from easy to more difficult pro-environmental behavior. *J. Environ. Psychol.* **2016**, *48*, 191–199. [CrossRef]
120. Jorgensen, B.S.; Martin, J.F.; Pearce, M.W.; Willis, E.M. Aligning theory and measurement in behavioral models of water conservation. *Water Policy* **2015**, *17*, 762–776. [CrossRef]
121. Rondinel Oviedo, D.R.; Sarmiento Pastor, J.M. Water: Consumption, usage patterns, and residential infrastructure. A comparative analysis of three regions in the Lima metropolitan area. *Water Int.* **2020**, *45*, 824–846. [CrossRef]
122. Corral-Verdugo, V.; Bechtel, R.B.; Fraijo-Sing, B. Environmental beliefs and water conservation: An empirical study. *J. Environ. Psychol.* **2003**, *23*, 247–257. [CrossRef]
123. Corral-Verdugo, V.; Frías-Armenta, M.; Pérez-Urias, F.; Orduña-Cabrera, V.; Espinoza-Gallego, N. Residential water consumption, motivation for conserving water and the continuing tragedy of the commons. *Environ. Manag.* **2002**, *30*, 527–535. [CrossRef]
124. Khodadad, M.; Sanei, M.; Narvaez-Montoya, C.; Aguilar-Barajas, I. Climatic Hazards and the Associated Impacts on Households' Willingness to Adopt Water-Saving Measures: Evidence from Mexico. *Sustainability* **2022**, *14*, 5817. [CrossRef]
125. Njoku, P.O.; Durowoju, O.S.; Uhunamure, S.E.; Makungo, R. Investigating the Attitude of Domestic Water Use in Urban and Rural Households in South Africa. *Water* **2022**, *14*, 210. [CrossRef]
126. Bruvold, W.H.; Smith, B.R. Developing and assessing a model of residential water conservation. *Jawara J. Am. Water Resour. Assoc.* **1988**, *24*, 661–669. [CrossRef]
127. Holland, D.; Janet, K.; Landrum, A. Experience is Key: Examining the Relative Importance of Factors Influencing Individuals' Water Conservation. *Water* **2019**, *11*, 1870. [CrossRef]
128. Long, H.; Shi, S.; Tang, Z.; Zhang, S. Does living alone increase the consumption of social resources? *Environ. Sci. Pollut. Res.* **2022**, *29*, 71911–71922. [CrossRef] [PubMed]
129. Makki, A.A.; Stewart, R.A.; Panuwatwanich, K.; Beal, C. Revealing the determinants of shower water end use consumption: Enabling better targeted urban water conservation strategies. *J. Clean. Prod.* **2013**, *60*, 129–146. [CrossRef]
130. Maas, A.; Goemans, C.; Manning, D.; Kroll, S.; Arabi, M.; Rodriguez-McGoffina, M. Evaluating the effect of conservation motivations on residential water demand. *J. Environ. Manag.* **2017**, *196*, 394–401. [CrossRef] [PubMed]
131. Grespan, A.; Garcia, J.; Brikalski, M.P.; Henning, E.; Kalbusch, A. Assessment of water consumption in households using statistical analysis and regression trees. *Sustain. Cities Soc.* **2022**, *87*, 104186. [CrossRef]
132. Domene, E.; Saurí, D. Urbanisation and water consumption: Influencing factors in the metropolitan region of Barcelona. *Urban Stud.* **2006**, *43*, 1605–1623. [CrossRef]
133. Fan, L.; Liu, G.; Wang, F.; Geissen, V.; Ritsema, C.J.; Tong, Y. Water use patterns and conservation in households of Wei River Basin, China. *Resour. Conserv. Recycl.* **2013**, *74*, 45–53. [CrossRef]
134. Syme, G.J.; Shao, Q.; Po, M.; Campbell, E. Predicting and understanding home garden water use. *Landsc. Urban Plan.* **2004**, *68*, 121–128. [CrossRef]
135. Rodriguez-Sanchez, C.; Sarabia-Sanchez, F.J. Does water context matter in water conservation decision behaviour? *Sustainability* **2020**, *12*, 3026. [CrossRef]

136. McKenzie-Mohr, D.; Schultz, P.W. Choosing effective behavior change tools. *Soc. Mark. Q.* **2014**, *20*, 35–46. [CrossRef]
137. Anibaldi, R.; Rundle-Thiele, S.; David, P.; Roemer, C. Theoretical underpinnings in research investigating barriers for implementing environmentally sustainable farming practices: Insights from a systematic literature review. *Land* **2021**, *10*, 386. [CrossRef]
138. Liberman, N.; Trope, Y. The role of feasibility and desirability considerations in near and distant future decisions: A test of temporal construal theory. *J. Personal. Soc. Psychol.* **1998**, *75*, 5. [CrossRef]
139. Wang, J.; Chermak, J.M. Is less always more? Conservation, efficiency and water education programs. *Ecol. Econ.* **2021**, *184*, 106994. [CrossRef]
140. Zhuang, J.; Lapinski, M.K.; Peng, W. Crafting messages to promote water conservation: Using time-framed messages to boost conservation actions in the United States and China. *J. Appl. Psychol.* **2018**, *48*, 248–256. [CrossRef]
141. do Canto, N.R.; Grunert, K.G.; Dutra de Barcellos, M. Goal-framing theory in environmental behaviors: Review, future research agenda and possible applications in behavioral change. *J. Soc. Mark.* **2023**, *13*, 20–40. [CrossRef]
142. Vazquez-Casaubon, E.C.; Cauberghe, V.; Van de Sompel, D. I conserve more water than others, do I? An exploratory study examining self-assessment misperceptions of water conservation. *Environ. Dev. Sustain.* **2023**. [CrossRef]
143. Balnave, J.; Adeyeye, K. A comparative study of attitudes and preferences for water efficiency in homes. *J. Water Supply Res. Technol. AQUA* **2013**, *62*, 515–524. [CrossRef]
144. Casaló, L.V.; Escario, J.J.; Rodriguez-Sanchez, C. Analyzing differences between different types of pro-environmental behaviors: Do attitude intensity and type of knowledge matter? *Resour. Conserv. Recycl.* **2019**, *149*, 56–64. [CrossRef]
145. Pérez Urdiales, M.; García Valiñas, M.T. Efficient water-using technologies and habits: A disaggregated analysis in the water sector. *Ecol. Econ.* **2016**, *128*, 117–129. [CrossRef]
146. Delistavrou, A. Water and energy conservation in Greece: The impact of values and attitudes. *Int. J. Sustain. Energy* **2021**, *40*, 602–615. [CrossRef]
147. van Valkengoed, A.M.; Abrahamse, W.; Steg, L. To select effective interventions for pro-environmental behaviour change, we need to consider determinants of behaviour. *Nat. Hum. Behav.* **2022**, *6*, 1482–1492. [CrossRef]
148. Jaeger, C.M.; Schultz, P.W. Coupling social norms and commitments: Testing the underdetected nature of social influence. *J. Environ. Psychol.* **2017**, *51*, 199–208. [CrossRef]
149. Sarabia Sánchez, F.J.; Rodríguez Sánchez, C.; Hyder, A. The role of personal involvement, credibility and efficacy of conduct in reported water conservation behaviour. *J. Environ. Psychol.* **2014**, *38*, 206–216. [CrossRef]
150. Dascher, E.D.; Kang, J.; Hustvedt, G. Water sustainability: Environmental attitude, drought attitude and motivation. *Int. J. Consum. Stud.* **2014**, *38*, 467–474. [CrossRef]
151. Schneider, C.R.; Zaval, L.; Markowitz, E.M. Positive emotions and climate change. *Curr. Opin. Behav. Sci.* **2021**, *42*, 114–120. [CrossRef]
152. Gkargkavouzi, A.; Halkos, G.; Matsiori, S. Environmental behavior in a private-sphere context: Integrating theories of planned behavior and value belief norm, self-identity and habit. *Resour. Conserv. Recycl.* **2019**, *148*, 145–156. [CrossRef]
153. Shahangian, S.A.; Tabesh, M.; Yazdanpanah, M. Psychosocial determinants of household adoption of water-efficiency behaviors in Tehran capital, Iran: Application of the social cognitive theory. *Urban Clim.* **2021**, *39*, 100935. [CrossRef]
154. Walter, N.; Demetriades, S.Z.; Murphy, S.T. Involved, United, and Efficacious: Could Self-Affirmation Be the Solution to California's Drought? *Health Commun.* **2017**, *32*, 1161–1170. [CrossRef] [PubMed]
155. Liu, H.; Zhao, Y.; Li, H.; Wang, L.; Wang, Q. Individual water-saving response based on complex adaptive system theory: Case study of Beijing City, China. *Water* **2020**, *12*, 1478. [CrossRef]
156. Abu-Bakar, H.; Williams, L.; Hallett, S.H. A review of household water demand management and consumption measurement. *J. Clean. Prod.* **2021**, *292*, 125872. [CrossRef]
157. Asprilla Echeverría, J.M. Cross-country evidence for social dimensions of urban water consumption during droughts. *J. Clean. Prod.* **2020**, *260*, 120895. [CrossRef]
158. Benzoni, N.; Telenko, C. A review of intervention studies aimed at domestic water conservation. In *Lecture Notes in Computer Science (Including Subseries Lecture Notes in Artificial Intelligence and Lecture Notes in Bioinformatics)*; Springer: Cham, Switzerland, 2016; Volume 9747, pp. 427–438. [CrossRef]
159. Carvalho, I.D.C.; Calijuri, M.L.; Assemany, P.P.; Silva, M.D.F.M.E.; Moreira Neto, R.F.; Santiago, A.D.F.; De Souza, M.H.B. Sustainable airport environments: A review of water conservation practices in airports. *Resour. Conserv. Recycl.* **2013**, *74*, 27–36. [CrossRef]
160. Grilli, G.; Curtis, J. Encouraging pro-environmental behaviours: A review of methods and approaches. *Renew. Sustain. Energy Rev.* **2021**, *135*, 110039. [CrossRef]
161. Hall, C.M.; Dayal, N.; Majstorović, D.; Mills, H.; Paul-Andrews, L.; Wallace, C.; Truong, V.D. Accommodation consumers and providers' attitudes, behaviours and practices for sustainability: A systematic review. *Sustainability* **2016**, *8*, 625. [CrossRef]
162. Hurlimann, A.; Dolnicar, S.; Meyer, P. Understanding behaviour to inform water supply management in developed nations—A review of literature. conceptual model and research agenda. *J. Environ. Manag.* **2009**, *91*, 47–56. [CrossRef] [PubMed]
163. Inman, D.; Jeffrey, P. A review of residential water conservation tool performance and influences on implementation effectiveness. *Urban Water J.* **2006**, *3*, 127–143. [CrossRef]

164. Jorgensen, B.; Graymore, M.; O'Toole, K. Household water use behavior: An integrated model. *J. Environ. Manag.* **2009**, *91*, 227–236. [CrossRef]
165. Koop, S.H.A.; Van Dorssen, A.J.; Brouwer, S. Enhancing domestic water conservation behaviour: A review of empirical studies on influencing tactics. *J. Environ. Manag.* **2019**, *247*, 867–876. [CrossRef]
166. Liu, A.; Mukheibir, P. Digital metering feedback and changes in water consumption—A review. *Resour. Conserv. Recycl.* **2018**, *134*, 136–148. [CrossRef]
167. Moore, H.E.; Boldero, J. Designing interventions that last: A classification of environmental behaviors in relation to the activities, costs, and effort involved for adoption and maintenance. *Front. Psychol.* **2017**, *8*, 1874. [CrossRef] [PubMed]
168. Ricart, S.; Villar-Navascués, R.A.; Hernández-Hernández, M.; Rico-Amorós, A.M.; Olcina-Cantos, J.; Moltó-Mantero, E. Extending natural limits to address water scarcity? The role of non-conventional water fluxes in climate change adaptation capacity: A review. *Sustainability* **2021**, *13*, 2473. [CrossRef]
169. Sanguinetti, A.; Dombrovski, K.; Sikand, S. Information, timing, and display: A design-behavior framework for improving the effectiveness of eco-feedback. *Energy Res. Soc. Sci.* **2018**, *39*, 55–68. [CrossRef]
170. Stankuniene, G.; Streimikiene, D.; Kyriakopoulos, G.L. Systematic literature review on behavioral barriers of climate change mitigation in households. *Sustainability* **2020**, *12*, 7369. [CrossRef]
171. Syme, G.J.; Nancarrow, B.E.; Seligman, C. The evaluation of information campaigns to promote voluntary household water conservation. *Eval. Rev.* **2000**, *24*, 539–578. [CrossRef]
172. Warren, C.; Becken, S. Saving energy and water in tourist accommodation: A systematic literature review (1987–2015). *Int. J. Tour. Res.* **2017**, *19*, 289–303. [CrossRef]
173. Weis, D.S. Systematic Literature Review on Impacts and Indicators for Measuring Costs and Benefits of Water Sector Related Interventions. *SSRN Electron. J.* **2019**, 18–20. [CrossRef]
174. Voskamp, I.M.; Sutton, N.B.; Stremke, S.; Rijnaarts, H.H.M. A systematic review of factors influencing spatiotemporal variability in urban water and energy consumption. *J. Clean. Prod.* **2020**, *256*, 120310. [CrossRef]
175. Gilg, A.; Barr, S. Behavioural attitudes towards water saving? Evidence from a study of environmental actions. *Ecol. Econ.* **2006**, *57*, 400–414. [CrossRef]
176. Lam, S.P. Predicting intention to save water: Theory of planned behavior, response efficacy, vulnerability, and perceived efficiency of alternative solutions. *J. Appl. Soc. Psychol.* **2006**, *36*, 2803–2824. [CrossRef]
177. Randolph, B.; Troy, P. Attitudes to conservation and water consumption. *Environ. Sci. Policy* **2008**, *11*, 441–455. [CrossRef]
178. Harlan, S.L.; Yabiku, S.T.; Larsen, L.; Brazel, A.J. Household water consumption in an arid city: Affluence, affordance, and attitudes. *Soc. Nat. Resour.* **2009**, *22*, 691–709. [CrossRef]
179. Attari, S.Z. Perceptions of water use. *Proc. Natl. Acad. Sci. USA* **2014**, *111*, 5129–5134. [CrossRef] [PubMed]
180. Kurz, T.; Donaghue, N.; Walker, I. Utilizing a social-ecological framework to promote water and energy conservation: A field experiment. *J. Appl. Soc. Psychol.* **2005**, *35*, 1281–1300. [CrossRef]
181. Gilbertson, M.; Hurlimann, A.; Dolnicar, S. Does water context influence behaviour and attitudes to water conservation? *Australas. J. Environ. Manag.* **2011**, *18*, 47–60. [CrossRef]
182. Aprile, M.C.; Fiorillo, D. Water conservation behavior and environmental concerns: Evidence from a representative sample of Italian individuals. *J. Clean. Prod.* **2017**, *159*, 119–129. [CrossRef]
183. Kantola, S.J.; Syme, G.J.; Campbell, N.A. The Role of Individual Differences and External Variables in a Test of the Sufficiency of Fishbein's Model to Explain Behavioral Intentions to Conserve Water. *J. Appl. Soc. Psychol.* **1982**, *12*, 70–83. [CrossRef]
184. Stewart, R.A.; Willis, R.M.; Panuwatwanich, K.; Sahin, O. Showering behavioural response to alarming visual display monitors: Longitudinal mixed method study. *Behav. Inf. Technol.* **2013**, *32*, 695–711. [CrossRef]
185. Suárez Varela, M.; Guardiola, J.; González Gómez, F. Do Pro-environmental Behaviors and Awareness Contribute to Improve Subjective Well-being? *Appl. Res. Qual. Life* **2016**, *11*, 429–444. [CrossRef]
186. Mondéjar Jiménez, J.A.; Cordente Rodríguez, M.; Meseguer Santamaría, M.L.; Gázquez Abad, J.C. Environmental Behavior and Water Saving in Spanish Housing. *Int. J. Environ. Res.* **2011**, *5*, 1–10.
187. Hamilton, L.C. Saving water: A Causal Model of Household Conservation. *Sociol. Perspect.* **1983**, *26*, 355–374. [CrossRef]
188. Moore, S.; Murphy, M.; Watson, R. A longitudinal study of domestic water conservation behavior. *Popul. Environ.* **1994**, *16*, 175–189. [CrossRef]
189. Torres, M.M.J.; Carlsson, F. Direct and spillover effects of a social information campaign on residential water-savings. *J. Environ. Econ. Manag.* **2018**, *92*, 222–243. [CrossRef]
190. Richter, C.P. Usage of dishwashers: Observation of consumer habits in the domestic environment. *Int. J. Consum. Stud.* **2011**, *35*, 180–186. [CrossRef]
191. Rajapaksa, D.; Gifford, R.; Torgler, B.; Garcia-Valiñas, M.; Athukorala, W.; Managi, S.; Wilson, C. Do monetary and non-monetary incentives influence environmental attitudes and behavior? Evidence from an experimental analysis. *Resour. Conserv. Recycl.* **2019**, *149*, 168–176. [CrossRef]
192. Martínez Espiñeira, R.; García Valiñas, M.Á. Adopting versus adapting: Adoption of water-saving technology versus water conservation habits in Spain. *Int. J. Water Resour. Dev.* **2013**, *29*, 400–414. [CrossRef]
193. Segev, S. Modelling household conservation behaviour among ethnic consumers: The path from values to behaviours. *Int. J. Consum. Stud.* **2015**, *39*, 193–202. [CrossRef]

194. Richter, C.P.; Stamminger, R. Water Consumption in the Kitchen—A Case Study in Four European Countries. *Water Resour. Manag.* **2012**, *26*, 1639–1649. [CrossRef]
195. Garcia, X.; Ribas, A.; Llausàs, A.; Saurí, D. Socio-demographic profiles in suburban developments: Implications for water-related attitudes and behaviors along the Mediterranean coast. *Appl. Geogr.* **2013**, *41*, 46–54. [CrossRef]
196. Chang, G. Factors influencing water conservation behavior among urban residents in China's arid areas. *Water Policy* **2013**, *15*, 691–704. [CrossRef]
197. Bhanot, S.P. Isolating the effect of injunctive norms on conservation behavior: New evidence from a field experiment in California. *Organ. Behav. Hum. Decis. Process.* **2021**, *163*, 30–42. [CrossRef]
198. Liobikiene, G.; Minelgaite, A. Energy and resource-saving behaviours in European Union countries: The Campbell paradigm and goal framing theory approaches. *Sci. Total Environ.* **2021**, *750*, 141745. [CrossRef]
199. Gu, D.; Jiang, J.; Zhang, Y.; Sun, Y.; Jiang, W.; Du, X.P. Concern for the future and saving the earth: When does ecological resource scarcity promote pro-environmental behavior? *J. Environ. Psychol.* **2020**, *72*, 101501. [CrossRef]
200. Bhanot, S.P. Rank and response: A field experiment on peer information and water use behavior. *J. Econ. Psychol.* **2017**, *62*, 155–172. [CrossRef]
201. Schultz, W.; Javey, S.; Sorokina, A. Social Comparison as a Tool to Promote Residential Water Conservation. *Front. Water* **2019**, *1*. [CrossRef]
202. Matikinca, P.; Ziervogel, G.; Enqvist, J.P. Drought response impacts on household water use practices in Cape Town. South Africa. *Water Policy* **2020**, *22*, 483–500. [CrossRef]
203. Goette, L.; Leong, C.; Qian, N. Motivating household water conservation: A field experiment in Singapore. *PLoS ONE* **2019**, *14*, e0211891. [CrossRef]
204. Lindsay, J.; Supski, S. Changing household water consumption practices after drought in three Australian cities. *Geoforum* **2017**, *84*, 51–58. [CrossRef]
205. Rogers, Z.; Bragg, E. The power of connection: Sustainable lifestyles and sense of place. *Ecopsychology* **2012**, *4*, 307–318. [CrossRef]
206. Tom, G.; Tauchus, G.; Williams, J.; Tong, S. The role of communicative feedback in successful water conservation programs. *Appl. Environ. Educ. Commun.* **2011**, *10*, 80–90. [CrossRef]
207. Wang, C.H.; Dong, H. Responding to the drought: A spatial statistical approach to investigating residential water consumption in Fresno. California. *Sustainability* **2017**, *9*, 240. [CrossRef]
208. Garcia, X.; Muro, M.; Ribas, A.; Llausàs, A.; Jeffrey, P.; Saurí, D. Attitudes and behaviours towards water conservation on the Mediterranean coast: The role of socio-demographic and place-attachment factors. *Water Int.* **2013**, *38*, 283–296. [CrossRef]
209. Tijs, M.S.; Karremans, J.C.; Veling, H.; de Lange, M.A.; van Meegeren, P.; Lion, R. Saving water to save the environment: Contrasting the effectiveness of environmental and monetary appeals in a residential water saving intervention. *Soc. Influ.* **2017**, *12*, 69–79. [CrossRef]
210. Sadalla, E.; Berlin, A.; Neel, R.; Ledlow, S. Priorities in Residential Water Use: A Trade-Off Analysis. *Environ. Behav.* **2014**, *46*, 303–328. [CrossRef]
211. Wang, Y.H.; Chang, M.C.; Liou, J.R. Effects of water-saving education in Taiwan on public water knowledge, attitude, and behavior intention change. *Water Policy* **2019**, *21*, 964–979. [CrossRef]
212. Katz, D.; Kronrod, A.; Grinstein, A.; Nisan, U. Still Waters Run Deep: Comparing Assertive and Suggestive Language in Water Conservation Campaigns. *Water* **2018**, *10*, 275. [CrossRef]
213. Chaudhary, A.K.; Warner, L.A.; Ali, A.D. Using perceived benefits to segment residential landscape irrigation users. *Urban For. Urban Green.* **2019**, *38*, 318–329. [CrossRef]
214. Hasan, H.H.; Razali, S.F.M.; Razali, N.H.M. Does the household save water? Evidence from behavioral analysis. *Sustainability* **2021**, *13*, 641. [CrossRef]
215. Aisa, R.; Larramona, G. Household water saving: Evidence from Spain. *Water Resour. Res.* **2012**, *48*. [CrossRef]
216. Lamm, A.J.; Warner, L.A.; Lundy, L.K.; Bommidi, J.S.; Beattie, P.N. Informing water-saving communication in the United States using the situational theory of problem solving. *Landsc. Urban Plan.* **2018**, *180*, 217–222. [CrossRef]
217. Cahn, A.; Katz, D.; Ghermandi, A. Analyzing Water Customer Preferences for Online Feedback Technologies in Israel: A Prototype Study. *J. Water Resour. Plan. Manag.* **2020**, *146*, 06020002. [CrossRef]
218. Daniel, D.; Pande, S.; Rietveld, L. Endogeneity in water use behaviour across case studies of household water treatment adoption in developing countries. *World Dev. Perspect.* **2022**, *25*, 100385. [CrossRef]
219. Warner, L.A.; Diaz, J.M.; Díaz, J.M.; Diaz, J.M. Amplifying the Theory of Planned behavior with connectedness to water to inform impactful water conservation program planning and evaluation. *J. Agric. Educ. Ext.* **2021**, *27*, 229–253. [CrossRef]
220. Graymore, M.L.M.; Wallis, A.; O'Toole, K. Understanding drivers and barriers: The key to water use behaviour change. *Water Sci. Technol. Water Supply* **2010**, *10*, 679–688. [CrossRef]
221. Ibáñez-Rueda, N.; Guardiola, J.; González-Gómez, F.; Ibanez-Rueda, N.; Guardiola, J.; Gonzalez-Gomez, F.; Ibáñez-Rueda, N.; Guardiola, J.; González-Gómez, F. The role of nature contact and connectedness to nature as determinants of household water use: A case study from Spain. *Water Environ. J.* **2022**, *36*, 282–291. [CrossRef]
222. Martinez, D.M.; Maia, A.G.; Martínez, D.M.; Maia, A.G. The Effect of Social Behavior on Residential Water Consumption. *Water* **2021**, *13*, 1184. [CrossRef]

223. Hodges, H.; Kuehl, C.; Anderson, S.E.; Ehret, P.J.; Brick, C. How Managers Can Reduce Household Water Use Through Communication: A Field Experiment. *J. Policy Anal. Manag.* **2020**, *39*, 1076–1099. [CrossRef]
224. Barberán, R.; López-Laborda, J.; Rodrigo, F.; Barberan, R.; Lopez-Laborda, J.; Rodrigo, F. The Perception of Residential Water Tariff, Consumption, and Cost: Evidence of its Determinants Using Survey Data. *Water Resour. Manag.* **2022**, *36*, 2933–2952. [CrossRef]
225. Jessoe, K.; Lade, G.E.; Loge, F.; Spang, E. Residential water conservation during drought: Experimental evidence from three behavioral interventions. *J. Environ. Econ. Manag.* **2021**, *110*, 102519. [CrossRef]
226. Gázquez-Abad, J.C.; Mondéjar-Jiménez, J.-A.; Vargas-Vargas, M. Factors influencing water saving behaviour for Spanish households. *Environ. Eng. Manag. J.* **2011**, *10*, 1873–1881. [CrossRef]
227. Vivek, V.; Malghan, D.; Mukherjee, K. Toward achieving persistent behavior change in household water conservation. *Proc. Natl. Acad. Sci. USA* **2021**, *118*, e2023014118. [CrossRef] [PubMed]
228. Bermejo-Martín, G.; Rodríguez-Monroy, C.; Núñez-Guerrero, Y.M. Water consumption range prediction in Huelva's households using classification and regression trees. *Water* **2021**, *13*, 506. [CrossRef]
229. Warner, L.A.; Turner, S.; Lundy, L. Comparing Linkages Between Descriptive Norms and Current and Intended Outdoor Water Conservation. *J. Ext.* **2020**, *58*, 1–9. [CrossRef]
230. Lyach, R.; Remr, J. Motivations of Households towards Conserving Water and Using Purified Water in Czechia. *Sustainability* **2023**, *15*, 2202. [CrossRef]
231. Thakur, R.; Onwubu, S.C.; Harris, G.; Thakur, S. Examining the factors influencing water conservation intentions amongst peri-urban communities of ethekwini municipality. South Africa. *Water Conserv. Manag.* **2022**, *6*, 81–88. [CrossRef]
232. Oğur Aydın, D.; Doğan, Ç. Exploring water-consuming personal care and hygiene practices in the bathroom environment and user intentions for improving effective water consumption. *Des. J.* **2022**, *25*, 828–848. [CrossRef]
233. Lameck, E.; Sesabo, J.; Mkuna, E. Household behaviour towards water conservation activities in Mvomero District in Tanzania: A convergent parallel mixed approach. *Sustain. Water Resour. Manag.* **2021**, *7*, 45. [CrossRef]
234. Sengupta, J. The Effect of Non-pecuniary-based Incentive Mechanisms to Reduce Water Usage at the Household Level and to Achieve Positive Environmental Outcomes. *Glob. Bus. Rev.* **2020**, *21*, 1232–1248. [CrossRef]

MDPI AG
Grosspeteranlage 5
4052 Basel
Switzerland
Tel.: +41 61 683 77 34

Water Editorial Office
E-mail: water@mdpi.com
www.mdpi.com/journal/water

www.ingramcontent.com/pod-product-compliance
Lightning Source LLC
Chambersburg PA
CBHW040800250926
51850CB00007BA/1042
9783725870486